Visionary Healing

Visionary Healing

Psychedelic Medicine and Shamanism

Alexander Shester, M.D.

Foreword by Charles Grob, M.D.

Preface by Cathy Coleman, Ph.D.

REGENT PRESS
Berkeley, California
2023

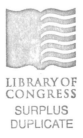

Library of Congress Cataloging-in-Publication Data

Names: Shester, Alexander, 1945- author.
Title: Visionary healing : psychedelic medicine and shamanism / Alexander
    Shester, M.D. ; foreword by Charles Grob.
Description: Berkeley, California : Regent Press, 2022. | Includes
    bibliographical references. | Summary:
Identifiers: LCCN 2022038526 (print) | LCCN 2022038527 (ebook) | ISBN
    9781587906343 (trade paperback) | ISBN 9781587906367 (hardback) | ISBN
    9781587906374 (ebook)
Subjects: LCSH: Hallucinogenic drugs--History. | Hallucinogenic
    drugs--Therapeutic use. | Hallucinogenic plants--History. | Shamanism. |
    Hallucinogenic drugs and religious experience--History.
Classification: LCC RM324.8 .S54 2022 (print) | LCC RM324.8 (ebook) | DDC
    615.7/883--dc23/eng/20221005
LC record available at https://lccn.loc.gov/2022038526

Copyright Disclaimer
My best intention was to use art images and photographs only with the permission of the artist, photographer, and publishers. I have attempted to contact each artist and publisher to obtain the consent of the copyrighted material, which is noted and credited. There are a few images I have not been able to track down to the original source or who have not responded before publication. If an image contributor objects that their material has been improperly used, please contact me so the copyright issues can be resolved. I value the work of other artists and creators in this book and strive to be fair.
— Alexander Shester, M.D.

Front Cover; *Peyote Vision* **— art by Alexander Shester, graphics by Geoffrey Shester**
This piece was done after a session with a Peyote shaman, Spirit Eagle, in 1989. It depicts the shaman's drum, from which the cupped hands contain the fire and the rose with a heart in the center and a star. It symbolizes the eros and love experienced when the heart chakra is opened during the experience. The butterfly emanates from the fire; representing the soul (Psyche from Greek mythology). The eagle symbolizes the freeing of the spirit as it flies freely into the cosmos to connect with the Creator of life.

Back Cover: *Emergence of the Anthropos* **— art by Alexander Shester, graphics by Geoff Shester**
Emergence of the Anthropos into the light from darkness, discovering and praising the godhead within. The birth of consciousness and love.

Table of Contents

Section Three / More Shamanic Lore: Other Sacred Medicines

Foreword by Charles Grob, M.D.

Over thirty years ago, while engaged in a clinical research project examining the effects of the visionary plant decoction ayahuasca among a religious group in the Brazilian Amazon, I learned a valuable lesson. It was customary in the ceremonial structure employed by the religious leaders, known as *maestres*, to present a sermon followed by a question-and-answer period with their congregation. One particular evening, during a lively exchange between the *maestres* and the congregants, my Portuguese translator lapsed into silence. As I was very interested in understanding the underlying psychology of the religion, and sensing there were valuable teachings to be learned from the discussion that my limited Portuguese could not quite grasp, I nudged my translator. She explained that they were discussing a crucial point raised by the *maestre's* sermon: if you agree to "show up" at a particular time and place, you be there.

The influence of such a highly suggestive plant hallucinogen no doubt amplified this message in the minds of the participants. I learned from my conversations with congregants afterward that the combination of the ayahuasca ceremony and the *maestres'* insight strongly impacted their sense of ethical conduct and responsibility. They were being instructed to lead more conscious lives and to proactively conduct themselves more responsibly and ethically in the various roles they had taken on, as spouses, parents, children, employers, employees, and members of the greater community. These visionary plants evoked, under the guidance of highly experienced and expert facilitators, a reinforced sense of responsibility and motivation to lead more ethical lives. But, for that transformation to happen, they were instructed by the profound altered state of consciousness they were immersed in to "show up." Showing up and paying attention were the critical determinants in the process of renewal and healing, the shared goals of participants in this modern iteration of the ancient art and science of ritual hallucinogen use.

I am honored to have been invited by Alex Shester to contribute a foreword to his delightful and highly informative new book, *Visionary Healing*. Dr. Shester, a senior psychiatrist and Jungian analyst, has contributed an insightful and comprehensive exploration of the range of plant and synthetic psychedelic compounds that have been available in one form or another to the inhabitants of this earth since the dawn of human existence. Inspired by his (and my) teacher, mentor, and close friend, Ralph Metzner — distinguished psychologist and pioneer of psychedelic research dating back to the early Sixties and prolific scholar of the diversity, value, and range of use of these extraordinary compounds — *Visionary Healing* arrives for our careful examination and appreciation at a pivotal time in human history.

The renowned Harvard ethnobotanist, Richard Evans Schultes, and his legendary Swiss colleague, medicinal chemist Albert Hofmann, in their valuable treatise, *Plants of the Gods*, identified for academic literature upwards of 120 hallucinogenic plants scattered around the world, though predominantly in South and Central America, that are still known to extant indigenous cultures and the anthropologists and ethnobotanists who have devoted their careers to their study. In these indigenous contexts, hallucinogenic plants are incorporated as ceremonial sacraments into rites of initiation, healing, and various divinatory purposes. They form the bedrock of many of these cultures' belief systems and in those contexts are culturally sanctioned, their ritual use elder-facilitated. Their use is never profaned for recreational purposes, and they are considered to be conduits to the realms of the spirits.

The shamanic model for plant-hallucinogen use is believed to predate the dawn of recorded history and likely forms the foundation for the subsequent evolution of culture and religion, though rarely have they been recognized as such. Many of these extraordinary plants have lately been incorporated into modern rituals, first deeply underground and clandestine and more recently emerging into the light of day. A case in point is the syncretic ayahuasca religions that first achieved legal sanction in Brazil in the late 1980s, followed by the U.S. Supreme Court voting unanimously in 2006 to uphold the freedom of religion rights of members of the União do Vegetal (UDV— the church led by maestres that I conducted research with in the 1990s) in the United States. That Supreme Court ruling allowed congregants in the U.S. to participate in twice-monthly, legally sanctioned religious ceremonies utilizing the potent plant hallucinogen decoction ayahuasca.

The legalization of plant hallucinogens in the modern era is the first time worldwide that government sanction has been granted in 1600 years, since the destruction in 395 A.D. of the Greek temple of Eleusis, where the sacred libation employed for the annual rites of Eleusis, the kykeon, is believed to have contained an ergot fungus containing lysergamides similar in chemical structure to LSD (lysergic acid diethylamide). Knowledge of these visionary plants and their ritual use has tragically eroded over the passage of time, their use often repressed and persecuted by invaders from distant cultures who perceived plant hallucinogens as heretical and punished with the harshest penalties mainstream secular and spiritual authorities could devise. Their very existence threatened with extinction, native peoples, particularly in South and Central America, over centuries disguised and concealed the continued active presence of these plants in ritual, often at great risk to themselves, their families, and their tribal cultures.

Today's modern world, teetering on the brink of global cataclysmic change, owes these cultures and their descendants a deep debt of gratitude, as yet unpaid, for preserving the sacred mysteries that hold great potential to facilitating a healthy realignment between the environment and the humans who inhabit the world, and who have brought us perilously close to destroying it. If we develop the presence of mind to show up and pay attention to the messages and lessons these visionary plants provide, there may yet be hope for deliverance into a safer and healthier world for those who will follow us. As our great friend and teacher, Ralph Metzner, once remarked, "Isn't it remarkable that by ingesting these plants we learn — we are taught — to be more human."

Charles S. Grob, M.D., *is Professor of Psychiatry and Pediatrics at the UCLA School of Medicine and the Director of the Division of Child and Adolescent Psychiatry at the Harbor-UCLA Medical Center. He previously held faculty positions at the Johns Hopkins School of Medicine and the University of California at Irvine. He has conducted approved clinical research with psychedelics since the early 1990s, including as Principal Investigator of the first study in several decades to examine the use of a psilocybin treatment model for patients with advanced-cancer anxiety.*

Preface by Cathy Coleman, Ph.D.

Ralph Metzner, to whom this book is dedicated, was Alex Shester's teacher, guide, and mentor, as he was to many others. Ralph was my teacher, colleague, and husband. When Ralph was Academic Dean, and then Vice-president at the California Institute of Integral Studies (CIIS) in the 1980s, I was the Director of Student Services. We worked alongside each other for nearly a decade; Ralph managed the academic side of CIIS, and I managed the administrative side. In the early 1980s MDMA was legal, and the small school was full of curious journeyers who were keenly interested in personal growth and transformation. During this time Ralph began to conduct visionary circles, as described in this book. He co-authored a compilation of personal experiences of people's MDMA journeys[1], under the pen name of Sophia Adamson in 1985 (re-published in 2013), followed by books on ayahuasca[2], psilocybin mushrooms[3], and a comprehensive compendium of work with various substances titled *Allies for Awakeninge*[4].

Alex Shester describes a Vision Circle, as structured by Ralph. The four phases of the circle journey are outlined, no matter what medicine is taken: first, the beginning when the body assimilates the substance; second, the visionary deep work; third, the wisdom teachings that emerge, and fourth, integration and awareness. He points out the important difference between insight and transformation—transformation occurs when behavioral changes, resulting from insights, are implemented and changed.

Alex notes the healing and transformative changes that can occur through serious, dedicated work with visionary medicines. Peter Faust wrote in his essay "The Teacher" in Intrepid Explorer: *Reflections on the Life and Legacy of Ralph Metzner*[5].

> "He [Ralph] took his role as teacher seriously, and expected you to take your role as student in kind … when the candles were lit and the ceremony began, it was time for business. As I saw it, a big facet of his business as a master teacher was two-fold … We were

there to seek healing and guidance. Healing the past and looking toward our future … Ralph would often ask during the integration rounds what we had been shown to do after we left the class. Then at the beginning of the next course he would check in and see if we had put our guidance into practice. Without integrating what you received, it was just an experience, he often said. Slowly implementing the guidance I received, during the years I studied with him, my life improved immensely."

Alex Shester was one such serious student. From his work spanning almost three decades, building on his experience as an M.D. and a Jungian analyst, he illuminates the promises and potential in *Visionary Healing*, offering individual chapters of information on numerous substances. Alex shares his own story of healing depression and transforming his work burnout, as well as his generating his creative unfolding that led to the writing of this book.

To help structure vision circles, Alex shares some meditations, including several from Ralph such as The Janus Model, The Cosmic Tree, and The Well of Remembrance. In addition, Appendix 2 describes nine meditations, taught by Ralph. Appendix 3 is a rich offering of music suggestions and inspirations.

Ralph always said that one must honor any vision, dream, or special message from the Divine and act upon it. By honoring the messages, he pointed out, one would continue to receive visions. Alex Shester has honored his visions and the transformative power of psychedelic substances by compiling and sharing the knowledge, wisdom, and experience that he has gained from working with many different medicines in visionary circles. *Visionary Healing*, an impressive volume of work, is a trememdous gift to both new and experienced therapists and healers.

1– Adamson, Sophia, With Ralph Metzner et al. *Through the Gateway of the Heart*, Solarium Press, 1985, 2013.

2– Ibid. *Ayahuasca: Sacred Vine of Spirits*. (Ed). Rochester, Vermont: Park Street Press. 3rd Edition, 2014

3– Ibid. *Teonanacatl: Sacred Mushroom of Visions*. (Ed). Rochester, Vermont: Park Street Press, 2003.

4– Ibid. *Allies for Awakening*: Guidelines for Productive and Safe Experiences with Entheogens. Berkeley: Regent Press, 2015.

5– Coleman, Cathy (Ed.). *Intrepid Explorer: Reflections on the Life and Legacy of Ralph Metzner*. Unpublished manuscript, 2022.

Cathy Coleman, Ph.D., *earned her doctorate in East-West Psychology at the California Institute of Integral Studies (CIIS) She worked at the CIIS as Director of Student Services and later Dean of Students. She later worked as Executive Director of EarthRise Retreat Center at the Institute of Noetic Sciences, as President of Kepler College (of Astrological Arts and Sciences) and is now working with CIIS' Center for Psychedelic-Assisted Therapies and Research. She was co-founder with Ralph Metzner, and is a current board member of, the Green Earth Foundation, and is the editor of a tribute book about the life and legacy of Ralph Metzner awaiting publication.*

Ralph Metzner, Ph.D.
(1936-2019)

Obituary and Dedication

I want to dedicate this book to my mentor and psychological and shamanic guide, Ralph Metzner.

Ralph Metzner died peacefully in his sleep at the age of 82, on March 14, 2019, at his home in Sonoma, California. He passed from idiopathic pulmonary fibrosis with an unknown cause. He was an excellent mentor who taught me how to incorporate deep psychological insights with indigenous wisdom and shamanic lore. He was able to make these ancient cross-cultural teachings accessible to the present Western psyche.

Metzner was a graduate student and a pioneer in psilocybin research in the early 1960s at Harvard, along with Timothy Leary and Richard Alpert (later Ram Dass). He dedicated his life to integrating shamanic techniques which alter consciousness and enable a deep awareness of the human psyche. He was a prolific author of many books about consciousness and mind-expanding hallucinogens and their role in visioning and healing. He also intensively studied yoga and meditation techniques to enhance life energy.

Although Leary and Ram Dass had other karmic trajectories, Metzner brought safe techniques using sacred plant hallucinogens from different cultures and parts of the world into a vision quest model. He held weekend and week-long ceremonies, called Vision Circles, with small groups of selected people. He would weave together both personal and mythological stories, guided meditations, as well as indigenous and trance-oriented music to carry the participants to extraordinary transpersonal realms. He taught how the use of entheogenic medicines, ritual chanting and drumming, and movement exercises could heal past wounds and help provide a participant a clearer sense of the future which could be integrated into daily living. He blended Eastern and Western thought with indigenous wisdom in a way that made it accessible to modern psychology.

In these Vision Circles, the participants came from all walks of life and were screened for appropriate preparation. Psychiatrists, psychotherapists, lawyers, teachers, actors, and secretaries all benefited from his wise, humble leadership. Metzner's books and tapes can be found at Green Earth Foundation, of which he was both the Founder and President. His work pointed to creating a greater appreciation of nature and the role of human beings interacting with it. He was an insightful contributor to the emerging field known as Ecopsychology.

He remains the most learned person I have had the honor to know as a mentor. His wisdom encouraged me to go from being a psychiatrist and Jungian Analyst to directly experiencing the transpersonal realm of consciousness. Through his guidance, these methods helped heal my depression and career burnout. The teachings launched me toward pursuit of my passions, further appreciation of science and the workings of the brain and mind, and manifesting my creativity in music and art. It is this work that inspired me to write this book.

He is perhaps the greatest pioneer and contributor to the present psychedelic renaissance. However, he is not adequately credited for his body of work in this field as an entheogenic shaman and scholar and advocate for preservation of the natural world. This book is an attempt to make his teachings known and more accessible.

In a word, Ralph was a true visionary. As of this writing, I was pleased to be informed that the neuroscience-based company Neuroscape and University of California, San Francisco (UCSF), my medical school alma mater, have joined in endowing a chair honoring Ralph Metzner as Distinguished Professor of Neurology and Psychiatry, with the purpose of promoting psychedelic research for the field of medicine.

Introduction

The human longing for exploration is an innate drive. This search continues in individuals through both outer and inner journeying. External pursuits can take one to new countries and cultures, from the heights of Everest to the depths of the oceans. One can travel to outer space to visit the moon, Mars, and the other planets. Humanity longs for adventures. Another person can take the inward path of discovery into the depths of the psyche and the outskirts of the infinity within to encounter the allies of the soul and spirit world. In these visionary realms, new relationships can be formed with ancestors and historical and mythical figures and guides, as well as with the intricacies of the natural and spiritual world. This inner exploration can open the *doors of perception* to heal the psyche and envision one's place within the earth and the cosmos.

The theories developed in the science of physics reflect the correspondence between the macro- and microcosms through understanding the expanding universe, the theory of relativity, and the sub-atomic, quantum domains. The search for a unified field theory between these two discoveries still continues.

However, as applied to human exploration, psychedelic medicines can reveal the intricate relationships between the personal and transpersonal psyche and the mystery of consciousness. In many ways, it can be more harrowing to take the inner "psychonautical" adventure than to be rocketed into outer space as an astronaut.

This book will instruct and prepare the reader for such a voyage through an introduction to several powerful psychedelic medicines, sometimes called *hallucinogens* or *entheogens* (for "god within"). It will also include personal memoirs describing the sacred usage of psilocybin mushrooms, ayahuasca, iboga, San Pedro cactus, and peyote for my own healing, revisioning of the natural world, and developing my relationship with the spirit domain. Other sacred medicines used in different cultures and historical times will also be described.

A psychedelic renaissance is happening worldwide for those who wish to develop a more comprehensive awareness of themselves and the planet. The proper usage of entheogens can lift the veil from our consensus reality and allow ordinary individuals to experience a larger field of awareness. These sacred medicines can expand insights and encourage behavioral transformation previously available only to privileged mystics.

Currently, so much new information is available about psychedelic usage that it can be daunting for anyone to sort through the deluge. How can you participate in this new period of human awakening and evolution while remaining grounded in integrity? Where can you obtain some accurate knowledge about psychedelics? Whom can you trust to listen to, or read? I hope that through the material in this book, it will become such a reference. I say this with the humblest intention. At my ripe age, I have been highly educated in science, medicine, psychiatry, Jungian analysis, and transpersonal shamanic methods. Under proper guidance over many years, I have undergone initiation through the crucible of experience with psychedelic medicines from around the world, using a vision quest model.

The intention for sharing my inner material is to create a living example of the profound psychological healing these medicines can promote. The visionary aspects describe my evolving relationship to the natural world as well as meetings with many ancestral and archetypal allies.

This book also contains accurate, valuable information about the various entheogens. Shamanic techniques will be described and explained as an aid in understanding the rituals necessary for safe and profound voyages to the psycho-spiritual realm, both with and without the use of psychedelics. These methods can help you prepare for the healing and visionary encounters you may be seeking.

This book's emphasis is on the sacred use of these substances to promote psychological healing of trauma and visioning to develop clarity about the future and your relationship to the transpersonal dimension of consciousness. I will also discuss the new emphasis in psychiatry and psychology on the use of psychedelics as medicines to treat various psychopathologies. However, the entertainment value, casual usage, and the present trend for micro-dosing psychedelics are not emphasized in this book.

Knowledge does not necessarily bring about change. The insights from nature may give you more choices related to redirecting your values toward preventing the extinction of humanity and all life on planet earth. When insights transform into behavioral changes, hope emerges. This type of exploration is a form of psycho-spiritual activism. It is my belief that when a critical mass of such inner exploration occurs, collective intelligence expands, bringing hope that it will break into our civilization's historical and political realities and humanity's future outcomes.

In what follows, you can expect to learn about all the major psychedelics from scientific, historical, mythological, and cultural perspectives. The first-hand accounts of my psychedelic adventures and accompanying imagery will provide an idea of what is possible during such an encounter for personal healing, as well as for meeting nature, spirit, and the divine within yourself.

Section One

Shamanism
and
Plant Medicines

Chapter 1
What Is Shamanism?

Shamanism is not a religion, but a method for healing and visioning since ancient times. The shaman learns to get in touch with the animistic spirits, or indwelling sentience, of the earth and the cosmos; where he or she believes healing remedies reside. The gods or spirits involved tend to be local to each culture. The animal spirits with whom the shaman makes connections are among those in that society's ecosystem. The gods and goddesses, whether those of Greece or of indigenous tribes, are relevant to the culture and generally polytheistic. The idea of monotheism, which maintains a more distant "One God" overseeing everything, is more representative of later religious traditions.

Shamanism represents an animistic belief system based on direct experience. In this way it is different than science, which is based on an observable method replicable in controlled studies. Spirit as sentience, as experienced by participants, inhabits not only human and animal forms but also the plant, fungi, and mineral realms. The shaman is able to communicate with stones, trees, elves, and fairies residing near trees, springs, and mountains, in order to receive help with healing and visioning. In the shamanic belief system, sentience is experienced as infused into everything; all things are interrelated: the *one in the many.*

Science is the modern mythology that governs what we consider to be truth, but it continues to leave many mysteries unanswered. In shamanism, animistic truths are viewed as valid since they have been in existence since ancient times and appear in all cultures. Carl Gustav Jung, as well as many other psychologists and teachers, believed that both the old and the new ways of knowing may coexist in the psyche of modern humanity, facilitating a more complete, deeper understanding of nature and our place in it.

Mircea Eliade (1907-1986), a Romanian historian of religion, called shamanism an "archaic form of ecstasy." Primarily it was a religious phenomenon, but based on direct experience rather than faith. The process of inner journeying to other worlds is distinctive to shamanism. This path is seen as necessary for participants to access help and knowledge, as well as to meet spirit allies who bring guidance in relating to this form of transpersonal intelligence.

The medicine man and woman in indigenous cultures generally functioned in a different role than that of shamans. He or she performed priestly activities through ceremonies and rituals in order to maintain the traditions of the culture. These rituals served the purpose of healing and binding the tribe and were often tied to dogmatic beliefs and rules. Shamans generally had more focus on bringing about ecstatic direct experiences connecting humans with spirits for healing, rather than seeing themselves as the agent of power behind healing. In other words, the power was in the spirits rather than in the person of the medicine man or woman.

Joan Halifax in *Shamanic Voices* states that the word shaman derives from the *Vedic Sram*, meaning "to heat oneself or practice austerities." (Halifax 1979, 3) This is reminiscent of the two main yogic paths: the lefthand ecstatic path of Tantra and the contemplative right-hand path of the ascetic approach. Of course, between these extremes exist many other practices of yoga, of which the earliest traces date back to the third millennium B.C.E. Eliade alternatively states that the word comes from the Russian Tungusic *saman*, meaning one who knows, or knows the spirits, of the Evenki culture in the Siberian region of Asia. Shamanism in the strict sense is preeminently a religious phenomenon of Siberia and Central Asia. (Eliade 1972, 4) The beautiful red and white *Amanita muscaria* mushroom was the common sacrament of these shamans.

The presence of the earliest shaman most likely dates back to cultures from the Upper Paleolithic period until possibly the times of the Neanderthals. The shaman was generally highly regarded within the tribe, but also feared. Shamans were typically viewed as outcasts, living away from the center of the community where the chief (leader) presided in authority. These healers lived on the outskirts, often at the boundary between the village and the forest or jungle. This was the boundary between the known and the unknown, between order and chaos, between the conscious and the unconscious, between the living and the dead, and between the human and the spirit world. It was at this boundary where the shaman was skilled with intercommunication. Often, shamans were perceived as *half-crazy* because of their vocal ramblings in the spirit world.

The shaman could embrace the concepts of illness, death, and resurrection and was able to realize illumination not privy to most others in the community. Often the power came to the shaman through his or her own near-death experience in childhood, which had left them wounded in some way. It might have been a physical, emotional, or spiritual experience that could have resulted in literal death, but, if the person survived this, he or she was often reborn into the world of a healer. This represented the initiation into their culture's magico-religious and healing realms. This experience often left the person with an intuitive window into the illnesses of others. It is said that "only the wounded healer can heal." This capacity represented the main power or gift of the shaman.

In broader terms, the experience of *death and rebirth* is a hallmark of the initiatory process. A person who looks death in the face becomes liberated from fear and limitations. It is the necessary way out of ordinary reality (or consensus trance) before transcendence can occur. For modern participants, this ritual death is the crucial experience in shamanic journey work. It is what humbles the ego in its attempts to become inflated when encountering the transcendent realm. Death of the ego is necessary before rebirth; this experience for humans mimics the changing seasons in nature. Often, between death and rebirth, there is an incubation period or *pregnancy* where one is utterly alone, orphaned from family, community, and old beliefs; until one is ready for rebirth into a new phase of life, at which time one is often given a new name and new responsibilities.

Mythologically, it is important to remember that the message was never to incur the envy of the gods by trying to become one in an act of hubris. Sooner or later, a leveling process would occur with a consequent fall from grace. In the Greek myth, the fall of Icarus and the story of the Phoenix represent the consequence of hubris, or *ego-inflation*. In Jungian psychology, this would be considered an ego identification, with the transcendent leading to inflation, rather than forming a *relationship* with the archetype.

The shaman's traditional role as healer pre-dated the treatment methods of Western medicine based in science, which became the prevailing belief system (or mythology) of the 20th century. The gods and spirits have completely disappeared in the practice of modern medicine, where shamanistic practices are seen as based in superstition and mysticism resid-ing in altered states of consciousness. Shamanic healing is still utilized in extant indigenous cultures, as will be described in later chapters.

It is interesting to note that as one result of the growing disillusion-ment with the Western medical model, shamanism is gaining acceptance once again. Additional alternative healing practices such as forms of med-itation, acupuncture, body movement and dance, drumming, and natu-ral supplements and herbs are all being incorporated into the integrative medicine approach. This approach is finding an increasing number of ad-herents in recent years.

Currently, due to the increased popularity of psychedelic-based sha-manistic quests, there are many neophytes, so-called "shamans." Many of these people have not done sufficient inner work of their own, yet wish to become known as sacred leaders or desire to exploit others financially (although they may be unconscious of these motives). These individuals are more concerned with self-interests, power, status, and getting on the "psychedelic bandwagon." Such people are found not only locally but also in villages in the Amazon, due to the growing popularity of Westerners seeking an ayahuasca experience. An aspect of modern eco-tourism is a travel adventure during which an uninitiated patron can meet a personal shaman and drink magical intoxicants. One can buy bottles of ayahuasca from street vendors in places such as Iquitos, Peru. Without proper prepa-ration and developing an appropriate mindset and setting, a life-changing or transformative experience is unlikely.

It seems that the psychedelic adventure has once again become wide-spread for those wishing a short circuit to the sacred realm. As in the days of Timothy Leary in the 1960s, when something becomes a collective phe-nomenon, the original value is very often diluted, becoming corrupted, then criminalized and made illegal. As with other forms of modern spir-itual practice, there are many "spiritual window shoppers" who are un-able to integrate the experience back into their daily life. The movement to decriminalize certain psychedelics such as psilocybin, MDMA, ayahuasca, and cannabis is occurring in some states, as more research into their med-ical and psychiatric use is becoming evident.

Chapter 2
My Background

Later chapters provide a subjective description of the major psychedelics in terms of experiences I have had with each of them, as well as from a scientific and historical perspective. So, who am I, and what are my qualifications for talking about psychedelics? I will tell you a little bit about myself before we take a closer look at preparation for journey work and each of the psychedelic plant medicines.

Early Days

Being a healer has been "in my blood" since I was a child. My fascination with doctors began after a surgery when I was nine years old. This would become my first introduction to the concept of the "wounded healer"—healers who themselves need healing. When younger, I thought about being a fireman, a policeman, or a soldier when I grew up, yet after the surgery, I felt a hero worship of doctors and intuitively knew my eventual fate was to become one. I started watching TV doctor programs (*Medic, Dr. Kildare, Ben Casey*), which consolidated my curiosity for this profession. My mother made me a surgeon's outfit with gown, hat, and mask. My sister and I started operating on her dolls, playing doctor and nurse. She eventually did become a nurse, just as I became a doctor.

At the time, I obviously was unaware of the difficulties to achieving such a goal. Many experiences

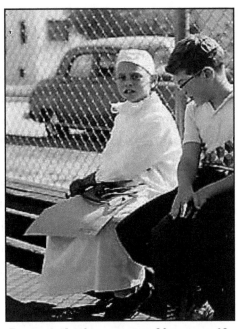

FIGURE 1. Author, young Alex, age 10, dressed as a surgeon for a Halloween parade at elementary school.

intervened in my life which created doubts that I possessed the necessary intelligence and perseverance to go through such a prolonged educational ordeal. It was in college that I re-experienced my scientific abilities to the extent that I believed that I was a capable candidate for this vocation.

Becoming a Doctor

I was eventually accepted into three medical schools, University of California, San Francisco (UCSF), University of California, Los Angles (UCLA), and University of Southern California (USC). I chose UCSF. I well remember my first day of school in the fall of 1967. I sat in a raised lecture hall, feeling a sense of pride as we students were inducted into the fraternity of medicine and heard the Hippocratic Oath recited for the first time. My initial vision was to become a cardiovascular surgeon.

I realized much later that to become a physician required much more than high intelligence. I have known many people more intelligent than I am who could never have become doctors. To endure the trials of training and practice takes a great deal of motivation, will, vision, and perseverance. Much self-sacrifice, loss of freedom, competition, debt, and mental and bodily stress are involved — especially impactful on persons who are still relatively young. Many arduous years of training with sleep deprivation and self-doubt are

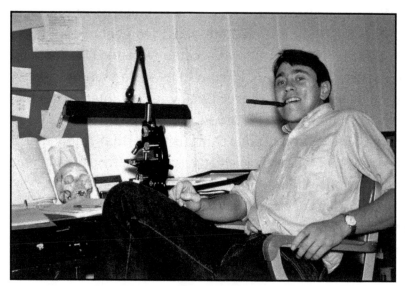

FIGURE 2. **First-year medical student, full of arrogance and hope, at UC San Francisco.**

inherent in the initiation process of becoming a physician. Many people want to be healers but have never subjected themselves to the crucible of integrating knowledge and responsibility to the degree required of a medical doctor.

I completed an extended trial of college, medical school, internship, and residency. While in school, my interest in becoming a surgeon waned. I had difficulty in identifying with the surgeon's mindset. There seemed to be a certain arrogance, competitiveness, and dedication to surgery at the expense of leading a more balanced lifestyle that did not attract me. My nature was more philosophical and artistic.

Since the time I began my career in the late 1960s, there has been a general societal evolution away from the prior hero-worship of doctors and a disillusionment with the medical profession as a whole. The sacred duty of a doctor has often been contaminated with greed, arrogance, and ignorance on the part of many of my colleagues. I grew increasingly aware that the healing values so important to me were not always shared. Often a disparity existed between raw intelligence (IQ) and spiritual awareness, between facts and wisdom, between rigidity and open-mindedness, and between science and religious faith. Having intelligence is not the same as developing consciousness.

I emerged at the end of medical school, unsure of my path. After a stint as a medical intern and a holdover year as a radiology resident, I was inducted into the Air Force as a medical officer during the last year of the Vietnam War. I was already interested in the philosophy of C.G. Jung and had read *The Teachings of Don Juan* by Carlos Castaneda. After my two-year term as a medical officer, I was accepted into the UCLA Department of Psychiatry residency program. My thoughts were that my interests in science and medicine would integrate well with my interests in philosophy, psychology, spirituality, and the study of consciousness.

As a resident, however, I soon came to realize that, rather than an exploration of the psyche, modern psychiatry was more focused on studying the aberrant neurotransmitters in the brain, which were seen as contributing to major mental illnesses such as psychosis, depression, bipolarity, addictions, and various anxiety disorders. There were essential things to learn about the neurochemistry of the brain, but it was reductionist in terms of thinking about consciousness.

C.G. Jung

My interest in the transpersonal psychology of Carl Jung then rose to the forefront of my interest and intellectual passion. During my psychiatry residency, I took some outside courses on Jung and dream interpretation. I was accepted into the psychoanalytic program at the C.G. Jung Institute in Los Angeles and began my training in 1981. With a few starts and stops, I finally was certified in April 1990. Typical of my over-idealization that this path provided the key to a more expansive consciousness, I slowly found myself again becoming disillusioned. To me the path felt dry, overly intel-lectualized, and somewhat cultish. I did learn how to interpret dreams and symbolism from a Jungian perspective and valuable techniques such as "active imagination" (a form of meditation and dialogue). I also had some outstanding Jungian mentors, but many of the analysts and conferences provided little nourishment for my soul's needs.

Shamanic Training

While I thought I was on the right path, as my intellectual interests increased, there was a growing inner feeling that I was drying up in an ivory tower of academic thought, missing the experiential realm of the psyche. I felt like *Siddhartha* on his journey in the novel by Hermann Hesse, stopping temporarily at various wisdom teachings, yet not sensing that I was reaching the essence of my being. So, I pushed onwards searching for passion in my life. As stated by one of my mentors from the Mythopoetic men's movement, Michael Meade, "It is better to stumble in the darkness alone, than to follow a roadmap made by tourists."

It was then that I continued my education by training in and then inte-grating shamanic techniques for transpersonal exploration. I do believe this range of training prepared me with an expansive knowledge to carry into my career. The difficulty of these integrative steps largely goes under-appreciated by patients, friends, and family. What is important is that I know how the hard work and sacrificing of comforts has been the key to becoming an effective doctor/healer, which was my goal.

I did find that my earlier study of Jung served to further my interest in healing, especially with the methods used by other cultures. Since the time humans first evolved on this planet, there have always existed healers using techniques, whether physical, psychological, or spiritual in nature, to cure illnesses as well as to provide a vision for the tribe. So, I found myself next pursuing this approach to expand my knowledge of healing traditions. In addition to modern, high-technology medicine, I learned about ancient and archaic methods utilized by shamans of various indigenous cultures, which have been brought to our present time and culture.

To help me along this path, I was fortunate to meet some wonderful teachers. One was a Navajo medicine man from Shiprock, New Mexico, known as Spirit Eagle, who used peyote as a teaching sacrament. But my primary influence was Ralph Metzner, Ph.D., a psychologist who was a life-long practitioner of shamanism and the use of sacred medicines, and to whom this book is dedicated. He was able to integrate these ancient techniques of other cultures and make them relevant to our modern Western mindset. He was sensitive about misappropriating indigenous cultures' sacred rituals and developed his own hybrid style for teaching. He remained grateful to these cultures but felt the need to make certain shamanic practices available for usage in our present traditions.

Indigenous literally means people who are original or who are descendants of a native culture of a particular region or country. It is crucial to know that this term not only applies to ancient or archaic societies, but also to present-day native people who are attempting to preserve their cultural integrity. It is why these cultures are sensitive to misappropriating their customs by Western-oriented people, such as vision quests, medicine circles, chanting, storytelling, sweat lodges, and sacred plant use. Present-day indigenous cultures are rightfully sensitive to the use of their terminology. Also, when we make use of native customs, what do we give back to them as a form of reciprocity? Credit and gratitude are necessary and important, but often we give little of substance in return for the wisdom gained. Perhaps we could provide better educational opportunities, health care, mental health, and addiction recovery centers to prevent further degradation of these cultures, as well as a heightened sensitivity to their plight, customs, and their land.

While on my path, I never abandoned traditional Western medicine and all that I incorporated from it. Instead I chose to expand my knowledge database by studying Eastern philosophical approaches and indigenous shamanism. Fortunately, in society at large, there has developed a current renaissance of interest in these ancient and indigenous forms of healing, many of which are becoming incorporated into the new field of integrative medicine. While I believe that the traditional medical model is based on the best that modern science can offer, so much yet remains unknown about illness and healing that it is now recognized to have significant limitations. Aldous Huxley notes, "As we all know, a little learning is a dangerous thing. But a great deal of highly specialized learning (higher education) is also a dangerous thing and may be sometimes even more dangerous than a little learning." (Huxley 1977, 1)

In the following chapter, I will describe the process of shamanic journeys that I have experienced and practiced in a modern context through the leadership of a guide. This preparation is the same regardless of whether or not sacred psychedelic medicines are to be used during a journey.

Chapter 3

Preparation for a Medicine Journey or Vision Quest

When an individual chooses to undergo an experience of leaving ordinary reality, it is important first to ask: Why go through it at all? For most people, it can be fearful to leave the known in order to venture into the unknown. An intention for the experience is necessary for orientation in the journey. This can arise through the person meditating upon what is needed for the psyche, the body, or the soul at that time.

Developing an Intention

Without a clear intention, the journey can become vague, chaotic, or meaningless. To develop an intention, it is best to ask a question as to what is needed or desired. It is important to view the intention as a bridge from this place to that place, from this world to that world. If the path is too narrow, one may be asking something too rigid or too literal and might miss out on other insights. It is best to develop a question with a wider path so that whatever emerges can be broader and, at times, surprising. The intention for a journey represents a path toward the altered state in order to receive and retrieve new information, but also provides the way back to normal, consensus reality with the insights gained that can be then used for transformation (e.g. the breadcrumbs of Hansel and Gretel).

Some aspect of the person may require *healing*, which commonly would be connected to an experience of past trauma or disappointment from childhood or the more recent past. The person may be facing something unclear in the future and then would need *visioning*, especially if there is a feeling of being stuck in the present situation or at a loss about how to develop more clarity in how to proceed in life. Often, the need might be for some combination of healing and visioning.

Often, no clear answer emerges during a journey, but other questions arise that lead to the next step. The answer may not come through directly but sometimes from the side, similar to peripheral vision, allowing one to notice aspects that central (inner) vision misses. Many times during a journey, one can become confused, lost, or seduced into places that are not part of the intention, making it necessary to remind oneself periodically to return to the main path. The shaman or leader may remind you that when you are unclear, have forgotten something, or are lost, it is important to "remember your intention."

Ralph Metzner would often say during a session: "A wise old owl told me, whatever your journey, wherever you are, don't forget your 1) intention, 2) your ancestors, 3) the light within you, and 4) remember the earth." It always had a calming and reorienting effect among the participants, especially if some fearful or chaotic experience was encountered.

This is a good metaphor for use in meditation and in daily life. An intention helps maintain concentration and focus in a journey, whether that be within a psychedelic or shamanic experience, or within everyday life. With all of life's distractions, one can become so scattered that goals or projects are never completed. Having an intention is also a good daily practice in communicating with other people in a more direct, clear manner, and coming from the heart.

Creating Sacred Space

Whenever there is to be a healing ceremony, the creation of a sacred space is necessary to separate the participant from ordinary life. This space provides a safe environment for exploration into the depths of the psyche, especially if an altered state of consciousness is induced by any means. A qualified leader or shaman who is experienced and familiar with the territory is essential to guide the individual or group in their journey and to assist if any problems arise. This space can be in a private home or a retreat center, or outside in a natural setting like the wilderness.

To begin to navigate the inner world, it is important to orient oneself to the outer environment. Often a circle is circumscribed along with the four main directions of the East, South, West, and North. There may be an invocation of the four directions of the compass to orient and align the inner world with the outer world. Each culture may have different invocations of the four directions, making them culture-specific or relevant to the individual. Sometimes it is called a *medicine wheel*. Invocations of various healing stories may be channeled by the shaman/leader. The main purpose is to create an orientation before exploration.

An example of orientation that I learned from my work with my guide, Ralph Metzner, is the following:

> *I invoke and would like to bring in the direction of the East—the direction of the rising sun, of new life, of new ideas; the seed which brings new things to us, the beginner's mind, the open mind, the child, and birthing.*
>
> *I invoke the grandmothers of the South, where there is growth and fertility, from which we are nurtured and sustained with food on this planet Earth, and all sustenance of the Great Mother Earth.*
>
> *I invoke the direction of the West, where the sun sets, the elders dwell; where all things go to die as all things do in nature. This is the place of the great transition where the great Pacific Ocean dissolves all of our old programs and allows us to bring back the water of life.*
>
> *I invoke the direction of the North, the place of Grandfather Wind, the winds of change that allow us to open to necessary changes; of breath, that which clears out the thoughts and feelings that are no longer useful to us.*

By invoking these four directions, the "Four-fold Way," the number four is constellated in the psyche. Four is the archetype of orientation representing the greater Self, according to Jung. It is from this deeper Self that one needs to navigate when one enters an altered state of consciousness. This quadrated circle is a mandala symbol. Jung stated that the circle represents the cosmos, and the four directions contain the physical and experiential elements of life on earth. Most native cultures intuitively create mandalas or

MEDICINE WHEEL

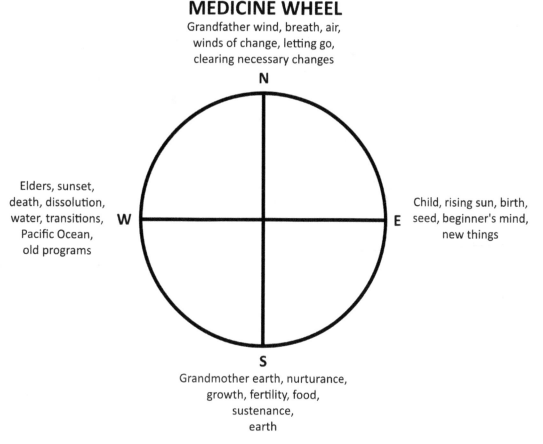

Grandfather wind, breath, air,
winds of change, letting go,
clearing necessary changes

N

Elders, sunset,
death, dissolution,
water, transitions,
Pacific Ocean,
old programs

W

E

Child, rising sun, birth,
seed, beginner's mind,
new things

S

Grandmother earth, nurturance,
growth, fertility, food,
sustenance,
earth

FIGURE 3. **Example of a typical medicine wheel.**
(As shared by Ralph Metzner)

medicine circles for orientation to reality; they appear in Tibetan, Chinese, Native American, Aboriginal, African, and European cultures. Frequently, ancient dwellings or townships would be erected in a circle.

Other invocations may be spoken to bring in the ancestors and the spirit animals that reside in the four directions to help as guides during a journey. (These and other invocations may be found in the Appendix 2.) The ancestors may take the form of the recently departed, such as family members or friends who have passed on, or of historical or mythical figures who are wisdom carriers. *They have been there before* and therefore may have some interesting insights about how to proceed in life. In an altered state, there is a reciprocal relationship that may be formed. One can inform them about what is going on presently in life, and the wisdom carrier can in return share wisdom from the past. In one of my own journeys, I have taken Abraham, Isaac, and Jacob on the thrill of a motorcycle

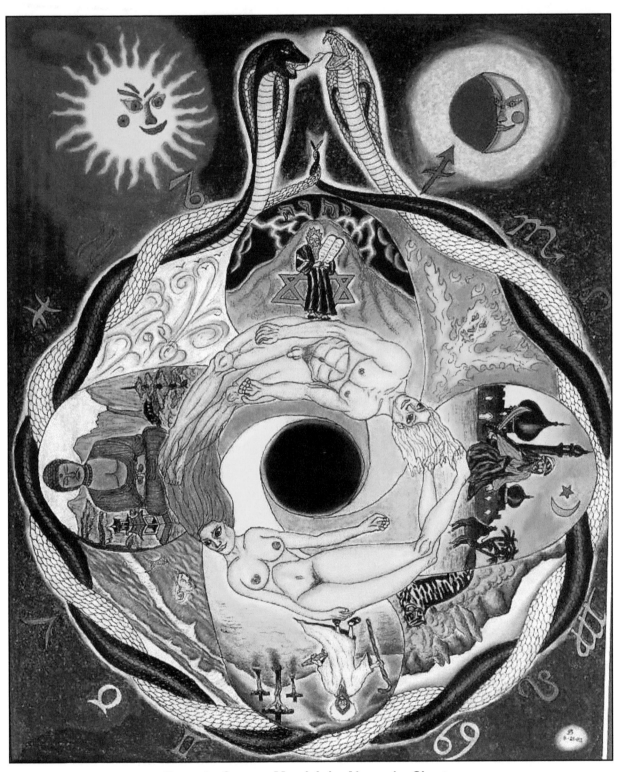

FIGURE 4. *Cosmos Mandala* by Alexander Shester.

ride, while they protected me from crashing and they spoke to me about Jewish history and mysticism. The ancestor may ask, "Tell me what you see," and one may then respond, "Tell me what you know."

You will see photos and artwork accompanying the descriptions of journeys in the following chapters. As the old saying goes, "A picture is worth a thousand words." Much of the artwork consists of my own colored pencil drawings. Other images are by visionary artists, with the vivid colors and symbols commonly seen during the psychedelic journey.

As you view these static images, I suggest you try to visualize them in constant motion, similar to what would occur during a psychedelic encounter. They are depicted in the vivid colors seen during a medicine journey. The art mimics the images seen with the various sacred medicines and can be appreciated by those people not inclined to using hallucinogens.

Try to be aware of your bodily functions and emotional states for each image presented. You might meditate on each image and see what arises for you. You might try to imagine not only the sights but also the sounds of nature, as well as other senses. View the image as a 3-D landscape that is alive; envision that you are participating in an extraordinary happening. Imagine the synesthesia with all the senses being driven by the music, the visions, and the teachings.

In Figure 4 are seen the entwined sacred serpents surrounding four of the great religions as well as the four elements. From within emerge the male and female. Outside the serpents appear the twelve signs of the zodiac and Sol and Luna depicting the opposites.

In the journey, human guides may appear as ancestors, present-day teachers, or historical or mythological figures. Various spirit animals may serve as guides or allies and can be very informative about nature, instinctual knowledge, and protection. These animals take different forms for each person or culture, depending on their location in the world and their ecosystem. For instance, a polar bear would not likely appear as a guide for a member of a tribe in the Amazon, whereas a jaguar or anaconda might. In addition, trees, forests, vegetation, rock formations, mountains, and bodies of water may serve as guides.

Set and Setting

The experience and outcome of any transpersonal journey are more dependent on the set and setting that are created than on the technique; or if being used, the dose or type of medicine. Please note that as a doctor and in situations when properly used, I am referring to these psychoactive substances as medicines as opposed to drugs, a term which has a negative connotation in society, especially when they are inappropriately used or abused. Other terms for psychedelic include *hallucinogen*, based on the Latin *hallucinatus*, meaning "wandering in the mind," and *entheogen*, based on the ancient Greek words meaning "the god within." I use these three terms interchangeably, although a shaman may prefer to use one term over another.

The "set," or mindset, is the attitude one brings to the session and is a part of the intention. One can approach the session either humbly with reverence, having an intention to heal or envision; or someone may participate primarily for purposes of recreation, entertainment, or getting high. Some people enjoy using certain psychedelics during the day while they venture out in nature in order to gain insights into their bodies and the environment. Others like to "party" with hallucinogens or the fantasy enhancer MDMA (Ecstasy).

While the primary concern of this book is with the intentional use of psychedelic medicines, their "recreational" use on occasion can have spiritual benefits as well. For example, experiences in raves and dance parties can correspond to the cosmic consciousness developed in the repetitive movements reminiscent of the Sufi Whirling Dervishes.

The "setting" of intentional journeys represents the place, surroundings, music, activity, time of day or night, season, and the people sharing the journey. Psychedelics or hallucinogens work as truth serum, bringing forth what is important for the person to know and understand. For an uninitiated or unprepared individual, the direction of the trip can be unpredictable, possibly turning negative, which may necessitate a change of setting. Although psychedelics are not physically harmful, one can become psychologically traumatized if the experience is approached without a sense of humility or with unrealistic expectations. With a calming guide or caring friends, often a "bad trip" can quickly shift to something positive. A change in music or environment can be helpful to facilitate that change.

It is essential for the person to remember that the medicine journey is time-limited; even a so-called negative experience, once integrated, can be seen to have delivered important lessons. It is also essential to remember that, while under the influence of medicine, the ego can be deconstructed, resulting in one feeling vulnerable, anxious, and suggestible to any input from the leader or others. If, for instance, one is using a medicine at a party or night club, there can be various destructive influences or people which can easily become absorbed, promoting a bad experience. Usually, the face (attitude) with which one approaches a journey is the same face that is reflected back to the person.

For instance, I personally experienced frightening imagery at times during journeys, such as a when a large snake displaying its fangs or a dragon with fire was coming to harm me. What helped me deal with this situation was to speak to the creature directly, saying something such as, "I came here to gain wisdom and teaching from you with respect and humility and not to be harmed." Instantly the imagery would change to a benevolent presence once the entity realized my true intention. It was as if I had to prove my worthiness before I could receive wisdom or healing from such transpersonal power entities.

I realize that the sharing of personal visions or dreams can be like going to a friend's home and sitting through a slideshow of their recent vacation. It is invigorating for the friend to recount their experience, but others can soon become bored; do skip through the sections that are uninspiring. Most soul journeys should be kept private or in confidence with someone close who understands the terrain of visions. This allows the contained soul work to continue transforming the person without becoming diluted by the feedback of others, however well-meant. I am opening up to share aspects of my own inner psyche, along with its pathology, to demonstrate the power of personal healing that potentially may be achieved by entheogenic medicines, shamanic techniques, and the vision quest model. Healing is different than curing. To cure means to abolish the pathology and permanently get rid of an illness, be it physical or psychological. My view of the meaning of healing is to confront the pathology, to work with it so that it no longer controls you, and to move on. Healing is the individual progress that occurs as one moves toward a genuine cure.

During life, certain illnesses and psychological material may emerge and recur. Each time this occurs, the person is presented with an opportunity to delve deeper into core issues so that the material can be reworked from a different perspective. For example, under various stressors, the wounded child-complex, low self-esteem, or the mother-complex (infantile/dependency needs) may present themselves again. The idea of ongoing work is to revisit these issues without identifying or becoming bogged down with them. Healing occurs when one goes into these past traumas and memories and returns to the present with a different perspective so that the person is no longer controlled by them. It is then possible to move forward and to feel the flow of life return with more hope and vision for the future.

Over fifteen years have passed since my last vision circle, and I now feel comfortable sharing these private moments to acquaint an interested person with the experiences and what can be accomplished by entering the *church of the transpersonal*. Each individual must decide whether this intense pathway is suitable for their own exploration. A warrior attitude is required to embrace this method of self-exploration. Many other options for growth exist that are less harrowing, yet the experience with a psychedelic can be profound and indeed a true spiritual experience. The use of medicines can amplify the effects of a powerful quest in a short period of time, a process which could take months or longer to experience through other means such as a spiritual retreat or intensive psychotherapy. Prayer and meditation are other longer-term methods of achieving awakening. The overarching issue for any individual, however, is what experience is integrated long-term, resulting in lasting positive behavioral transformation.

To be invited into a vision circle is indeed an honor. One requirement is that participants must respect the structure and boundaries set forth by the shaman, which may vary for different leaders. The one common ground is that it is a sacred ceremony and not for entertainment. If medicines are used to enhance the experience, it must be understood that it is still illegal to possess or use hallucinogens or entheogens in most places in our society, so utmost confidentiality must be respected by the participants. As did the alchemists of old who needed to go underground to practice their art, those who journey in present-day exploration with medicines become part of a "secret society" of people on the cutting edge, experimenting in a new form of healing and visioning to enhance an expanded consciousness.

Many have wondered if using such medicines result in an artificial spiritual experience, or a true one. Huston Smith (1919-2016), a friend of the psychedelic pioneer Aldous Huxley (1894-1963), is one of the most respected and beloved authorities on world religions and has taught at such universities as Massachusetts Institute of Technology (MIT), Syracuse University, Washington University, and University of California, Berkeley. In his book *Cleansing the Doors of Perception*: *The Religious Significance of Entheogenic Plants and Chemical*s, he concludes that the psychedelic spiritual experience is truly mystical in nature.

Some vision quests or circles may last a week or more, but more commonly they involve a weekend or even a one-night experience. The shaman/leader must be experienced with the medicines that are used, techniques to properly guide participants to the other world and back, and methods to deal with disturbing psychological material that may emerge for an individual. That is why it is very important to have an experienced shaman or leader as a guide.

Chapter 4

An Earth Vision Circle Structured by Ralph Metzner

Following is a description of a vision circle which took place in Joshua Tree, my favorite desert ecosystem. A similar structure is used in other places such as forest or mountain habitats, or even in private home settings. Ralph would call his gatherings "vision circles" rather than "vision quests." The latter is an overused term appropriated from indigenous and native peoples and does not usually imply the use of psychedelic plant medicines.

It is always interesting at the initial gathering to meet both veteran experienced explorers and new participants coming for the first time. We would gather in the late afternoon or early Friday evening in a safe place such as a home or cabin in the wilderness. The places I have experienced circles have been in desert and mountain locations. These cabins were not being used by those not participating, in order for the group to experience undisturbed sessions that enhanced our confidence in the safety of the setting.

My preferred setting is the desert. It is a rugged environment with interesting boulder formations, washes, cactuses, tortoises, rabbits, lizards, and bird creatures. Different animals appear during the day and night. The temperature can vary from very hot to cold, windy or rainy. I found that one must be prepared to encounter whatever nature offers at that season or time of day. The sunsets in the desert offer a spectacular display as day turns to twilight and then to night with the expanse of stars, planets, and the Milky Way.

Prior to arrival for the vision circle, we were encouraged to fast for the entire day except for water hydration, and no alcohol was permitted.

After the first evening session, the fasting would begin in earnest until the end of the main medicine journey on early Sunday morning. For anyone using SSRI antidepressants, it was encouraged (if possible), for the person to taper them or stop using them a week or two before the main session. These drugs can saturate the receptor sites with serotonin, the same sites in the brain that the tryptamine-based psychedelics use. This effect could dilute the experience or cause *serotonin syndrome*, potentially harmful, occurring when too much serotonin floods the brain with the combination of the antidepressant and the psychedelic. The syndrome is experienced as marked flushing, hyperthermia, tachycardia, sweating, and muscle rigidity.

Of note, other than this warning, sacred medicines have been shown to be extremely physically safe and non-addictive. As a psychiatrist, I have treated patients in whom use of a psychedelic drug unleashed a psychotic experience, but this is extremely rare. The most dangerous aspects of psychedelic use can happen when there is not an experienced guide to oversee what is happening during the journey. For example, I know of a situation in which a "wanna-be shaman" who had become inflated with self-importance was not paying attention, and a person using ayahuasca drowned while submerged in a hot tub.

Friday

At the Friday evening session, after the introductions, there would typically be some group drumming and perhaps a trial of a short-acting medicine known as toad slime, a form of DMT which comes from the Colorado River toad, *Bufo (Incilius) alvarius*. The leader, Ralph, called this *Jaguar medicine*. Its chemical name is 5-methoxy dimethyltryptamine (5-MeO-DMT), the organic form of the more-commonly synthesized DMT. The toad secretion used had been desiccated, crystallized, and chopped so that it could be intra-nasally snorted. The purpose was to "open up" channels in our brains as preparation for the longer journey the next day. DMT-derivatives would only last about five to ten minutes, after which one would return to a near-normal state of consciousness within fifteen minutes.

The DMT experience tends to bring about a rapid dissolution of both ego and body awareness to a state of pure energy during which, for example,

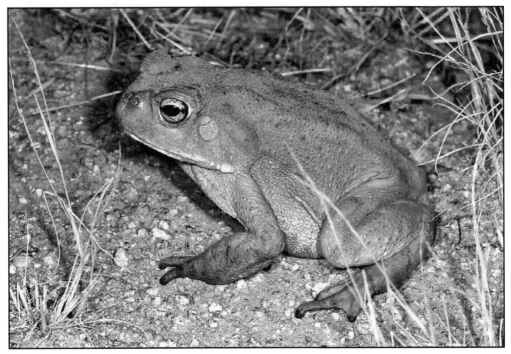

FIGURE 5. *Bufo (Incilius) alvarius* – The Colorado River Toad.
(from Wikimedia commons)

either extra-terrestrial beings are encountered, or spark-like scintillas and geometric swirling energy are perceived. One is blasted into a new space of reality which can cause some temporary anxiety, but the experience is over very rapidly. For some, it can be an overwhelming experience of joy. On no occasion did I personally receive anything transformative from such an intense and rapid experience, except the sense that it prepared my neural channels for the main journey with less apprehension. It was like Drano that cleared out the sludge in my brain networks. However, there was a sense of amazement and awe from retaining my sense of awareness but being launched into a cosmic space of pure formless energy.

Saturday

On Saturday of each weekend circle, a day-long vision walk would take place during which each member would hike alone in nature to meditate and to clarify his or her intention. At this time there was an opportunity for the psyche to interact with the surrounding environment. I found that I developed a deep appreciation for both the desert and the forest habitats during these times.

After a day of solitude, we would all gather again outdoors at a prescribed spot and time to share our experiences and our intentions with the group. At this time, each participant would choose among the medicines being offered by the shaman/leader (Ralph). Usually, such medicines as ayahuasca (or analogs), psilocybin mushrooms, San Pedro cactus extract (*Trichocereus pachanoi*), and occasionally iboga would be available. On occasion, synthetically synthesized LSD, 2C-B, or DMT would be offered as adjuncts to enhance the primarily plant-based medicines. The choice of medicine for each person would be determined by the intention of that individual consolidated by the day-walk.

The Saturday evening session would usually take place indoors, although occasionally outdoors. A contained space added to a sense of safety and unity among the group members. Typically, the circle for the journey included between eight to twelve participants. Such a size represented a particularly intimate circle allowing much to be accomplished. I have also participated in larger circles of twenty or more, but the experience for me was diluted with this number of people. Besides the leader, each circle included two to four *sitters* who would not take any medicine and would therefore be available to assist any group member. Of course, sitters would often experience a contact high in addition to absorbing the teachings of Ralph as well as the music during the evening. They would also participate in the circle when we paused our journeying for the rounds of chanting and sharing.

The medicine sessions would begin around sunset. Ralph would start by having us each in turn imbibe the prescribed medicine. He would bless each of us with sage and a feather-prayer dusting, wishing us a good journey. We would then all seat ourselves quietly in a circle. In the center of the circle would be prayer rug altar to which we had each contributed an object of significance that we had brought from home; for example, a crystal, small figurine, a feather, poem, or a symbol. This contributed to the creation of sacred space.

We would then lie down with our heads toward the center of the altar while Ralph spoke an invocation orienting us to the four horizontal

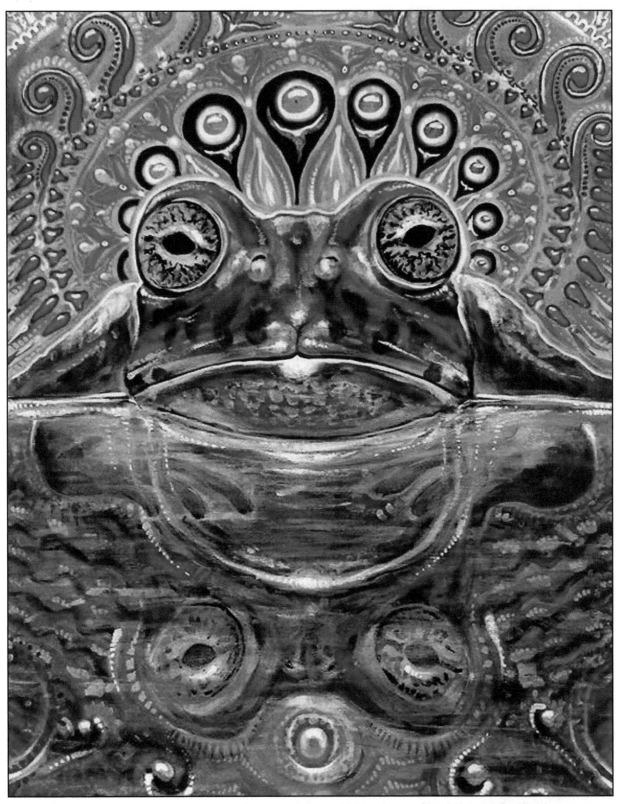

FIGURE 6. *Zabka* (Representation of a 5-Meo-DMT Journey) by Michael Garfield.

directions as well as toward the two vertical directions of the cosmos and the depths of the Earth. At times, he would then offer a short induction meditation or tell a story which included a myth or historical event, to activate our psyches as we all waited for the medicine to be absorbed and begin to take effect. Gentle indigenous or electronic music would be played at low volume as a vehicle to help carry us to the other realm and to enhance a calm mindset. After we had meditated in this state for about an hour, Ralph would offer a small booster dose for those who needed it to be further launched into the journey.

Music is an interesting auditory sensation that carries deep into the psyche. Often as one deepens, the music transmutes into visual patterns or other sensory phenomena and emotions, known as *synesthesia*. In a journey, multiple senses can be activated and engaged to expand the experience. The musical aspect of a journey was very important in that it could induce different visions and emotions. If the music was too loud, one could get absorbed in its own beauty and get off-track with the intention. If the music was too soft, its ability to serve as a boat in the journey was lost. Ralph had an intuitive way of knowing what pieces to play for us during the induction phase, the psychedelic/visual stage, the teachings aspect, and the ending of the session. I found that the music alone created a wonderful setting and was enough to make the sessions worthwhile.

In the Journey

Generally, each psychedelic journey can be seen to involve four phases, no matter which medicine is taken. It must be noted that sometimes, not much at all occurs during a journey, leaving the individual frustrated and disappointed. But generally, there is an initial phase of body sensations as the body assimilates the medicine, often accompanied by the physiological changes of increased heart rate and blood pressure, dizziness, nausea, or general discomfort. Often there is a brief period of anxiety or fear (sometimes of death) as the ego-body attempts to hold on to consensual reality until it is able to "break through the veil" to the expanded, transcendent realm. This involves a letting go, going with the discomfort and trusting the body to manage the sensations and keep oneself alive. This can often be facilitated through breathing and relaxation techniques, reassurance, and beautiful music. Often a good purge (vomiting), especially with ayahuasca, relieves all these tensions.

One then proceeds to the second phase of the psychedelic journey, which often involves an intensely multicolored, luminescent visual display of kaleidoscopic, mandala-like, or rapidly-changing expanding patterns seeming to emanate from a center point, akin to a beautiful firework. Depending on the medicine involved, these visuals can also appear as slowly changing arabesque patterns, swirls of lights, or three-dimensional serpentine images. During a journey when I had taken iboga, the visuals I experienced were arrays of highly detailed Baroque, Persian, and Egyptian patterns of intricate bejeweled artwork, rugs, or architecture, which would change every few seconds. With San Pedro or peyote, common are *mescaline visions* in which spacious and multicolored landscapes appear and then fade from one to another, much like breathing. The changes are slower, more like a sunset that corresponds to breathing in and out. During this phase, everything can only be described as stunning, unlike anything experienced in actual reality. It can be worthwhile to simply lie back, observe, and appreciate.

As time passes, these visuals become less predominant, and in the third phase, the wisdom teachings from the allies and ancestors emerge, and the answers for the initial intention are revealed. Often there is no direct answer but only another question to lead one further into exploration. Often an insight does not appear directly but from the periphery. This comprises the main teaching phase of a psychedelic journey.

The fourth phase occurs as the medicine wears off and these meditations diminish. This is the period when the integration of the lessons begins. This awareness may start right from the very beginning but usually continues for days, weeks, or months as the insights trickle in from one's memories of the powerful journey.

Notably, many psychedelic adventurers attempt to take high doses of medicine in order to maximize their journey. Often, this can result in their being launched into such a far-reaching realm (the outskirts of infinity) where they only experience ego-dissolution into pure energy. Either a pleasurable or a negative experience might occur, depending on the mind-set and setting. No psycho-spiritual work can really take place until the medicine is metabolized, when the ego and the body can again communicate and reintegrate with the various transpersonal teachers. However, sometimes a phase of total ego dissolution may have a healing effect at a molecular level without conscious involvement. It is in this relationship, the ego/transpersonal/Self axis, where transformational work occurs. The experience is actually driven less by the particular medicine or the dose than by the purity of the person's intention, the set, and the setting.

Methods to prolong the acute changes resulting from a journey, such as mindfulness, meditations, visiting nature, active imagination, journaling, and deeper and more genuine relationships, become necessary for a more lasting transformation. After a few months, this experience of deep truth may feel like simply an unreal drug-induced fantasy, therefore it is important to note what actual changes persist in one's personality and behaviors, or all is for naught. The visions and the immediate teachings can be wonderful, but how they deepen the individual over time represents the true wisdom. One must practice the teachings in ordinary life to fully integrate plant wisdom. It is the difference between insight and transformation.

It is crucial to note this difference. Insight comes easily with the visions and teachings in the altered state. Transformation refers to behavioral changes of the individual and is much more difficult to achieve. Dysfunctional and habitual behavior patterns tend to be ingrained over many years of living. To change a negative behavior to a more positive one, repetition and reinforcement are necessary. A new and more functional habit needs to be established. The distinction between insight and transformation is also valid in traditional psychotherapies. The bottleneck for change resides between these two concepts, as all psychotherapists and patients know. Creativity is more glamorous than the hard work of manifestation.

Chapter 5
Meditations to Structure a Vision Circle

A medicine journey can be disorienting and overwhelming. There are many different ways a leader may structure a journey to make it more comprehensible, positive, and retrievable to memory after the experience. Guided meditations during a vision circle help establish the set of a journey. I will describe several used very effectively by Ralph Metzner.

Six-Direction Medicine Wheel

The following diagram depicts the Six-Direction Medicine Wheel as a globe and demonstrates the possible directions with different attributes in each quadrant. The sacred medicine helps the traveler's journey to any direction depending on their intention. The participant sits in the center of this sphere, balancing the six parts, and can venture to any direction along the horizontal or vertical axis. The *coniunctio* (conjunction) represents the union of opposites between the masculine and feminine component. The four directions are a way for participants to orient themselves on the horizontal earth plane. The vertical axis represents the shamanic tree, with visioning at one end of the axis and healing at the other. With the participant (pilot) sitting in the center of these six directions, during a journey it is possible to travel into any of the directions to experience the intention through conscious will. For the pilot, there is an observing aspect of the transpersonal journey as well as an ability to move to different domains for exploration. By asking questions along the chosen path, various insights emerge in the form of an answer or another deeper question.

SIX DIRECTIONS JOURNEY

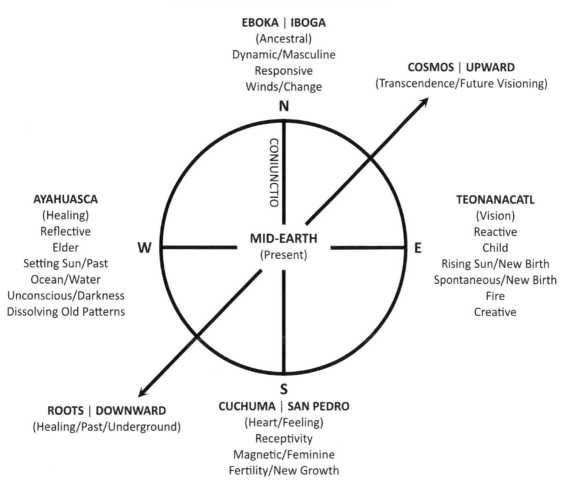

FIGURE 7. Six direction medicine wheel.
(As shared by Ralph Metzner)

Janus Model of Integration

In the figure on the following page, the Janus Model of Integration is diagrammed and named after the Roman god of two faces; one facing the past, where healing takes place, and the other facing the future, the place of visioning. We cycle through the past and future, always returning to the present, our life's work, with new insights gained by traveling in those two directions.

JANUS MODEL OF INTEGRATION

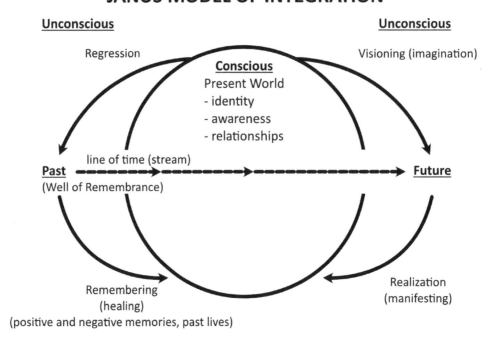

FIGURE 8. Janus model of integration.
(As shared by Ralph Metzner)

When using medicine, as a general rule, higher doses are required for healing. In these journeys, the ego is more obliterated or dies, and the medicine itself is able to "do its work" on a more cellular level without intervention of the participant directing how they think they should be healing. Visionary figures may be observed participating in the healing. As the healing progresses and the medicine begins to wear off, the ego-consciousness may return and become more involved in the healing. A helpful metaphor is of the visionary surgeon performing healing in the depths, and as one is coming out of anesthesia, the assistant (ego-participant) is being asked to close the wound and stitch up the patient to complete the process.

For journeys in which the intention is traveling to seek a vision of the future, a lower psychedelic dose is usually sufficient. This allows the person/ego to participate more actively with the incoming visions and insights, and to direct the storyline, much as in lucid dreaming. Those people who are gifted with lucid dreams find themselves able to direct the dreams in which they find themselves involved.

These dosing guidelines are only general, since healing may also be profound with low doses and envisioning can occur with higher doses. Much may also depend on the set and setting of the experience as to what happens. Some journeys incorporate both healing and vision. The Janus model figure displays schematically these two types of possible shamanic journeys of past, present, and future. Most crucial is that the healing (past) or visionary (future) insights of the journey will need to be brought back to the present time and be integrated if transformation is to occur in daily life. Also important is that while certain medicines can lend themselves to specific directions, any of the medicines used can potentially take one to any of the directions for exploration. Although there are qualitative differences in each entheogen, all roads lead to the transpersonal realm of experience; the direction is correlated to the participant's intention and mindset.

Tree Meditations

The tree is a universal symbol or archetype suitable for shamanic visionary work. It represents both the central vertical axis and the *anima mundi*, or world center, with its roots leading to the underworld and the crown of the tree reaching for the sky or cosmos. Often the participant, depending upon the intention, may choose a downward journey to the roots, to explore the past, or an upward journey to the treetop to gain a far-reaching vision. One can also choose to remain on the horizontal plane of the present and journey in any of the four directions. Often the individual will open a doorway at the base of the tree and enter, and follow a stairway downward to the roots, or climb upward. There are many different tree-like vertical meditation themes that come from many different traditions: Nordic, Jewish, and Indian. Here are a few:

Yggdrasil

The World Tree is considered sacred and found in numerous cultures. *Yggdrasil* (meaning Odin's horse) in Nordic mythology is a sacred ash tree supported by three roots and branches extending toward the heavens. Often a bird or spirit is found at the top of the tree, where one can catch a ride to some other place for exploration, usually for a divinatory perspective of the future.

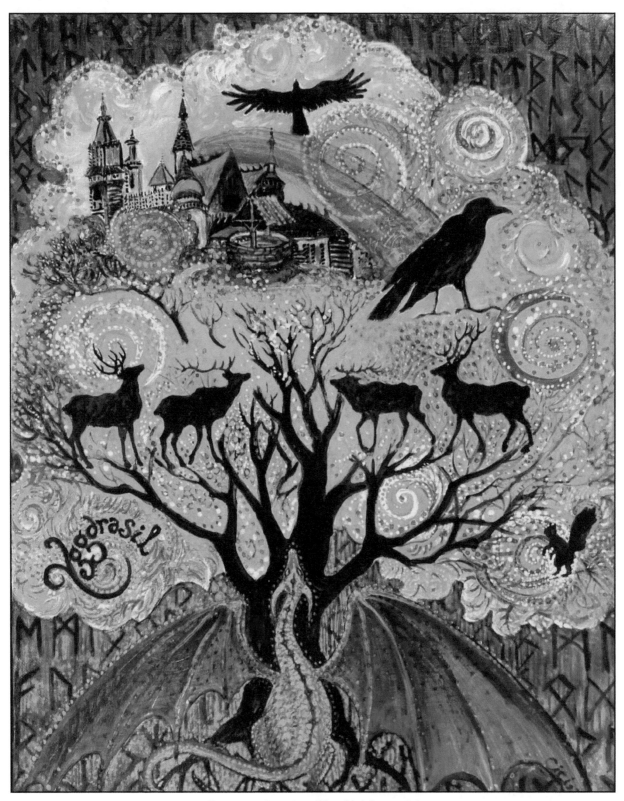

FIGURE 9. *Yggdrasil* by Cici Artemisia.

COSMIC TREE
Correspondences between cultures & the Chakra system

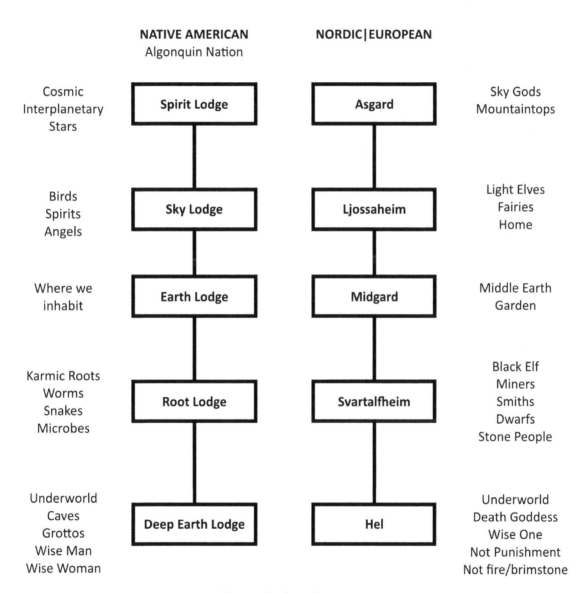

FIGURE 10. Cosmic tree.
(As shared by Ralph Metzner)

The Nordic tree is also represented in Figure 10, depicting five levels that can be explored. These levels have archetypal correspondences to the tree of the Algonquin Native Americans. Note that this structure allows for an exploration of the cosmos, the earth we inhabit, and the underworld, as well as all points in between.

Kabbalah

A similar symbol of the archetypal tree is found in the Jewish mystical tradition, the Kabbalah. The mystical tree is comprised by the ten *Sephiroth*. There are two aspects of God. The *En-Sof* is the hidden God that is insensible, and unintelligible, and can never be known. It is like the trying to conceive of what existed before the "big bang," before time and space were created 13.7 billion years ago. The other is the ten branches of the Sephiroth, which are the known attributes or manifestations of God. From the unknown God, energy spills downward into the containers of each Sephiroth (similar to chakras). As the energy falls, different spiritual attributes of God become known until lastly the Kingdom of God manifests on the earthly plane of mortal existence. This is sometimes described as the community of Israel, or as the *Shekhinah*, the feminine aspect of God. This becomes the power and divine life within a human.

One of the tasks in mystical Judaism is to implement the redemption of fallen humanity from its earth manifestation back to the original spiritual reality. This is done by completing the 613 commandments of the Torah. The *Shekhinah* returns to God, much like Shakti to Shiva (explained further below). There are many spiritual, cultural, and shamanic correspondences depicted in tree symbolism representing the vertical axis of the medicine wheel. Below is a diagram of the Kabbalistic Sephiroth tree. Notice all the interconnections and communications of the branches.

Tantra / Chakras

A similar archetypal constellation of the vertical axis also occurs in the Tantric Kundalini, Hindu, and other Asian systems as the various chakras. Here the coiled serpent, *Shakti*, sits at the base of the spine. Once activated, the serpent-goddess travels up the spinal tree through the various

TEN SEFIROTH - MYSTICAL TREE OF GOD

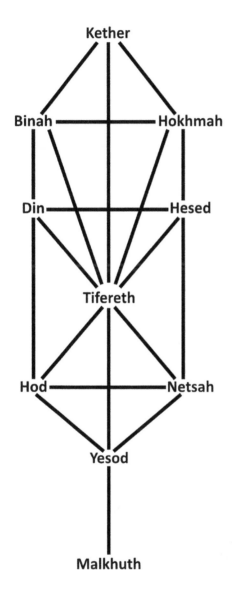

1. **Kether Elyon** - supreme crown of God

2. **Hokhmah** - wisdom or primordial idea of God

3. **Binah** - intelligence of God

4. **Hesed** - love or mercy of God

5. **Din or Gevurah** - power of God chiefly the power of judgement and punishment

6. **Tifereth or Rahamim -** compassion of God, beauty, mediates Hesed and Gevurah

7. **Netsah** - lasting endurance of God

8. **Hod** - majesty of God

9. **Yesod** - foundation of the active forces of God

10. **Malkhuth** - kingdom of God, Israel's community, Shekhinah

FIGURE 11. Kabbalistic Sephiroth tree representation.

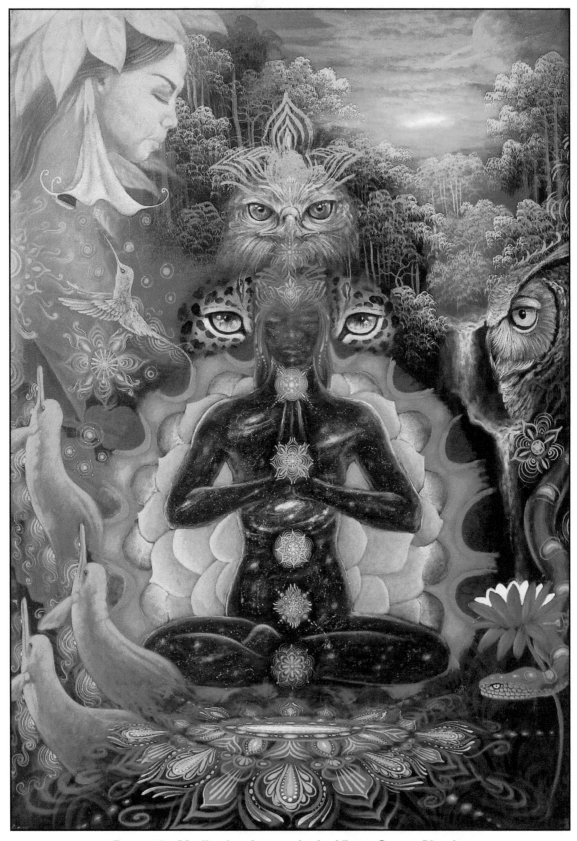

FIGURE **12.** *Meditacion Amazonica* by Victor Guerra Pinedo.
Chakras represent different forms and levels of consciousness.

38

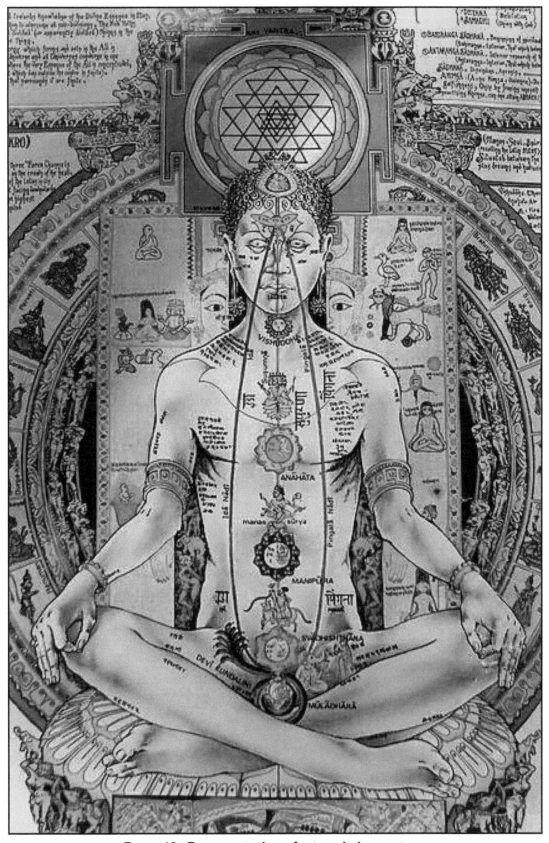

FIGURE **13. Representation of a ten-chakra system.**

39

chakras until she unites with god *Shiva* who inhabits the crown. These chakras are regions located along the spinal cord (akin to a tree trunk); the chakras are centers of consciousness with different attributes upon which adherents meditate.

Using a seven-chakra system and moving upward, the base chakra *Muladhara* (Sanskrit), represents the anal region at the base of the spine and connects one to the earth and roots. The next chakra, *Svadhisthana*, corresponds to the pelvic region, sexual organs, and the bladder, representing the water element. Ascending further leads to the solar plexus, navel, gut, and power chakra, *Manipura*, also the water element. The serpent rises next to *Anahata*, the heart center of feelings and emotions, the fire element. Then comes *Vishuddha*, the throat chakra, giving voice through the wind. Higher up still, the serpent-goddess meets the third eye of all-seeing wisdom, the region of insight and vision known as *Ajna*. Shiva sits atop at the crown chakra, *Sahasrara*. This is known as the spiritual center of pure consciousness beyond the body where self-realization (*samadhi*) occurs. The union of the masculine Shiva and the feminine Shakti represents a union of opposites (*coniunctio*) known as the Great Bliss. The crown is considered the place where spirit enters the body and flows downward. The soul flows upward from the earth through the anus and other centers and meets the spirit at the throat, where it projects human manifestation through the voice and the arts.

In *The Serpent Power* Sir John Woodroffe says, "Divine power Shakti, is coiled like a serpent (Kundalini), asleep at the base of the spine (Muladhara). The Sadhaka pronounces a mantra and awakens the Kundalini. She moves up the interior of the spine (Shushumma) to each lotus or chakra. Shakti, after her ascension through all the lotuses of the Shushumma unites with Shiva and achieves fulfilment and dissolution of the world." Tantra corresponds to the cosmic tree and can be used for the Tree of Life Meditation as seen below. In this path, the individual begins as a seed in the ground and moves upward. During the process, the various stages are suitable for visionary examinations of our life's memories.

TREE OF LIFE DIAGRAM

Serpent	Life Fire / Earth Wisdom
Birds	Thoughts from others outside us Teachings
Fruits	Creativity / Productivity Children / New Life
Leaves / Flowers	Inner Thoughts and Images
Sap	Soul
Branches	Relationships / Places / Projects Self Extensions (branches can break off and die but the tree continues)
Trunk	Course of life extending through time
Emergence	Birth
Roots (3)	Maternal / Paternal / Ancestral + Past Lives
Seed	Original Nature / Origin

FIGURE 14. Tree of life diagram.
(As shared by Ralph Metzner)

WELL OF REMEMBRANCE MEDITATION

Drink from it | Look down into it | Step into it | Go back in time

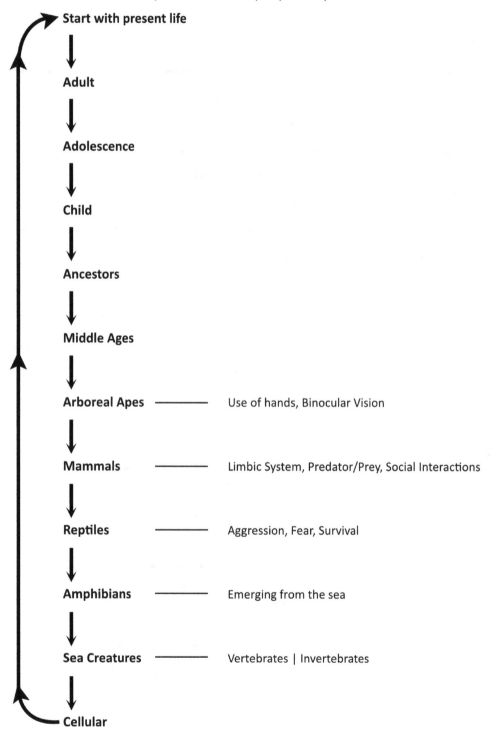

Start with present life

Adult

Adolescence

Child

Ancestors

Middle Ages

Arboreal Apes ——————— Use of hands, Binocular Vision

Mammals ——————— Limbic System, Predator/Prey, Social Interactions

Reptiles ——————— Aggression, Fear, Survival

Amphibians ——————— Emerging from the sea

Sea Creatures ——————— Vertebrates | Invertebrates

Cellular

Figure 15. Depiction of the Well of Remembrance Meditation.
(As shared by Ralph Metzner)

Well of Remembrance

Another journey shared by Ralph is one he called the Well of Remembrance meditation, which is also the title of one of his books (a must-read). The meditation begins at the top where one drinks from the well at the base of the tree Yggdrasil. As one descends, one passes through reverse evolution (regression) from the adult through various ages to the cellular level of existence and then cycles back to the present.

Any of the above active meditations can be presented by the leader during a shamanic journey or can be utilized later for individual reflection. These journeys, in addition to the described horizontal plane ventures, are used to help orient the participant from the daily reality to the transpersonal, visionary realm. With this orientation, the participant can begin to navigate to the needed direction, following their intention. During a journey, several directions may be explored. The intention always is the bridge to and from consensus reality and to the other world of wisdom teachings. What we learn from any journey needs to be brought back through memory into daily existence and then integrated into a behavioral change.

The following prayer often is chanted at the end of the ceremony:

PRAYER TO THE FOUR ELEMENTS

We thank you Grandfather fire who gives us Warmth
We thank you Grandmother ocean who gives us Peace
We thank you Grandfather air who gives us Change
We thank you Grandmother earth who gives us Life

Chapter 6

The Shadow Side of Psychedelics

With the new wave of popularity of the psychedelic experience, there are an increasing number of charlatan shamans proliferating in the collective population. More cases of dangerous malpractice are being reported in an unregulated environment under false pretenses of "shamanhood." (Lawlor 1991) Disguised as mystical and healing ceremonies, psychedelic use can fuel and inflate the ego of the untrained leader and participant into self-promotion and delusional-grandiose patterns reminiscent of cult status. It becomes a spiritual inflation of the ego and remains unintegrated into the deeper core Self.

Many seek transcendent experiences or enjoy the "high" and the colorful visions of psychedelics as a form of recreation but not for attainment of wisdom. People are quick to seek a shaman or guru, project authority onto such a figure, and then worship the guide. These charlatan shamans bypass scrutiny by the participants for their unethical behavior under the auspices that they hold the key to ancient wisdom. Some of these so-called healers will abandon their client if a negative experience occurs or the session time has ended, which is unconscionable behavior. They rarely screen incoming clients and provide no on-call medical help if needed. They can also charge enormous sums of money for the experience.

Unfortunately, some participants delude themselves and declare they have been healed—although this is premature—without adequate integration and follow-up. For the person who feels healed by such a mystical experience, often in the wake of such a fusion with the leader and lacking protective boundaries, the ego's deeply rooted troubles reemerge without any lasting transformation. (Lawlor 1991) Inflation by the experience often is expressed as a higher-than-thou, judgmental attitude: "I now have higher wisdom than you." The short side of such an experience is that, with time, all the old neurotic patterns of behavior return unless follow-up therapy continues to integrate the gains perceived. Even though psychedelic-based treatments are potentially helpful, there must be further longer term reinforcement for positive changes to fully integrate and be maintained.

Such circumstances are reminiscent of the Timothy Leary era of the 1960s, when a collective cult-like following of unrestricted psychedelic usage developed, resulting in many people following the mantra, "Turn on, tune in, and drop out." Yet, the world was not saved. Sidney Cohen, a leading psychedelic researcher from UCLA, dating to the 1950s, once debated Timothy Leary. Cohen warned that psychedelics "expand one's gullibility" and produce "completely an uncritical" state. It caused many unsavory people and adulterated drugs to enter the marketplace with consequent suffering. Timothy Leary's propaganda about LSD led to an undifferentiated counterculture, which ironically promoted Nixon's new war on drugs. These negative effects led to the criminalization of psychedelics and the abrupt stoppage of all research into their potential use as legitimate medicines. They were relegated to Schedule I status, the same class as opioids, amphetamines, and other dangerous and addictive drugs.

This type of self-aggrandizing inflation has also been seen in the stories of a number of spiritual gurus who developed cult followings but were not using psychedelics. The difficulty with following leaders lies in the reluctance or ignorance of people in general to engage in the challenging work of self-examination and integrating the shadow side of the personal and collective psyche, as described by C.G. Jung. Often, the uninitiated person projects their own inner authority on to another charismatic individual who seems to hold all the answers. In doing so, people disempower themselves. On a collective level, the shadow is typically involved with politics or religions, especially when there is division into tribes such as in our present time. The dark or evil side is projected onto the other political party, race, or different religious point of view. There is no self-scrutiny or reflection regarding opposing differences or values, and one's position becomes intolerant of the others.

The shadow can be a great teacher if it is realized as such, puncturing the inflation leading to grandiosity and holding a person or group accountable for any excesses in their attitude or behavior. The narcissists of the world in positions of power are a result of the lack of integrating the shadow experience. The hallmarks of a narcissistic personality are: a lack of accountability, projection of negative material onto other people or groups (blaming), a self-inflated opinion of oneself, striving for power, and lack of compassion for others. All connote the absence of integration of the shadow aspects of the psyche. Before authentic spirituality can occur, there must be a descent into the dark realm, much as in Dante's *Inferno,* in which the poet travels to the lower circles of Hell before his ascent to Paradiso is possible. This corresponds to the ritual death experience in shamanic initiation rites, or the ego death during a psychedelic experience; which can be fraught with fear, anxiety, and negative content. The psychedelic experience often forces a person to confront their shadow issues as a gateway to a higher spiritual realm. They earn entrance to transpersonal wisdom by the journey through the shadow.

In my work during the Mythopoetic men's movement, the primary founder, Robert Bly, called this phase "enclawment." He associated it with being pounced upon from behind by a panther and pulled down to the ground to face unintegrated aspects of reality that a person has buried and does not want to face. Usually these are painful or traumatic experiences that a man or woman encountered in childhood, or during life adversities. Only after facing these can the ascent to a more profound, authentic, and positive reality be integrated. The shadow is a potent teacher.

Unfortunately, there are numerous descriptions of psychedelic therapy abuse by well-known, seasoned, and credentialed psychedelic therapists conducting underground circles. The underground shamans/gurus are not held to the ethical standards to prevent exploitation of boundaries required of legitimate researchers and psychotherapists. When you add in psychedelics, defenses are lowered as the ego dissolves and dissociates, making the client highly suggestible to the input of the leader, who is often idealized. There is an obvious power imbalance between the shaman/leader and the client, which is a dynamic that can lead to potential abuse. There have been multiple reports of sexual boundary violations by psychedelic therapists, usually with the old excuse that it is done with a healing and loving intention. The sexual boundary issues include not only intercourse, but also snuggling, kissing, nurturing touch, and spooning. Any leader offering touch during a session needs to distinguish beneficial nurturing and touching from a sexual-boundary violation, with the former incorporated into treatment protocols with client consent.

Other reports of psychedelic abuse have occurred in sessions in which a person has a negative or frightening experience, and the therapist rationalizes that it is the client who is "crazy." The problem is "not the leader's fault." In a vulnerable altered state, many buried or traumatic contents from the client's unconscious may come to the surface and re-traumatize the person with strong emotional content. Often, an untrained or unscrupulous leader will claim that it is the patient's diagnosis that led to a traumatic outcome, rather than that the client was victimized by the leader. This is experienced as a profound betrayal by the participant. Such a leader may hold him or herself above the fray with an inflated sense of spiritual authority.

When such leaders do not offer follow-up after sessions, a client who is having a difficult time during or after the session can feel abandoned. Another abuse is that often clients are not screened for medical issues or concurrent drug usage that may contraindicate psychedelics. Participants should be aware of the plan if a medical complication occurs during a session. It is imperative to know how is it to be handled and what emergency procedures are available.

I have indirectly known two people who died while in a hot tub, one on MDMA and another on ayahuasca. Also, serotonin syndrome, which can be dangerous, may occur with people on SSRI antidepressants who take tryptamine-containing or MAOI-containing psychedelics. When choosing a practitioner, do interested individuals ask legitimate questions of the leader and are they answered? For example, are there proper preparation, intention, and follow-up sessions being offered?

As hallucinogens are becoming promising once again in psychiatric treatment, as well as common in psychedelic underground circles, "Big Pharma," with its profit-driven motivation, has begun getting involved. Both licensed, credentialed practitioners and charlatan guru/shaman types are all participating in this renaissance period. This creates a dangerous mixture to sort out for those wanting to experience the new age of psychedelia.

It is important to remember that academic credentials and experience do not screen for the ethics of any individual practitioner. Having a M.D. or Ph.D. degree does not screen for the power drives or competency of the doctor/healer. One personality trait that I highly value in a potentially enlightened person is humility. Financial exploitation of vulnerable people who are seeking enlightenment and healing also is prevalent, with some practitioners charging thousands of dollars for promises of cures for chronic and serious medical conditions. Also of serious concern is that at present, there exists no oversight over the purity and standardization of the various medicinal compounds used outside research institutions. The saying *caveat emptor* applies, and yet silence about these abuses persist. Even Michael Pollan's groundbreaking book promoting psychedelics, *How to Change Your Mind*, does not adequately describe the hidden dangers and abuses that have occurred.

At present, I have found the best description of the shadow side of hallucinogen use discussed by Will Hall, M.A., who describes his disturbing personal abuse encounters in an article in *madinamerica.com* (September 25, 2021), titled "Ending the Silence Around Psychedelic Therapy Abuse." It has caused me to pause and think about the prevalence of psychedelic usage in these times. (Google this article)

Despite the above shadow and abuse concerns, the future effective use of psychedelic therapy will depend on developing a group of transpersonal facilitators and clinicians who are highly trained. This new community of entheogenic practitioners will ideally be taught accurate empathy and shadow-integration techniques to help the client heal from destructive patterns and become free from delusion. Psychedelic treatment shows great promise for healing and visioning for many people. It is important for participants and practitioners alike to maintain awareness of the potential for misuse. Another aspect that will require further inquiry is the current popularity in micro-dosing for cognitive enhancement, and creativity. The future of psychedelic therapy depends on better integration of the above-described shadow aspects and will only be as good as its weakest link; ethics matter.

Section Two

Psychedelic Medicines and Experiences

In earlier chapters, I presented some basic concepts regarding shamanism and described how this approach can be helpful in expanding our modern understanding of healing as well as realigning our relationship to "Mother Earth" and the natural world. One aspect of shamanism involves the use of sacred plant medicines, which I will describe in detail in this section. The chapters that follow will combine research and descriptions of entheogenic medicines with my personal visionary experiences. It is focused on the plant medicines with which I have the most experience. Each account of one of my experiences with a medicine will be followed by an in-depth look at the medicine's properties and history.

Chapter 7

A Personal Ayahuasca Medicine Journey

In the autumn of 1991, I decide to ride my Harley Davidson out to a Joshua Tree home as part of the adventure I was embarking on. When I arrive, I am welcomed by Ralph Metzner and several other participants. I am feeling a bit apprehensive, which is common prior to any psychedelic experience into the unknown. The journey is held within a house on the outskirts of the town which abuts boulder formations in back. As twilight approaches, the subtle and beautiful colors of the desert landscape intensify as the rabbits emerge to forage outside the window. All is calm, quiet, and natural, lending to a feeling of safety and security.

The Journey Begins

The medicine choices being offered that night are San Pedro cactus, psilocybin mushrooms, and ayahuasca. Each person makes the choice of which medicine to take on the journey, based on their intention and aided by the vision meditation in the desert earlier that day. I review my own intention for the evening: to understand my relationship to my career, which has seemed dry and unfulfilling, as well as my relationship to the earth and my family. I also want to address my times of depression and understand more about the dynamics causing them.

We start the evening with a round of *Mr. Toad's Ride medicine* (5-MEO DMT) which we all insufflate nasally in turns. This secretion comes from the Colorado river toad, *Bufo alvarius*. First, I feel a dizziness, followed by a rapid disintegration of ego-consciousness into pure energy with the appearance of flickering light scintillas against a dark background of outer space. I had no significant insights, and the experience ends in about ten minutes. It had the overall effect of "cleaning the pipes," opening up my neural pathways, and diminishing any anxiety about the upcoming journey with ayahuasca.

Around 8:30 p.m., Ralph measures about 90 ml (milliliters) of the molasses-like ayahuasca for me. I drink it in about three or four gulps, followed by some tea to wash it down and dark chocolate to abate the horrendous aftertaste. After Ralph blesses me, I go to prepare my bedding site in the circle with my Pendleton Chief Joseph blanket, pillow, and the purging bowl at my feet. I then put on my eyeshade to block out the external ambient light and the scene of my surroundings.

After all of us have taken the medicines, we settle into the circle with our heads toward the altar and feet extended outward. Ralph begins an induction meditation of breathing and rebirthing, but I soon feel myself withdrawing from his words into my own inner space. I am finding it difficult to move about as I feel gravity pressing me to the ground. After about twenty minutes appear some early visions of darting snake heads and a multitude of eyes observing me. Ralph then puts on some music with drums, which takes me further inwards, and slowly some very colorful visions appear, somewhat reminiscent of LSD but without the ego dissolution or fear state and with an accompanying sense of relaxation. The visuals are abstract three-dimensional matrices with a serpentine quality and are extraordinarily beautiful. They are experienced by all my senses and I shift into an increasing state of ecstasy.

I lie quietly and just observe as the music syncs with the visual display. Although I cannot move, I become aware of others in the circle entering their own individual spaces but all with a connection to the group. Someone has already purged, although as yet I feel no nausea. Another person is sobbing uncontrollably, but there is no judgment. Soon I witness a collage of iridescent green snakes and other reptilian creatures intertwining with the abstract visuals. Vegetation is everywhere, lush with greens, rich blues, and with dark black and purple spaces in between. Colorful snakes appear and are beautiful. Then some Amazonian natives appear, all looking at me with their faces painted, bones through their noses, and feathered headdresses. Serpents appear and bare their fangs to me in attempts to frighten me. I comment to them that they are not frightening and ask them for wisdom teachings. They instantly change into luscious, sensual female snakes with long eyelashes and large red lips. Water is everywhere, flowing in streams and waterfalls, and dripping off leaves.

Despite this all taking place in the desert, I feel I am in the midst of an

Amazonian rainforest. I am overwhelmed by the awareness of the immense beauty, sensuality, the holiness of nature, and the interconnectedness of everything. Even the dark creatures are beautiful. No image lasts long, but they flow kaleidoscopically from one to another. If I think a thought, it turns into an image. I see black panthers with blazing eyes stalking the forest. The vegetation is near swampy waters with creatures, all neon, iridescent, and luminescent, crawling in and out of the morass. Snakes turn into phalluses, which appear everywhere and turn into mushroom-like stalks with red tips which are constantly penetrating the surrounding vegetation, appearing like moist vaginas. The vegetation keeps opening up and spreading, receptive and accepting to being penetrated by the phalluses in this giant dance of fertility and fecundity. The phalluses then turn back into snakes and reptiles of a thousand species. Intense colors are everywhere with glowing lights against a dark background. I briefly think that this might all be lost when the rainforest is lost to the world. I am observing all of this with a sense of awe, as if I am present and part of the scene.

Following are several ayahuasca paintings that are representative of this awe-inspiring vision.

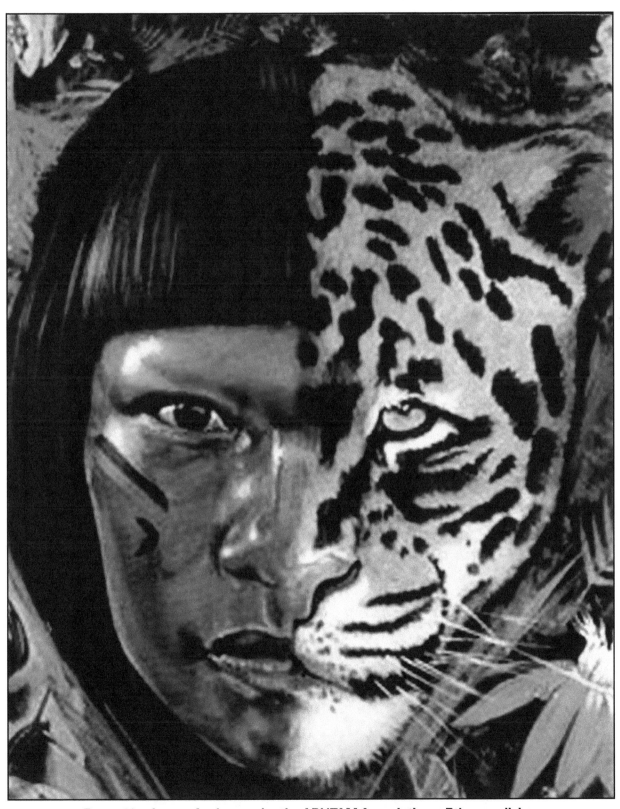

FIGURE **16.** *Jaguar Ayahuasca* by the ARUTAM Association – Ethnomedicine.

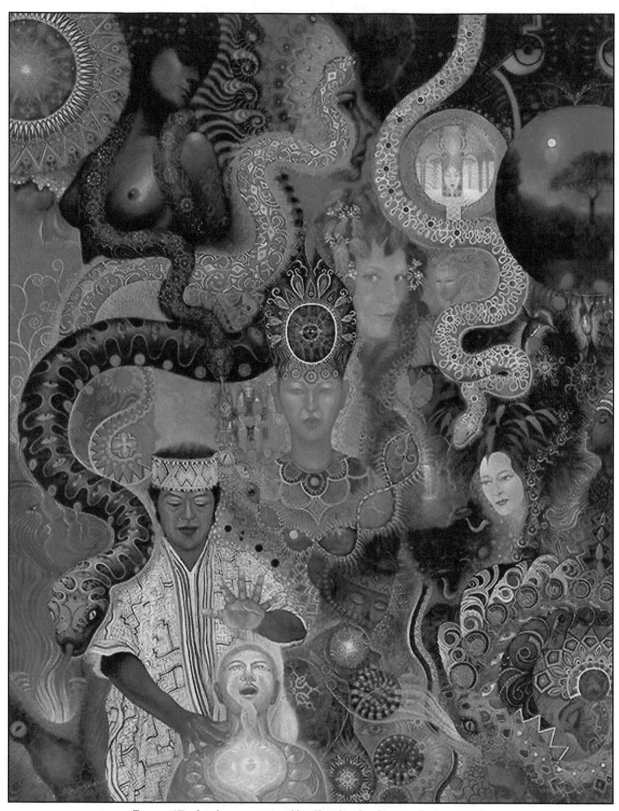

FIGURE 17. *Ayahuasqueros Healing* by Anderson Debernardi.

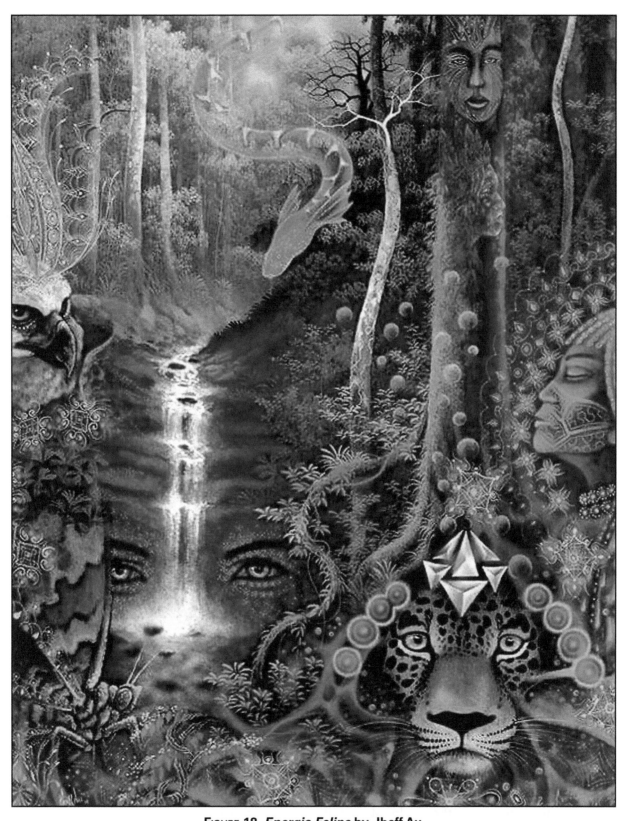

FIGURE 18. *Energia Felina* by Jheff Au.

The goddess of fertility is everywhere. Her face appears seductive, her shape taking Aphrodite/Cleopatra forms with beautiful bodies all around her. The whole forest is a mass of moving fertile creatures, bodies and forms, which are bending, changing shapes, kissing, and embracing. Nature appears seductive but without any sense of manipulation, domination, or hierarchy—one enormous ecstatic dance of receptivity and penetration. I observe all this and feel extremely erotic but not sexual. I ask myself whether this is just all a wonderful psychedelic journey and wonder, to what end? It is all seductive and I now feel stuck in this phase of the erotic. The images following drawn by me, are expressions of these visions.

I then hear the voice of Ralph breaking through saying, "A wise old owl told me that in the midst of a journey, it is important to remember your intention." I then remember, and I ask the creatures surrounding me to teach me their wisdom and to help guide me to heal my depression and deepen the work I do in my career. I ask for wisdom that I can remember and take back with me.

The First Round

The structure of the circles was always to lie down while going on our individual journeys with the medicine and music. Typically, every ninety minutes during a session, Ralph would have us all sit up facing the altar and participate in some form of vocal but non-verbal expression, which was called round one. Round two would consist of short vocal or verbal vocalizations. Then we would return to our individual time lying in a circle. The third or final round would consist of each sharing one or two sentences about the experience. Then we would end the evening session. In the integration session the following morning, we all would discuss the experience in more detail and how it applied to the initial intention.

Ralph asks us to sit up and connect as a group for round one of the circle. First, I realize I have to get up for a purge of watery diarrhea in the bathroom, and when I return, I feel extremely nauseated and vomit a brown liquid into my bowl. The purge comes from deep down inside me and feels like a welcome release. I still feel some residual queasiness in my solar plexus regions. The sitters are there to help us with all of these physical aspects. It is explained ahead of time that these purges are normal and everyone in the circle takes these purges in stride.

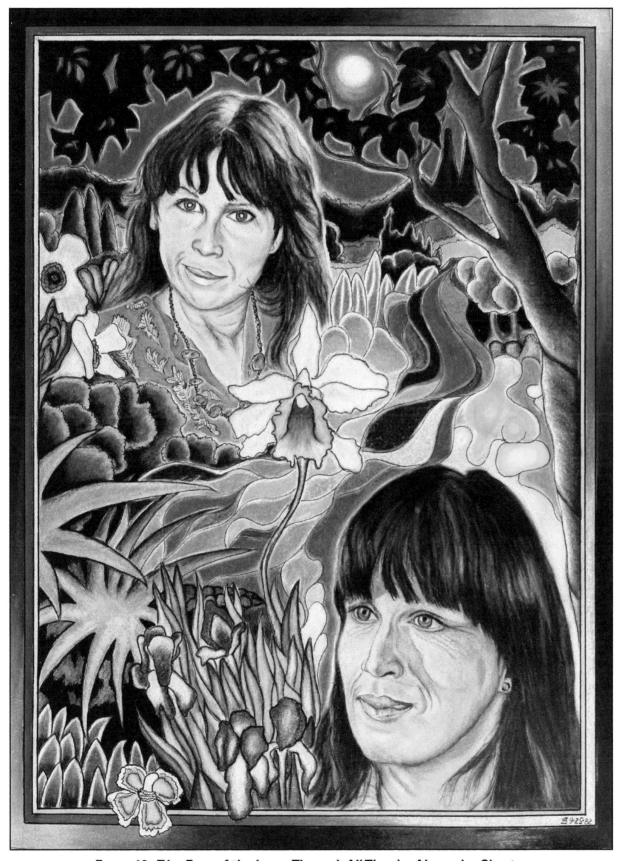

FIGURE **19.** T*he Face of the Lover Through All Time* by Alexander Shester.

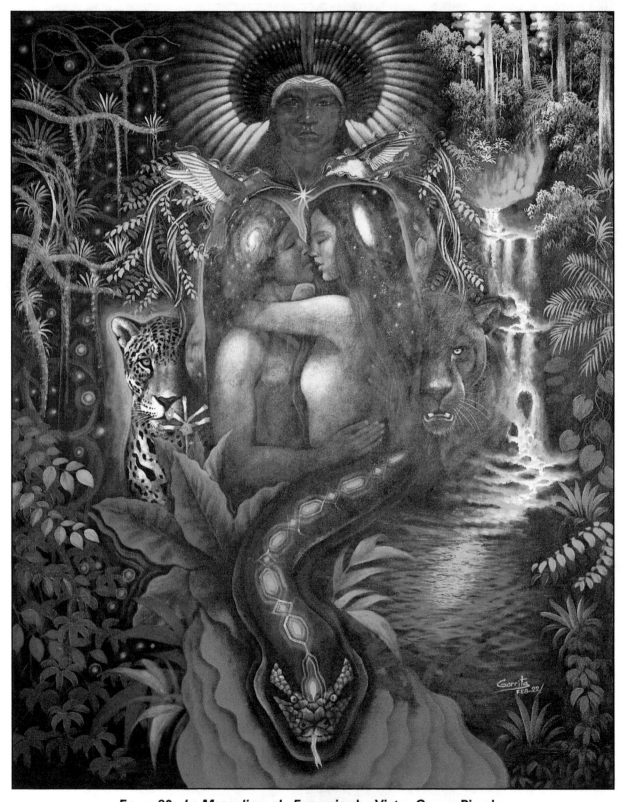

FIGURE 20. *Lo Masculino y lo Femenino* by Victor Guerra Pinedo.

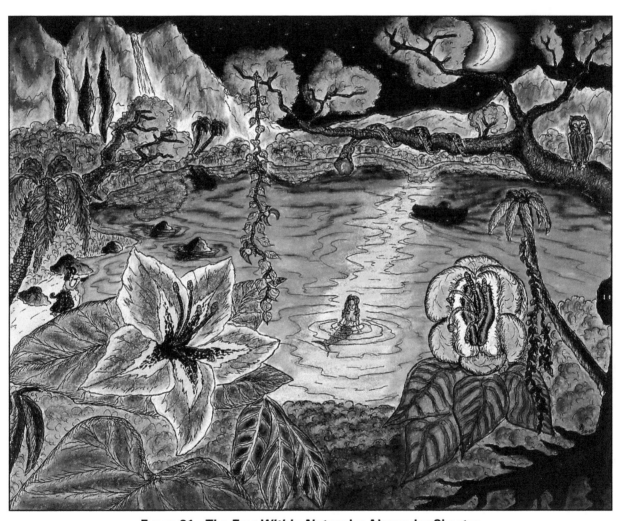

FIGURE 21. *The Eros Within Nature* by Alexander Shester.

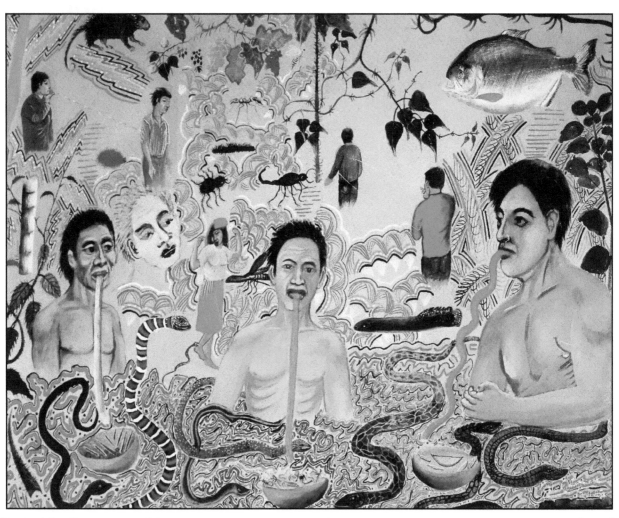

FIGURE 22. *Three Types of Sorcerers* by Pablo Amaringo, Luna, and White. A depiction of Purgativo. (1989)
(by permission of North Atlantic Press)

Ralph asks all of us if we need a small booster of medicine. At first, I think not, but I feel that the animals in my images are still embedded in a technological matrix and are asking to emerge more completely. I am feeling well and that the medicine is giving me a splendid journey, so I tell Ralph that I would like to go inward more intensely. At first, I am reluctant to leave my inner journey to rejoin the circle of fellow travelers. I realize only later that these rounds serve to help us maintain connection as a group and provide a sense of how others are progressing on their journey. Additionally, Ralph and the sitters have an opportunity to check up on us to make sure no one is lost or having a very difficult time.

For round one, Ralph asks us to sit up and vocalize or chant with a rattle or drum, but without verbalization. The Vine medicine makes it difficult for me to sit up or relate with the other attendees. I have an overwhelming need to lie down, close my eyes, and go back to inner space. I feel the full gravity of the earth pushing me down. Those who have taken mushrooms and San Pedro cactus are all sitting up without difficulty. I do manage to vocalize non-verbal sounds, which seem to start in my lower chakras and ascend through my solar plexus, which is still churning, then up through my heart chakra and into a voice that comes out beautifully.

As I return to my own journey, I have images of being in a swampy, boggy area with reptiles everywhere. I look into the water and see numerous fish and cold-blooded creatures crawling out of the water onto land and beginning to breathe. It is as if I were witnessing evolution. The fish turn into greenish amphibians which then display their fins as they fan out. I am realizing that because they are cold-blooded, their activity level is dependent on the outside climate and environment. The music is powerful and continues to synergize the experience.

The teachings then begin for me as I realize that the reptile brain in me is a metaphor for when I am not in harmony with the natural or psychological climate of my surroundings, for instance, in my work. In humans, the reptile brain consists of the brain stem and sub-cortical structures governing the instinctual and unconscious physiological phenomena linked to survival. When this disharmony occurs, there is a desynchronization of my entire nervous system, which, when not working efficiently, leads to negative thoughts and depression. This insight is instantaneous as I realize that my instincts are not in harmony with my cerebral thought patterns,

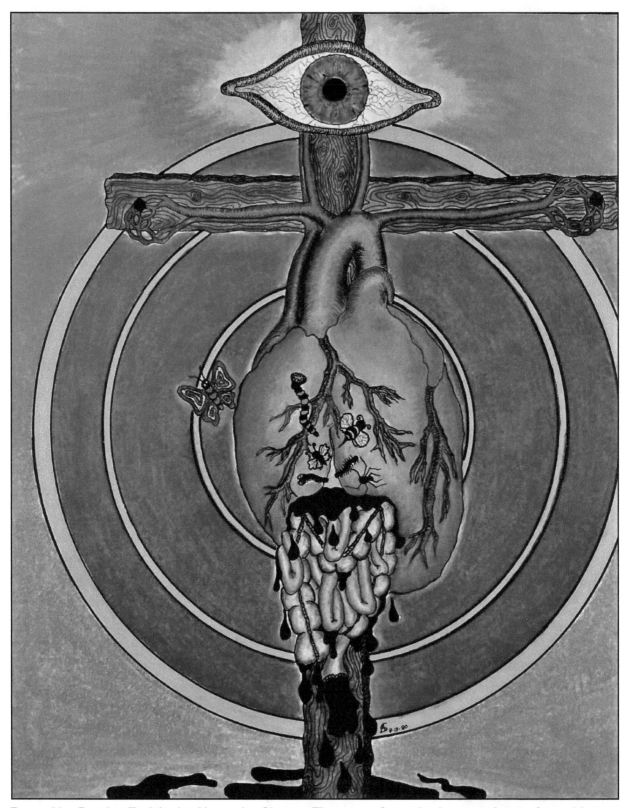

FIGURE 23. *Purging Toxicity* by Alexander Shester. The purge from the heart and gut of psychic toxicities, freeing the soul. The all-observing eye of consciousness is on the cross, which has both the horizontal and vertical axis to which the body is pinned to in life, expressing a form of vulnerability.

emotions, and consciousness. The medicine is attempting to resynchronize my entire nervous system by putting me in touch with the ways of the natural world.

In other words, I have been living too much in my head and not with my gut, heart, and passion. Our higher brains enable us to observe and analyze, but they can disconnect us from the instinctual ecological nature of our brainstem, our "inner reptile." Brainstem health is essential for vitality, purpose, drive, intention, and wakefulness. Otherwise, the lizard is detuned to a lower frequency and becomes sluggish and underactive, as when living in a cold environment. In my vision, I eventually become a reptile and experience that level of life.

I continue to observe the reptiles and amphibians in the jungle, which are in perfect harmony with the moist, warm climate. Their movements are tuned toward focused intention with purpose, keyed to surviving, eating, and procreating. The lizard keeps appearing in the visions as a powerful spirit animal. It asks me for help in allowing it to live again more fully by breaking through the imprisonment of my technological, medical mindset and any suppressing medication. The lizard reacts like an impulsive force, not trying to gratify itself as instincts often do in humans, but as a force for survival in the natural world. When the lizard is in touch with nature, it has pure intention, functioning without any waste, inefficiency, or indulgence. It just "does its living," aware of the lushness of its surroundings with all the color and beauty, but not needing to respond cerebrally. It eats, is eaten, protects territory, reproduces, and moves. It is the life force itself, pure instinct. I feel the lizard entering my being and becoming part of me.

Next, I see a crocodile. It is swimming in the river, and then, I actually become it. I am hungry and focus my attention on the fish that I eat. My eyes are ever watchful of my surroundings. I enjoy the experience of being a crocodile, which seems to be my reality at the moment. The experiential truth aspect of mind-expanding medicines is like the difference between watching a movie and being an actor inside that movie. It all feels so real. It is similar to having a direct three-dimensional experience of an archetype, either relating to or becoming it. It brings to mind the saying that somehow "the plant knows more about me than what I know about myself." Either the godhead wisdom resides in the plant itself, or its chemicals open up the gateways to the transpersonal receiver in the brain, removing the veil that keeps us unaware of our own hidden inner wisdom. Perhaps both are true.

The teachings are direct and straightforward during the experience. Only later one might cynically second-guess what occurred and conclude that the insights were false information from the wanderings of an intoxicated brain. Yet it really does not matter if the vision is a truth or a falsehood if a positive behavioral change results from it. Is a dream or active imagination any less real because of our participation in creating it? The value lies in just accepting and understanding what is being presented without a judgement regarding veracity.

This session has been an experience that cannot be replicated by psychotherapy, which I conclude has become too cerebral for me. On one journey, during a brief break, the person next to me rolled over and whispered to me, "reptiles are where it's at" and "this concentrated session was worth six months of intensive psychotherapy." I realize that this represents the disconnect I feel at work. The cerebral observational context has become overemphasized at the expense of direct experience and instinct. Analyzing what a lizard is doing in a dream symbolically is very different than becoming that entity and experiencing what it is doing and how it actually functions within my psyche.

When one encounters a spirit animal or plant, asking it for help and guidance can lead to answers one is seeking through the initial intention. I realize that the help I am really asking for in this vision is that of resynchronizing my body and brain, my instinctual world and my cerebral world, and moving toward valuing direct experience over academic knowledge. I view it as returning to nature and becoming a snake with a light beam shining from it: conscious instinct as the force that will illuminate my path. So, these encounters become my spirit guides into this instinctual realm.

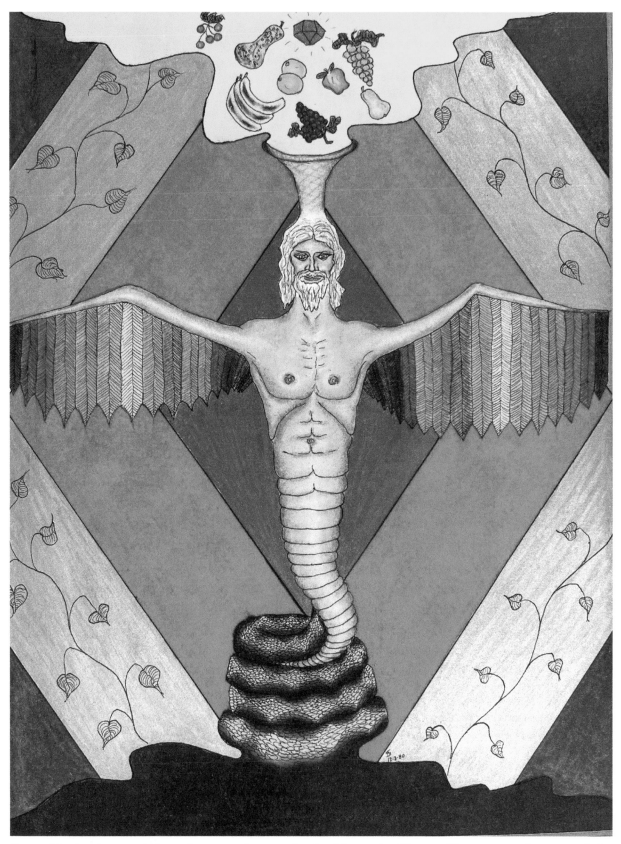

FIGURE **24.** *Instinct and Consciousness Integrating* by Alexander Shester. The serpent rises out of the primal darkness and ascends to manifest the fruitfulness of awareness.

The Second Round

Ralph then calls us back for a second group round. I am still having difficulty raising up my body, while those who took mushrooms or San Pedro are relating more from a heart and mind level with a better degree of social awareness and verbal capacity. "Ayahuasca is gravitas." After the round, I return to my journey.

The music being played is now a choir of Christian monks and a woman's voice chanting something spiritual, which raises my consciousness to a higher chakra frequency, out of the swamp and jungle of my solar plexus and root chakras. I have an observation about the importance of the music provided during the circles. Ralph usually brings some exquisite ethnic music, which serves as a vehicle to carry us on our individual journeys. Often it is some combination of electronic and indigenous music, both meditative and rhythmic. He is aware of how easy it can be to become seduced by the music alone while journeying, so frequent reminders to remember our intentions are given periodically to help each of us get back on track.

I then see the image of a beautiful White Goddess in the heaven above, with a veil and wings spread out like an umbrella over the dome of the sky. She is protecting all of the Earth below, including myself. A feeling of unconditional grace and love flows through me. I experience what life without fear and with total trust is like. I, my children, and the world are all protected if only we are able to let go of negative preconceptions and to be receptive to all the values that nature has to offer. I recognize the interdependence of all creatures, plants, and minerals. I realize that this type of peace exists within my psyche and that I need to cultivate it in further meditations. Developing trust is essential. I feel the truth of its existence as a pervasive consciousness in the external Universe.

By 2:30 a.m., all the participants have left the circle and are socializing, except for the *ayahuasceros* among us. Many are now eating soup, nourishing themselves after a long fasting period and journey. I am not yet very sociable or hungry and feel a sense of physical fatigue from the adventure I just went through. I eventually do eat and go outside for a short walk with two others in the dark desert. Although I am still a bit dizzy, the night air and glorious sky with all the stars slowly bring me back to this world. I chat for a while and am told by the more experienced travelers that this incredible feeling will remain clear for two or three weeks as a psychedelic afterglow. Avoiding such parts of life as TV, freeways, and the news will help prolong the vividness of the journey.

Closing Circle: Integration

After a few hours of sleep, we all awaken on Sunday morning and eat a hearty breakfast. We gather again around the altar and Ralph leads us with chants using his shaman's drum and rattle. We then go around the circle, each of us in turn expressing our individual experiences, which differ from very powerful to minimal, ecstatic to difficult. We each relate the experience to the individual intentions we had brought into the journey. Ralph offers minimal interpretation of the experiences shared to avoid intellectualizing them.

Despite the intense journey being over, we are told to expect persistent new insights arising for us over the next weeks. We are reminded that it is important to take the insights and use them to make behavioral changes in order for transformation to occur. Otherwise, the visions would diffuse, and we would likely retain our old habits and return to our previous state of consciousness without much gain. The psychedelic experience would then become merely recreational rather than a format for gaining wisdom, healing, envisioning, and change. After the integration round is over, Ralph plays some upbeat, ethnic music that we all dance to in a circle of joyousness. We then break the circle, clean up the house and surrounding grounds, say our goodbyes, hug, and head back to our homes and lives.

Aftermath and Retrospective

In the following weeks, I continue to contemplate the lessons of the vision quest. I make efforts to learn more about my own local bioregion, both environmental as well as social, and the influences it has on me, both positive and negative. I initially thought my return to work Monday morning would be a shock, needing to deal with the pathologies of my patients, but I found it to be an easy transition. I found myself able to quickly focus on each patient's psychodynamics and help them with acute insights and understanding.

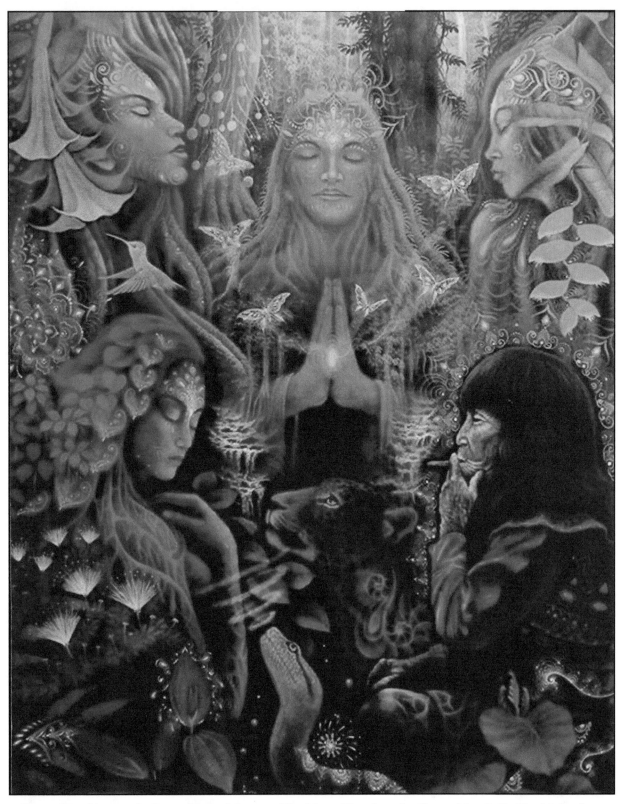

FIGURE 25. *Shamanic Sacra-Mental Spaces* (Goddess Blessing the Forest) by Felix Pinchi Aguirre.

The lessons of fertility within nature, stewardship with the earth, and the presence of the Goddess, with her receptivity and loving-kindness, remain with me. I recognize the dryness of my approach at work with its emphasis on intellect, masculine values, and the technological, scientific, medical model. I realize that my connection to the interdependence of the ecological/Gaia realms in my psyche needs to be reestablished. I also contemplate the power of my Harley Davidson motorcycle—a symbol of my "Wild Man"—but am aware that I need to mix this masculine power with more gentleness, stewardship, and caring. The "Green Man" archetype has also been awakened and will become a new symbol for me to meditate upon, as a balance to that dynamic wildness within.

In relating my experience to that of others, I find that a majority of those taking ayahuasca experience a clearing out all the "psychological toxins" that accumulate in the mind and body, leaving the person feeling cleansed, lighter, and energized. This *purgativo*, which some people find distasteful and uncomfortable initially, tends to leave one feeling revitalized, ready to return to the more routine issues of daily life. Whatever one feels burned-out about, in career or relationships, is now imbued with clarity and a sense of hope. One feels like a "clean machine," at least for a while, until the "creepy crawlers" of stress, old habit patterns, and disappointments recur in the body and psyche, clogging up the filters of experience and blocking psychic energy again.

In retrospect, I found that the visionary aspects of the use of this plant medicine quickly, and with great intensity, propelled my psyche into truth-bearing insights. However, the physical and psycho-spiritual aspects were demanding on my body and soul and a period of restoration became necessary. I felt that such journeying was not something I could do again soon. However, I learned on a future week-long vision quest in the New Mexico mountains that the medicines could be utilized every night without harm. More will be discussed about this later.

Lessons Learned

One major lesson of my ayahuasca journey was that one aspect of depression is a desynchronization of the primitive, instinctual brain from the higher cerebral functions, partly due to a loss of connection with the natural world. Instinct and passion are connected concepts. The medicine can have the effect of retuning the brain by waking up the instincts and harmonizing them with thought processes. It can dissolve ingrained habitual and dysfunctional structures of the neural pathways and allow for new connections to occur. In science, this is called *neuroplasticity*. An outcome can be letting go of negative cognitive functioning. A renewed sense of hope can occur, not only for oneself but also for Mother Nature, as valuing stewardship of her, rather than an attitude of dominance and abuse.

The psychedelic experience can be humbling in that it can burn away narcissistic aspects in the psyche by a confrontation with the shadow drives. Psychedelics can help to penetrate an individual's grandiosity and self-inflation as aspects of a false sense of self, acting like a personal truth serum. Shadow material emerges that either frightens the person into a bad trip, or the confrontation causes a reckoning of the true self. The person then has an opportunity to become more grounded, compassionate, and authentic. Most of us have some degree of narcissistic traits that require reexamination; but when one has a significant narcissistic personality disorder, any single insight may or may not make a dent.

The second major lesson learned from my ayahuasca journey involved the beauty and fertility that abounds in the natural world. Nature in its creative element can be quite erotic during a journey. I discovered that one could become over-identified with or stuck in the world of sensuality. The attractiveness of experiencing the presence of nature this way can become an obstacle to further exploration of intentions in which the allies and spirits can teach wisdom about conducting a more fulfilling life. It can also prevent recognizing all the interconnections within a biological and psychological ecosystem. Additionally, I learned that the immersion in the experience can be truly spiritual, one which can help us remember the godhead nature of the cosmos as well as of the earth. For me, the allies represent the polytheistic pagan nature forces of earth, and the ancestors connect us to the past wisdom of humanity.

Chapter 8
About Ayahuasca

Ayahuasca is a plant medicine from the Amazonian regions of Columbia, Brazil (Tukano tribe), Peru (Conibo-Shipibo and Campa tribes), and Ecuador (Jivaro and Zaparo tribes). It is an admixture of a liana or vine, *Banisteriopsis caapi*, and the plant *Psychotria viridis*. In the Quecha language, the *Psychotria* plant is called Chacruna. The *Psychotria* is a tryptamine-containing plant (like DMT) that is activated by the vine, which is a monoamine oxidase inhibitor (MAOI).

Chemically, the *Banisteriopsis* vine is rich in indole alkaloids of the beta-carboline type called harmaline. This chemical is an MAO inhibitor, which prevents the tryptamine derivative from being metabolized and rendered inactive before it can reach the brain and create its hallucinogenic effect. When this combination is mashed together and boiled, it becomes a potent visionary hallucinogen (see included artwork renderings of the visuals produced by ayahuasca).

Recent studies in neuroscience imaging, as reported in the ayahuasca segment of the Netflix series *Unwell*, show that ayahuasca, and possibly other psychedelics, activate three parts of the brain. These include the occipital cortex, where vision occurs; the limbic region associated with episodic memories, and the frontal cortex, presumably where insight is processed. As these three areas communicate, the visions and memories combine to account for the profound teachings and visual displays.

There exist other ayahuasca analogues using two synergistic plants, such as the mimosa plant, which contains tryptamine, along with Syrian rue, an MAO inhibitor (*Jurema*). Other names for ayahuasca are Yaje, Caapi, Natema, Dapa, Mihi, Kahi, Pinde, la Purga, and Daime. It is also referred to as the "Vine of the Soul" or "Vine of the Dead." Sometimes it is called "the ladder to the Milky Way" or the "Spirit Vine." Among aboriginal tribes, it is often employed for prophecy, divination, sorcery, and as a healing medicine. It is used as a shaman's tool to diagnose illness, to ward off impending disaster, to guess the wiles of the enemy, and to prophesize

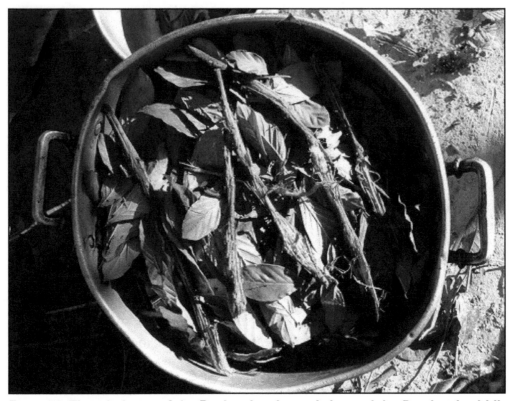

FIGURE 26. The admixture of the *Banisteriopsis caap*i vine and the *Psychotria viridis* leaves, mashed and brewed together to make ayahuasca.
(photo – Awkipuma – Wikimedia commons)

the future. (Schultes 1992) As a physical medicine, it can combat intestinal parasites and is effective in killing malaria protozoa.

Ayahuasca can produce a rich tapestry of colorful visual hallucinations susceptible to being driven by sounds, especially vocal sounds. The *ayahuasceros* (shamans) have a large repertoire of *icaros* (magical songs) that they chant to direct the sounds to heal specific parts of the body and the unexamined mind. These can be used on individual patients or to create a group mind through telepathy, as used in the Santo Daime shamanic religion. (McKenna 1992) There are church groups, such as the Santo Daime and the União do Vegetal in Brazil, that utilize ayahuasca as a sacrament along with a combination of traditional Christian dogma and the nature values of the region's indigenous people.

There is no known addiction nor harmful effects within the cultures that have used this medicine frequently and over the long term. In fact,

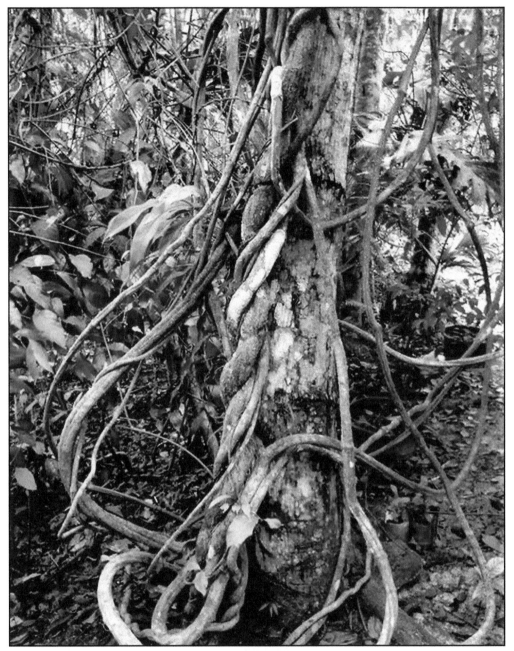

FIGURE 27. *Banisteriopsis caapi* – Vine of the Soul.
(photo – newsweek.com)

these cultures seem to demonstrate extraordinary states of health and psychological integration with a low incidence of serious mental illness or alcoholism. There is a high potential for its future positive use in the field of psychiatry.

The effects of ayahuasca are described as follows:

> There is a magic intoxicant in northwesternmost South America which Indians believe can free the soul from corporeal confinement, allowing it to wander free and return to the body at will. The soul, thus untrammeled, liberates its owner from the realities of everyday life and introduces him to wondrous realms of what he considers reality and permits him to communicate with his ancestors. The Kechua (Quecha) term for this inebriating drink—Ayahuasca ("vine of the soul")—refers to this freeing of the spirit. (Schultes, Hofmann, Rätsch 1998, 120)

Pablo Amaringo, the visionary artist and shaman warned, "Ayahuasca is a drink, although not toxic, if it is used incorrectly, it can cause the body to not be able to withstand the vibrations of the spiritual world that it enters through visions." (Luna and Amaringo 1991)

Since this plant originally came from the Amazon, it frequently creates lush jungle visions within the partaker, even if it is imbibed in a setting away from this habitat. Common visions include serpents of enormous power, jaguars and other forest animals, as well as indigenous natives. Hummingbirds and other bird-like creatures are also often seen. At times, underwater creatures emerge like dolphins. Multiple eyes observing the person are often experienced.

Interestingly, spaceships, flying saucers, and otherworldly and ancient creatures may appear, giving a cosmic dimension. Perhaps this is why it is sometimes referred as "the ladder to the Milky Way." Common visions that many participants report involve encounters with the *Divine Feminine* in all her splendor and beauty. Although there are incredible visionary images and colorful displays, ayahuasca is known primarily as an agent for healing. After a session, a person usually reports feeling totally cleansed in mind and body for some weeks later. The above also applies to ayahuasca analogs such as *Jurema*.

A common archetypal vision is that of the sacred serpent, a giant anaconda called *Sachamama* by the natives. It is said to live at the bottom of the forest, often in a river, where it remains still, sometimes for many

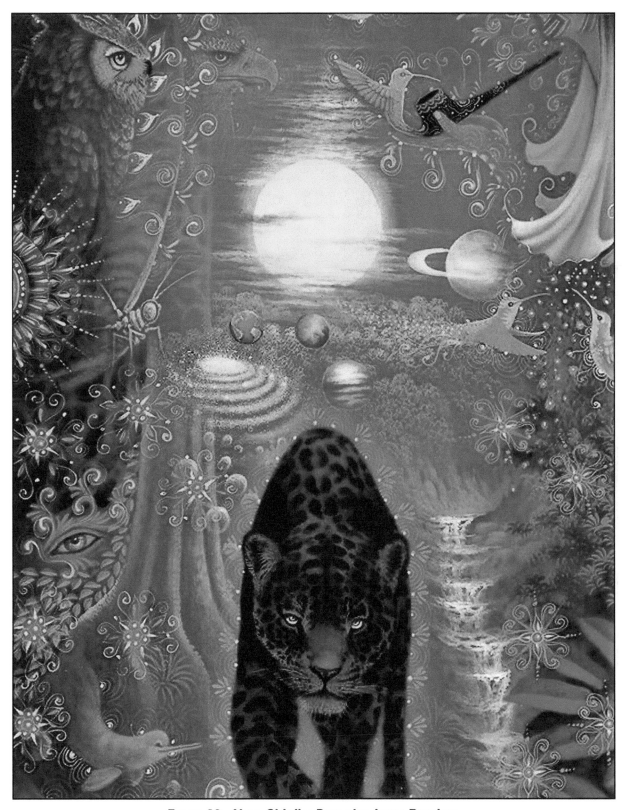

FIGURE 28. *Yana Shipiba Puma* by Jorge Ramirez.

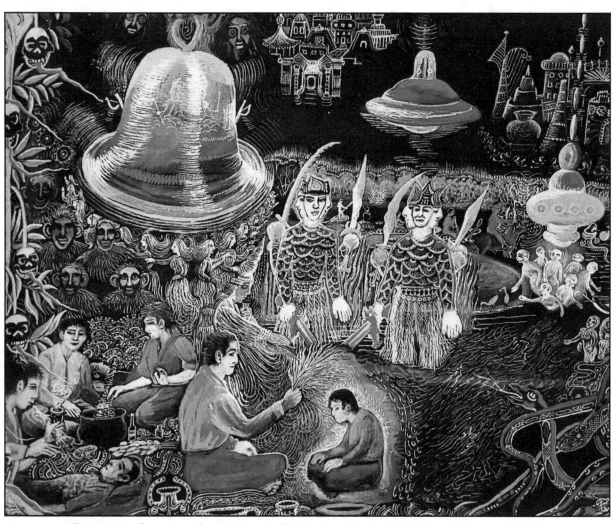

FIGURE 29. *Campana Ayahuasca* by Pablo Amaringo, Luis Eduardo Luna. *(*1989)
(by permission of North Atlantic Press)

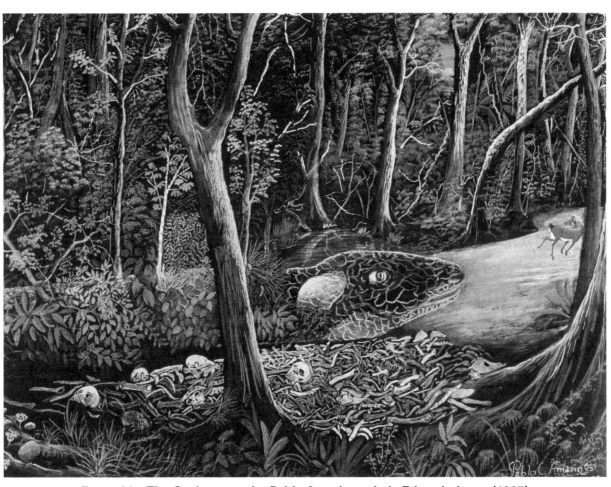

FIGURE 30. *The Sachamama* by Pablo Amaringo, Luis Eduardo Luna. (1985)
(by permission of North Atlantic Press)

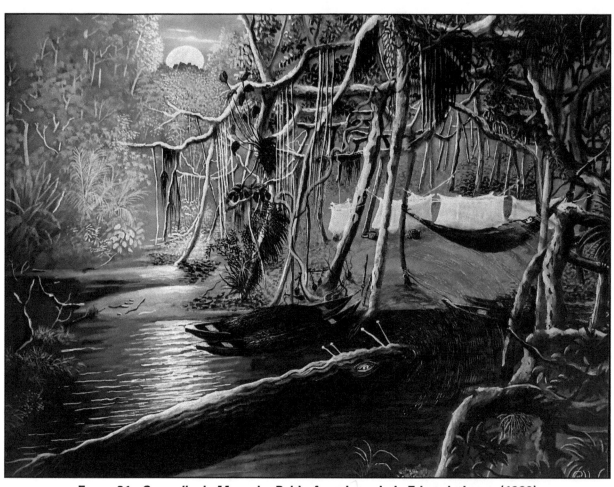

FIGURE 31. *Sanguijuela Mama* by Pablo Amaringo, Luis Eduardo Luna. (1989)
(by permission of North Atlantic Press)

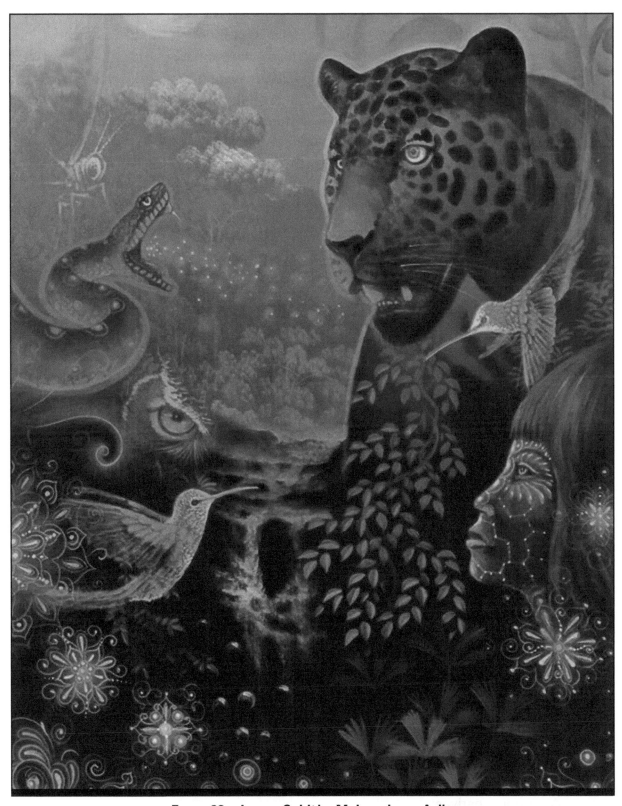

FIGURE 32. *Jaguar Spirit* by Moises Josue Avila.

years. The serpent may appear as a large fallen or rotten tree and is usually considered harmless unless an animal, like a deer, appears before it. Then Sachamama may hold it in a paralyzing gaze, attracting it toward its mouth. Sachamama is considered the "mother of the jungle floor." In visions these serpents can also be seen flying. If someone comes near the serpent, they must swiftly leave since Sachamama can produce strong winds, lightning, and rain capable of knocking down trees. (Luna and Amaringo 1991, 76)

The jaguar is another powerful spirit of the Amazonian rain forest that may appear in ayahuasca visions and is associated more with the power of the earth. The serpent and jaguar are apex predators and are considered the guardians of the forest.

A Map of the Ayahuasca Journey

The chakra system provides a good analogy for the primary centers where the effects of each plant medicine are experienced. Ayahuasca centers in the belly or solar plexus chakra, with its swamp-like feelings and images of reptiles, jaguars, and indigenous natives. It involves more watery images and lush foliage, as seen in the jungles and rivers of the Amazon basin where it originated. The images also can be of ancient undersea, strange-looking creatures, but again often may include flying saucers and outer-space scenes.

The ayahuasca experience can also travel down the spine to the base chakras of the bowel, bladder, and anus and ultimately can connect one to the earth and underground. Rapid excretion of bowel and bladder contents are part of the purgative effect, having a cleansing function for the gastrointestinal tract by eliminating accumulated toxins both physical and psychological. The base of the spine, where one sits on the earth, is very grounding for the individual. This medicine tends to pull a person low on the ground, making them feel heavy and immobile.

The medicine can also travel up the spine to higher chakras, to the heart center and voice center. The *icaros*, or ayahuasca songs, of the Amazonian shamans have a loving lullaby quality to them, and along with the rhythm, the vocal expressions drive the visions. The calm phrasings and vocalizations come more from the gut with deep resonances.

Below are some amplifications of the ayahuasca experience as told by Amazonian natives:

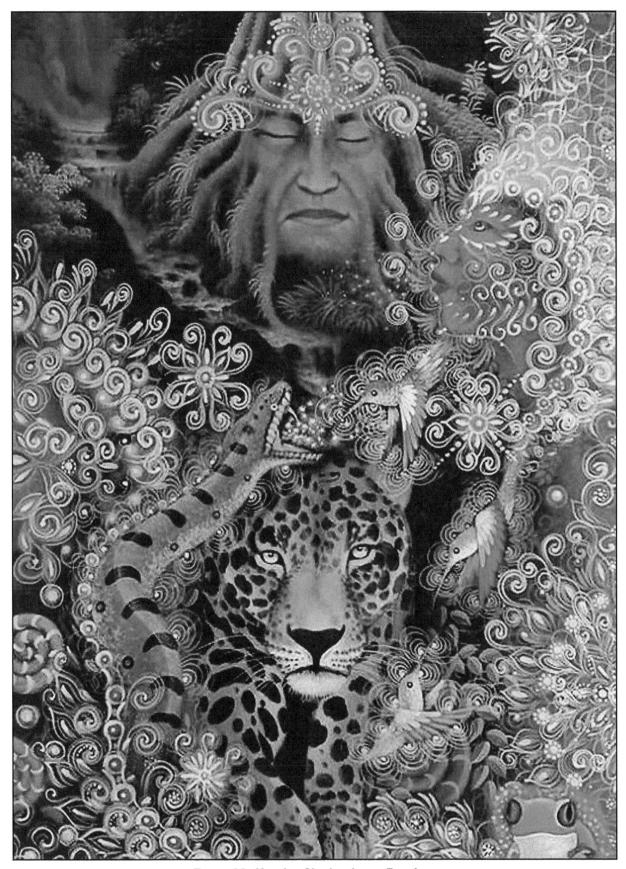

FIGURE **33.** *Kambo Cito* by Jorge Ramirez.

Ayahuasca Meditation and Story

"Spirits of the forest
revealed to us by honi xuma
bring us knowledge of the realm
assist in the guidance of our people
give us stealth of the boa
penetrating sight of the hawk and the owl
acute hearing of the deer
brute endurance of the tapir
grace and strength of the jaguar
knowledge and tranquility of the moon
kindred spirits, guide our way
O most powerful spirit
of the bush with the fragrant leaves
we are here again to seek wisdom
give us tranquility and guidance
to understand the mysteries of the forest
the knowledge of our ancestors
Phantom revealing spirit of the vine
we seek your guidance now
to translate the past into the future
to understand every detail of our milieu
to improve our life
reveal the secrets that we need"
—Manuel Cordova-Rios (Lamb 1974, 88-90)

Another story describing ayahuasca use appears in this Tukano native myth from Colombia and Brazil:

There lived among early Tukano, a woman – the first woman of creation – who 'drowned' men in visions. Tukanoans believe that during coitus, a man 'drowns' – the equivalent of seeing visions. The first woman found herself with child. The Sun-Father had impregnated her through the eye. She gave birth to a child who became Caapi, the narcotic plant . . . The woman – Yaje – cut the umbilical cord and, rubbing the child with magical plants, shaped its body. The Caapi-child lived to be an old man zealously guarding the hallucinogenic powers. From this aged child, owner of Caapi or sexual act, the Tukanoan men received semen. For the Indians, wrote Gerardo Reichel – Dolmatoff, 'the halluci-natory experience is essentially a sexual one . . . to make it sublime, to pass from the erotic, the sensual, to a mystical union . . . attained by a mere handful but coveted by all.' (Gerardo Reichel-Dolmatoff, 1971; Schultes, Hofmann 1998, 131)

A number of artists have been able to capture and to paint the images experienced while taking ayahuasca. For reference, one of the best books of visionary art is *Ayahuasca Visions: The Religious Iconography of a Peruvian Shaman*, by Luis Eduardo Luna and Pablo Amaringo. (Berkeley, CA: North Atlantic Books, 1991)

Chapter 9

Jurema and "The Surgeon from Outer Space"

The following describes an experience I had with the medicine *Jurema*, considered an ayahuasca analog. It is a combination of the tryptamine-containing mimosa species along with the MAO inhibitor, Syrian rue.

I again attended a vision quest retreat weekend lead by Ralph in Joshua Tree, this time in the winter. Ralph introduces Jurema, a new medicine for those in the circle inclined to experiment. Along with myself, other veteran psychonautical explorers will be trying this medicine. My intention for the night is to receive deep healing, to reconnect with my inner healer, and to gain wisdom on how to become a better doctor in my medical practice. In essence, I hope to have a renewal experience.

I take the first dose of Jurema at 7 p.m. I ask to go further and deeper after about an hour and take a booster dose. The visions then quickly intensify with serpentine, luscious, sensual imagery. Yet the visions do not seem as organic as those associated with ayahuasca. I know from my past experiences to try to relax and enjoy this erotic part of the journey, but do not want to get seduced by this entertaining and beautiful phase. For me, it seems that this erotic phase is always a gateway to deeper insights, so I press on, keeping my intention in mind.

Mythologically, I am reminded of Odysseus's men, who are seduced by Circe and her goddess entourage and then turned into swine (the pig nature of male sexuality). The men then must be rescued by Odysseus after being stranded on the island of enjoyable love-making in order to proceed on their journey as warriors to return to their homeland. One must have warrior energy to do this intense medicine inner work.

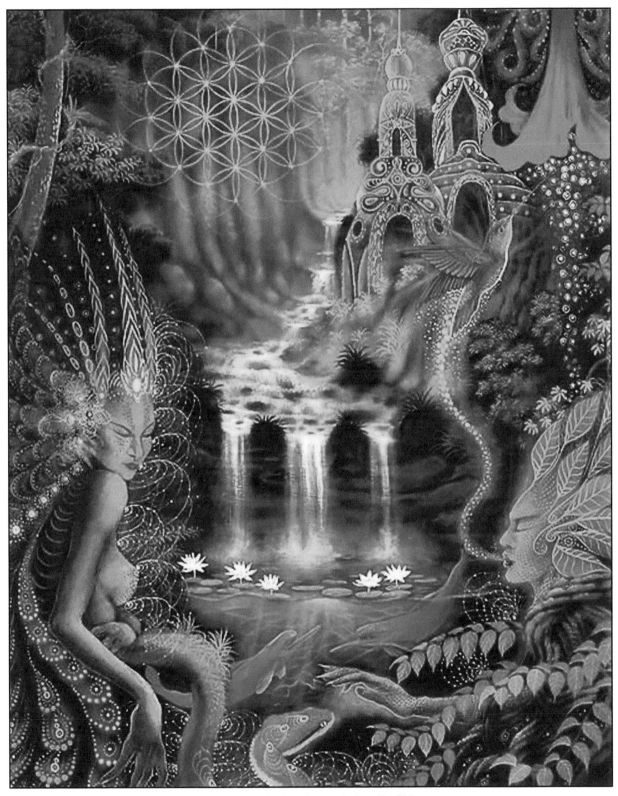

FIGURE 34. *Poder Sagrado* by Jheff Au.

The visions continue. First appear an array of eyes looking down upon me, then emerge the ancestors with their quiet, benevolent observation. Then I find myself on an operating room table looking up at four surgeons who have an otherworldly appearance, somewhat like a pre-historic *Triceratops* dinosaur with three horns protruding backward from each of their heads. Their eyes are piercing and very focused on me. I realize they are the cosmic healers, the "surgeons from outer (or inner) space." I let go of any fears and allow these healers to operate on me. They dissect me using their instruments with meticulous precision, proceeding first with my heart region. They expose and splay apart all the surrounding vessels and begin to unclog the arteries, clearing out all the old, crusted, rigid patterns and sludge surrounding these structures. These otherworldly surgeons are highly trained, super-intelligent, and very good at their work, which they seem to enjoy.

They then proceed to work on blockages in my lungs to open up my breath. The look on their faces is of "objective compassion," not emotional or personal, but very purposeful in their healing efforts. This healing seems to come from a higher source of energy without form, but with unconditional benevolence. They are so skillful that I become receptive to further and deeper surgery, finding myself completely dismembered yet without fear in this vulnerable state. The Jurema surgeons then begin to work on a molecular level, rearranging the atoms and molecules to clean out any toxicities; flushing the spaces in between the molecules with some type of new, pure, organic fluid filled with healthy neurotransmitters.

They then start polishing all my synapses until they are "platinum-tipped." As this is happening, I experience deep healing within and a spaciousness in my breath channels. I ask how I can bring all this back to my work. I am told that healing requires crystalline-pure clarity of the mind. What is necessary is to perfect the concept of objective compassion. Following is an image representing the *Jurema* surgeon from outer space.

These surgeons as healers bring back memories of my childhood surgeries, which initially activated my vision of becoming a doctor. I am told to hold this vision of the surgeons as deep psychic entities, allies available to guide me further in my work. I realize that I need to improve my clarity, to read more for increased knowledge, and to become more objective and less waterlogged by negative, subjective emotions. It becomes apparent

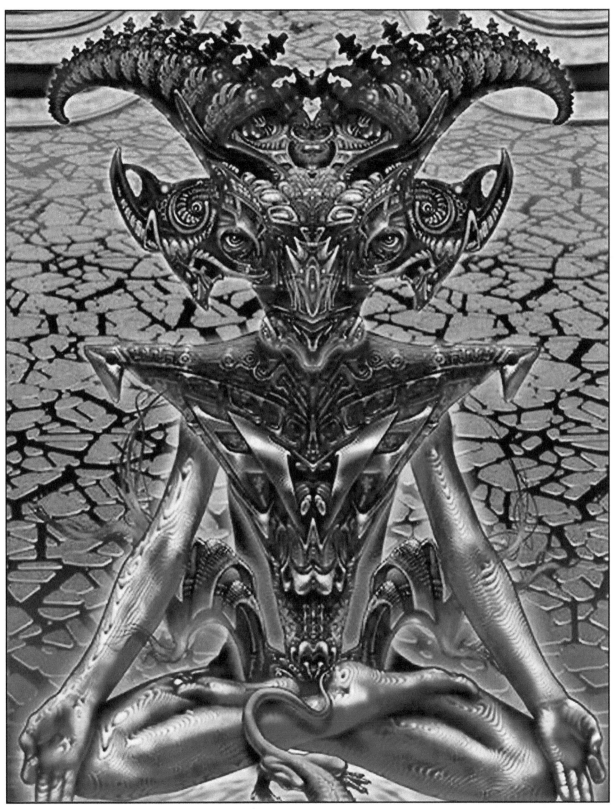

FIGURE 35. *Jerrestrial* by Luke Brown.

that compassion and nurturance can be non-personal and less touchy-feely.

I am told to be more particular in who I choose to work with as patients while also respecting and accepting those who are not open to their deeper psychological structures due to their fears and rigidity. Such intervention tends to be perceived by these people as intrusive, and they could then feel violated. I am reminded to respect their resistances and perhaps just allow the traditional medicines used in psychiatry to do some of the work of healing.

I am also told that objective compassion prevents a power inflation of the healer's need to rescue a person without their permission. Compassion further reconstructs the elements that have become dismembered in the psyche. A positive attitude in my work means to take pride in my purpose and skillfulness as a healer, yet without inflation. The failures and disappointments occur at work to keep me humble, not to humiliate me. Humility needs to be cultivated because it is the healer's truth. Objective compassion and humility are the two factors at the healer's core.

I ask *Jurema* about a dream I had earlier in the week. In my dream humanity as we know it was soon to end because humans were being assimilated and overtaken by alien beings. I think of my sons, about this dilemma, and I see on their forehead a series of question marks. Somehow these questions marks turn upside down and the alien predator beings are not able to read this new coded message. They just pass through and the earth and humanity are saved.

The medicine wisdom reveals that these aliens represent the corporate, soulless, computer-driven, digital culture machines trying to destroy us. To prevent assimilation by these entities, we must stand on our heads and see everything upside-down and inside-out in order to gain new perspective and thus remain intact in the new millennium. While everything is topsy-turvy, turned around, and exposed, we are able to clean out the nooks and crannies of our psyches from the accumulated negative structures that have become embedded through the effects of these collective alien entities.

During this organic dismemberment period of my journey, Ralph begins his wisdom talk in which he invites the Council of Beings to the circle to meet in the *Cave of the Heart*. He invites the past and present teachers and ancestors, which include all the members of our present family, our mothers and fathers, children, and even pets. He then invokes the presence of the inner child, the wise elder, the masculine and feminine energies, the angry self, the grieving/sad self, as well as the shadow self, all the aspects of ourselves we have rejected. All must be invited into this greater family. The inner self-helper facilitates this Council for healing by asking each of us to review intentions and to give voice and speak. While I am disassembled and vulnerable, I experience all these entities within myself, asking to obtain a deep, molecular healing. At the end of my vision-ary experience, I ask Jurema, the healer, to help strengthen my confidence; to help me grow and empower me as a doctor in the service of others.

Another Jurema Journey

During a week-long retreat with Ralph in Ocamura, New Mexico, I had another experience with Jurema. The memories start by leaving the child of the East and heading North toward adolescence. The gateway is through the pain experienced by one of my sons in pre-adolescence, when he was bullied in junior high school because he was skinny and smart. My paternal bond to him intensified as I dealt daily with his tears and demoralization with encouragement, telling him it would get better in time.

The scene then morphed into my own adolescence, to a time when I was injured in football, and my father took me to the hospital to treat my dislocated shoulder. I then remembered him taking me go-karting on week-ends when I was thirteen years old and helping me to soup-up my engine to customize my go-kart. He also enjoyed helping me put on hootenannies at the house when I was in high school and took me to a downtown L.A. pawn shop to buy a guitar and, later, my Pete Seeger model long-neck Vega banjo. He took me to USC for free career counseling as a senior in high school where I was told to consider becoming a doctor. I remember how he would take me on Saturdays with him to make rounds with some of his engineering customers in the industrial area of Los Angeles, where I saw the high level of respect these customers had for him. We would go out to lunch together afterwards. These were all reconciliation memories of my bonding with my father; they brought tears to my eyes. I became aware that in my adult life, I tended to focus on the negative and trau-matic aspects of my relationship with my father and to disregard all of his supportive influences.

I then shifted back to childhood again and reexperienced a significant dream I had as a three-year-old in India, that of a black angel descending into my bedroom. My father had come in and wrestled with the angel, protecting me when I was terrified. Only much later did I realize that this may have represented the archetypal descent of Shiva, the Hindu male god presence, into my life. I recalled that my father took great pride when I became a doctor and how appreciative he was when he later developed heart disease and I stood by him during his last heart attack. At that time while in his hospital bed, he had a premonition that he would die and wrote a letter of blessing to me and my sister the night before he perished. I now felt moved by these many wonderful thoughts about him, which I now realize I had integrated, and all that I owe to him in my own role of fatherhood. The revisiting with my father was very healing in that instant.

Young adult memories then flooded me, and I recalled my relationship to a family friend about six years older than me, Jack Ginsburg, who introduced me at age seventeen to fine literature, such as Hesse, Kafka, Camus, Kazantzakis, Sartre, Durrell, and the existentialists. I resonated with Hermann Hesse in particular and his classic book *Siddhartha*, which became a roadmap of inspiration for my life's path. This inspired a love of literature and philosophy in me and a feeling of a deeper intellectual ability and curiosity. To be exposed to this at such a young age was a true gift.

Jack never finished college but was one of the most brilliant intellects I have ever met. He also taught me about fine cigars, pipe smoking, and alcohol. Jack even helped me get through the loss of my first love in college, who had left me. He was a role model in my initiation from being a teenager into a young adult.

The positive memories continued to flood me. One in particular was the time I was introduced to the music of Bob Dylan as a senior in college, when a young woman approached me from a distance as I was polishing my Triumph motorcycle. I took her for a ride into the mountains. When we returned, she took me to her home and turned me on to Bob Dylan, which opened me up to being musical again. Unfortunately, I never saw her again after that day, but it is a lovely memory.

As the medicine fully took effect, the flood of personal memories shifted to the transpersonal realm. I became a lion-predator stalking an antelope-prey. I felt the lust of the hunt as well as fright and the fight for survival as I aggressively tracked down the now terrified victim. I was experiencing the eternal struggle of life and death within nature, with both sides as two parts of the whole. For a moment, I became associated with the male rapist and the blood lust of dominance, as well as the scream of the woman at the moment of unwanted penetration. This is the moment of resignation and soul loss when the victim is still alive but knows the chase is over. At that moment I experienced a great sense of sadness, mourning, and compassion for all who perish or are sacrificed in this archetypal battle and personal trauma.

This male predation and dominance then shifted to Kurgan warriors on horseback descending through the steppes of ancient Russia, conquering villages, killing, and raping women. This imagery represented the power principle as it came to dominate peaceful agrarian cultures. Then, I shifted into being a warrior myself and met a beautiful woman. My first impulse was to violate her, until I gazed into her eyes and saw the "face of my lover" throughout all time (illustrated in my art piece included previously). She taught me about relatedness and falling in love, as well as learning to respect, adore, protect, and feel compassion for all living beings. In this scene, I experienced firsthand the transformation from the berserker-warrior mentality of uninformed toxic masculinity to that of the protector-warrior preserving life through the influence of love. The eternal struggle between love and power is a theme that I see requires increased understanding. I remember the saying by Jung, "Love never has its seat in the center of power."

The scene again changes from the angry warrior to the image of a glorious god with long gray hair and a beard sitting on a throne of flames while I lie naked and prostrate at his feet. He is a strong and guiding figure blessing me. The flaming god, Agni, sits looking benevolently at my vulnerable life. I feel he is supportive, yet firm, with a purpose of inspiring me to go onward in my work as a doctor/healer and in my creative life to play music, draw artwork, and write. He encourages me to let go of my fears and financial worries. This was the bond of the positive aspect of the archetypal father with me as the son. I understood the notion of the son of God.

In the background Ralph emerges into my awareness as he retells the story of Osiris-Set, the struggle between the vegetative god Osiris of the flooded fertile Nile plain and the fiery Set representing the Sky-warrior cult of the hot desert, in the region's annual struggle between wet and dry. Isis, the goddess, reconstructs Osiris yearly, including the phallus she shapes for him, to bear Horus who continues the struggle with Set. This death and rebirth image occurs with the seasons and in the myth of man becoming magnificent through the efforts of loving the goddess. This story has a powerful synchronicity with my own journey.

In summary, the theme of this medicine journey was the archetypal reenactment within myself of the father/god bond, both personal and archetypal, as well as the evolution of the strong male, who is transformed from the shadow warrior through love and relatedness. It could be said that I was looking "through the eye of God" at the world, particularly the world of men. It brought to mind something Ralph said, "Gravity on a cosmic scale is what love is on a personal scale."

Chapter 10
Jaguar Medicine

Ralph called the psychedelic toad *jaguar* medicine, which he often administered at the beginning of our evening sessions. The active agent of the magical toad is 5-MeO -DMT. This medicine contains the slimy venom of the Colorado River Toad, *Bufo (Incilius) alvarius*, which contains the highest naturally occurring concentration of 5-MeO-N, N-dimethyltryptamine. The synthetic equivalent is N, N-dimethyltryptamine (DMT). There may be subjective differences in these similar compounds, but both are ego-obliterating and rapidly dissolve a sense of self (bodily identity).

Each jaguar session I attended was about fifteen minutes in length. The short journey was accompanied by Tibetan bowl sounds from the music "Magnificent Void" by Steven Roach. This mellow sound allowed us a gentle, yet rapid catharsis of ego dissolution into pure energy of observing awareness without an accompanying body. One is transported to a non-dual experience of "pure consciousness, a sense of "inherent belonging to all the energy of the universe." (Lawlor 1991)

The experience was like surviving an explosion which had disintegrated the body but left consciousness intact. I felt as though I were being shot into outer space amongst the stars. The experience was imbued with swirling, scintillating lights accompanied by non-human, yet highly conscious round beings overlooking me with compassion. It was amazing how quickly it began and then dissipated. Then I returned to my body where this incredible energy could circulate and heal. Within fifteen minutes, all felt normal and my sense of self returned, although there was a feeling that something extraordinary had occurred, and I was not the same.

It is noteworthy that, as is true for other psychedelics, this medicine is being studied for use in treatment-resistant depression. Recent research shows evidence that the *mystical experience* commonly encountered by those taking various hallucinogenic medicines has positive results in treating multiple mental health disorders, including depression, anxiety, addictions, and PTSD. A study published in 2018 included twenty participants who took the psychedelic toad medicine, of which about 75 percent reported a mystical experience, as verified by the standardized Mystical Experience Questionnaire (MEQ) used in other psychedelic research. (Lawlor 2019)

The purported value of using DMT substances is their relatively short duration of action, making them valuable for use in adjunct psychotherapy. This contrasts with longer-duration medicines such as psilocybin or MDMA where the effects can last seven to eight hours, therefore requiring the assistance of two psychotherapists for administration. It has been estimated that MDMA-assisted psychotherapy could cost between $13,000 and $30,000 to achieve optimal results. As noted, MDMA is called Ecstasy, or X-stasy when used for recreational purposes at raves and parties, but it is gaining momentum for use in treating psychiatric disorders such as PTSD.

Even if these substances were to become legal, there is doubt as to whether insurance companies would authorize their use. DMT therapy would allow more frequent and economical use by patients who may require multiple sessions in a controlled setting. It is also simpler to synthesize than MDMA and other medicines. One limiting factor for using "organic toad," as reported by Sean Lawlor in *Psychedelic Times* (2019), is the amphibian's dwindling population due to its recent popularity, which will necessitate using the synthetic form. Intramuscular injection, as opposed to nasal insufflation, would serve to slow down the onset of action, bringing about a gentler experience, alleviating the potential for terror reactions.

DMT is also found in the beans of the Yopo tree plant, *Anadenanthera peregrina*, which was used as a hallucinogenic snuff among the Waika Indians in southernmost Venezuela and northern Brazil, where it was known as *Yupa*. (see Chapter 24) The shaman would blow this snuff into the nostrils of the recipient through a long tube made from a stem of a plant. This served to invoke the *Hekula* (spirits) with whom they would be communicating during the period of intoxication. Its uses were for prophecy and divination, protection of the tribe against epidemics or sickness, and bringing more alertness to the hunters. (Schultes, Hofmann, and Rätsch 1992, 116-119)

The issue remains as to whether a peak ego-obliterating (and speechless) mystical experience is necessary, or if a lower-dose regimen, referred to as psycholytic as opposed to psychedelic, as is practiced in Europe, would be sufficient to obtain the desired positive effects. A question also remains about the necessity of having a therapist/patient relationship when this medicine is used. More research is needed, since the use of DMT-derivatives is relatively new, whereas the practice of taking medicines such as ayahuasca has been carried out by indigenous tribes for thousands of years without apparent harm.

Chapter 11

A Psilocybin Journey

Below is a description of one of my personal journeys with the sacred psilocybin mushroom, with augmentation using the Syrian rue plant, *Peganum Harmala*. Syrian rue, a type of birdseed, is not psychoactive by itself but acts as a monoamine oxidase inhibitor (MAOI), which prolongs and enhances the effects of the tryptamine in psilocybin on the brain. It does this by preventing the rapid metabolism of the tryptamine derivative, allowing more of it to be transported across the blood-brain barrier into the brain. As discussed previously, Syrian rue is also used with other psychedelics, such as Jurema, the admixture of Syrian rue and the tryptamine-containing plant mimosa.

Intention

My intention for the evening ceremony is to replenish my psyche due to its depletion from traumas I have encountered in my work setting as a psychiatrist. These traumas include patient suicides, angry patients, and suffering, treatment-resistant patients whom I am unable to help. I ask for guidance in penetrating deeper into the mysteries of illnesses suffered by my patients and in following the guidance "heal thyself" in order to return to work with a renewed sense of vigor.

I ingest three grams of the Syrian rue placed into capsules one hour before taking the psilocybin mushrooms. One hour later, the beginnings of sensual and beautiful female images appear, but I feel stuck at this threshold and ask for a booster. I am quickly catapulted into the psychedelic experience, first finding myself dealing with bodily anxiety. I feel as though I might die of a heart attack or stroke as I experience pressure in my head, skipped heartbeats, tachycardia, mental confusion, and dizziness.

I try to let go of the successive layers of fears, knowing that I must pass through this gate of the uncomfortable somatic phase before I am able to transcend to the visionary experience and relaxation. I realize that this is a type of death/rebirth experience in and of itself. I concentrate on continuing to let go by using my breath. I also say to myself, "If I die, so what," but I begin to trust that I will survive and continue living.

Induction

Ralph begins with an induction he calls the *River of Time* meditation. He suggests that we are floating down a river on a raft, letting our baggage float next to us. We decide what we need to take with us on the journey and are to let go of any baggage we no longer need. He reminds us of the story of Osiris, Isis, Set and Horus, and relates this to the ecological/climatic aspects of ancient Egypt, with its periods of flooding and fertility, heat and drought. Osiris, the green-skinned god of vegetation, becomes dismembered by the desert heat represented by Set, the hot one. Isis, through her love for Osiris, gathers thirteen of the fourteen dismembered pieces, but Osiris's phallus remains lost. She then fashions a stick and fertilizes herself, then gives birth to the one-eyed Horus.

Osiris represents the god of corn, fertility, the agrarian and cooperative mode, and the water element. Set represents the male-dominator warrior mode, who dismembers the peaceful hunter-gatherer stewards of the land. Set destroys this fertility by degrading the land to a desert (the fire function). Isis, the great goddess, remembers the "old ways" and rejoins the vegetation god Osiris and the desert god Set. This can be seen as a metaphor for the present climate crisis and our alienation from the natural world.

Ralph then suggests that we each relate this story to our own needs for healing our dismembered parts. We could recall our pain and struggles in life and then venture on a journey to find that which has been lost to us as a result of our disconnection from nature through male-dominated cultural attitudes. A part of our soul has been lost. The journey is to find and remember (opposite of dismember) the part in order that fertility can again be experienced in our psyche. This is the essence of "soul retrieval" work.

The Experience

At this juncture for me, the mushroom visual experience is very strong. Colorful emanations emerge from a central point as a firework display, like a mandala that is alive and changing form. The music creates a synesthesia of rhythm morphing into intense colors and emotions. My visions then expand as I experience a sense of deep grief about all the suffering I have witnessed in my life and work. This has settled into my body, a feeling of clogging up of the filters down to my bones, blocking the flow of energy. I experience the frustrations and resentments I continue to carry as baggage in my relationships with people. I let them go into the stream as I have a good, cathartic cry. I then recall my intention, and the ancestors appear in a vision. A tribunal of wise Jewish elders hear my sobbing and begin to speak directly to me:

"We [ancestors] are here for you. We understand your suffering and thank you for remembering us and asking for our help. We have been through the suffering in the world and we want you to thrive and to carry on our legacy. As you remember us, we ask you to carry us in your heart as we are able again to live through you. We speak with the authority of all the ancestors of the ages, the wise ones, who have suffered before you. We have lived in the desert land and know the suffering and hardships of an oppressed, exiled people. We have been liberated from the oppression in Egypt and have experienced the Exodus, the hardships of the harsh desert, and the joy of the 'promised land'. We speak to you with full authority and vouchsafe to you the responsibility of being a prophet of the spirit and a carrier of the present space-time in life. You are to speak and carry on the faith and belief in our God that unites our community against dissolution and dismemberment. We speak to you with the full authority of the ages, that we recognize you, Alexander, as a potent carrier of wisdom and as a prophet of our spirit to inform and to help others evolve. We will help you manifest this." (Archetypes tend to speak in this language form.)

They continued, "But you must 'wake up;' this will occur through remembering us, our story, and our journeys as a metaphor in your own life. Your suffering and transcendence can speak to your descendants so that they will also know the potency of their birthright and their identity with the Jewish culture. You are a person of light, like Moses and the prophets, and are a Jew at root, but you have disdained us by forgetting us. Put

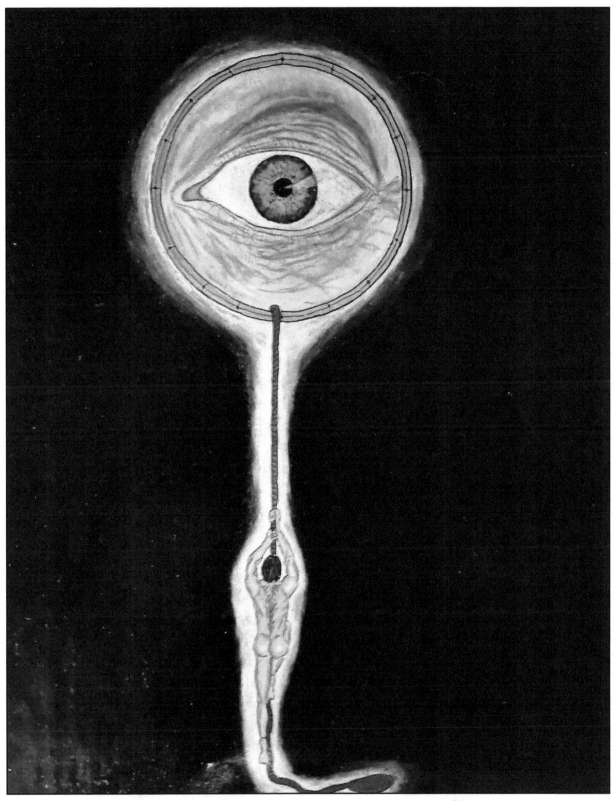

FIGURE 36. *Connecting with the Eye of Awareness* by Alexander Shester.

aside your dislike of our warrior-king mythology, for we have had to survive in harsh climes and have been under attack by many who have tried to dissolve our faith in God and community. Do not become anti-Semitic by avoiding this part of your nature. Your deepest self is a prophet seeker and healer. Go out and be a healer with an awakened and open 'eye,' with mental clarity and perspective to deeply penetrate the illnesses affecting others; as well as to heal yourself. Your ability to continue depends on your health and remaining awakened; remember that as a Jew, your suffering and joy will help you succeed in healing and inspiring others. It is what you do and who you are."

They go on to say, "Your strong spirit is renewed. You are being born into an elder. Your bones are continuing to grow older with the gravity of time, and the aches and pains are part of becoming older and wiser. The gravity of enduring aging goes into the bones, and the body is the filter of life's hardships."

This meeting with my Jewish ancestors felt very powerful and true for me. The strength of their message placed a responsibility on me to carry onward. A reciprocal relationship with the ancestors was again established. They say, "Tell me what you see, and we will tell you what we know." I carry them with me in this space-time so that they can continue to live, and they will promise to guide me if I can remember this message. They dressed me down and humbled me, yet in a constructive manner. This allowed that I might let go of my insecurities, fears, defensiveness, and pettiness. I am a Jew, but the message was that I do not have to practice it within an organized religion. The ancestors know that I am different and have my ways of believing; I must only express my Jewish roots with humility and integrity. I can sing the message strongly with a purposeful heart and, in so doing, heal myself. I do decide that I should read the Bible and Jewish history, especially the story of the Exodus.

The music in the vision circle changes to a Native American chant with rattles. They sing the songs of their ancestral wisdom and I am encouraged to chant along with them to remember my Jewish roots. As the circle comes to a close, I ponder that my shadow-self is someone who sleeps, who is in hiding and thus avoiding the deeper issues of life. I will need to strengthen my will to awaken, be present, show up, and participate in being a leader. (see figure above) I close with an insight that comes to me,

"Passion is not a momentary experience or a memory of extreme pleasure or pain but is rather a way of life. Ride on." I take away from this experience a feeling of calmness, joyfulness, centeredness, renewal, and motivation for my work. I look forward to seeing patients come Monday morning and to participate more fully in the healing venture.

Afterthoughts

The teachings that came to me from Teonanacatl (psilocybin) in the session just described were powerful and second to none. Each medicine teaches in different ways, yet each can serve as a truth serum acting in the best interest of the partaker with respect to vision and healing. I found the mushrooms were a bit more aggressive in their approach to me, humbling me, but in a caring way.

The imagery was fast-moving, and I understand why mushrooms have a mischievous reputation. The imagery and insights were not subtle, but had a tricky quality of teaching through cunning. In different ways the wisdom comes through; ultimately it seems that the mushrooms want to helpfully communicate. *Los niños* (the "little children," as mushrooms are sometimes called) can be playful and mischievous with a person. But in this experience, they did confront me with my laziness, my failure to carry on the visionary messages about our planetary state, and my prior disdain of the Jewish religion and thus my roots. To awaken and find my soul loss, the missing phallus of Osiris, is necessary in order to give forth fertility in my relationships and career and to age more gracefully.

In addition to the teachings, I found the visual aspects of the entire trip to be extremely erotic. There were many colorful images of sensual, beautiful women with lavish buttocks and legs. They were all receptive, unfolding, glistening, lubricated, and inviting penetration. It was nature unfolding her fertility, the Divine Feminine mixed with the "sacred prostitute," open yet loving to any weary person, as well as myself. Such visual images seem to be a recurring theme for me no matter what medicine I use. I have learned to enjoy them without getting seduced away from the teachings. For a while during my journeys, they served to indulge my passionate nature in the arts of loving, sensuality, and pleasure without judgment, a gift to me as it counteracted the suffering I endure in my life.

In the past, the cosmic experience of the godhead was open only to the occasional mystic-philosopher or the practitioner of deep meditation. With entheogens, the spiritual component is now open to all people. My experiences have been confirmed by many other partakers as well. One does not have to be brilliant to understand what is happening. The transformative effects can occur with anyone having basic intelligence who properly prepares for the journey. However, the long-lasting integration of spiritual insights into everyday behavior does require motivation, a degree of intellectual insight, and perseverance.

A beautiful image of sacred sexuality is depicted on the next page in the illustration of Shiva and Shakti facing each other embracing.

Another Mushroom Journey

I had another similar psychedelic mushroom experience some months later during a week-long retreat led by Ralph in Ocamura, New Mexico. Each night of the retreat was devoted to a different plant medicine.

The medicine for this particular evening is psilocybin mushrooms; each participant is given two grams of dried mushrooms augmented with Syrian rue. My intention is to explore the divination from the ancestors, old age, and dying, which are all aspects of the direction of the West. As the medicine begins to take effect, I am being led to the West by a large bumble bee spirit guide to meet with the elders.

Once I meet my ancestors, they tell me they would like me to peer into the realm of the dead. They are the guardians at the gate to "Hel," the underworld. The gates are very gothic, made of large iron doors guarded by gargoyle creatures who honor my presence and open the doors. I walk inside downward to a space that looks like a giant underground beehive. Here the souls of the dead are placed in the honeycombs. They glow like luminescent green globules that are being tended to by bees and other insects. The souls are being repaired from their previous lives on earth, with all the traumas and wounding experiences, and they are being prepared for their next incarnation. In the Buddhist tradition, the belief is that at death, we are born into another plane of existence. In this transpersonal realm, we await rebirth physically or transcend the wheel of reincarnation. *Samsara* is the karmic cycle of reincarnation. If one's karma is completed,

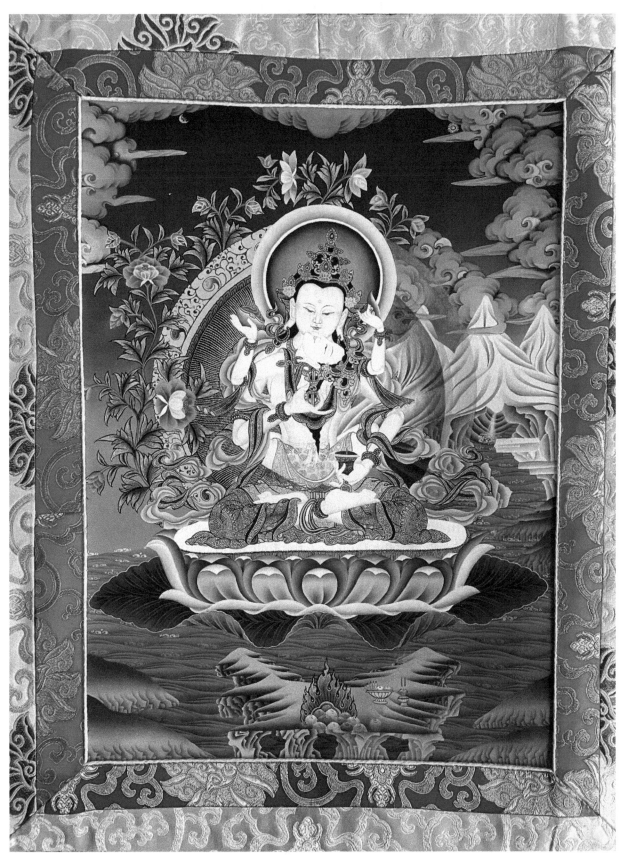

FIGURE 37. Shiva and Shakti Embracing
(Thangka in author's collection)

then *Nirvana*, or liberation and enlightenment, occur and reincarnation is no longer necessary.

The ancestors appear, sit quietly, and wait for people to come to them for help. They first listen and then speak; it is clear that one should always be respectful of them. I ask them about my work problems, especially with the patients who become upset with me. These patients have come to me for help but express their distress in ways that I feel disrespected by. The ancestors tell me that I first need to just listen to such a patient without reacting. But, if the disrespect continues, then to speak up and set limits. If the person continues to be disrespectful of me a third time, then I need to turn around and drink from the "Well of Remembrance" and to remember my "radiant child." I need to have the "elder" therapist within me connect with the radiant child in order to preserve my self-esteem and core essence as a good, competent doctor. This is the protective warrior function of my inner healer.

Synchronistically, I then hear Ralph begin to speak. He discusses the path of the healer in the life cycle in which 1) one must do repair work of various psychic structures (heal thyself); 2) activate the warrior function to protect those healed structures; then 3) the explorer/adventurer aspect of the healer is invoked and may extend outwards, taking new risks creatively with less need for protection. Continuing on the path, 4) the artist is allowed to enter to manifest visions through beauty and appreciation. Then finally, 5) the healer can communicate these teaching to others. This process is exemplified in the figure on the following page.

As this Circle comes to a close, as a group we are reminded to remember the four directions and reconcile the child of the East, the mother/goddess of the South, the father/god of the North, and the elders/ancestors of the West, that all within us may join the circle in the Medicine Wheel of Life. It is important that we need to work toward cultivating an extended tribe of healers, artists, warriors, adventurers, and teachers to ultimately show more kindness in life. We end the circle singing "Amazing Grace" as a group.

THE HEALER'S JOURNEY

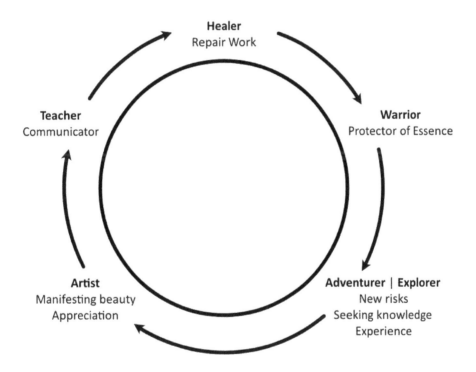

FIGURE 38. The Healer's Journey.
(As shared by Ralph Metzner)

Chapter 12

About Psilocybin Mushrooms

Teonanacatl, meaning divine flesh, was the name given to one or more species of the Psilocybe mushroom in the Nahuatl language of the Aztec people. Tribes in Mexico, such as the Mazatec, Mixtec, and Zapotec, knew these mushrooms as *holy saints* and "little children (*los niños*) that spring forth" with ecstatic visions. (Metzner 2004, 1) The Mazatec Indians sometimes call the mushrooms *Nti-si-tho*, a term of endearment meaning "that which springs forth," since no one knows when or why they emerge from the ground. These mushroom ceremonies have taken place for centuries in Mexico, and there is present evidence to suggest that the mushroom cult flourished in prehistoric times, from 100 B.C. to about 300-400 A.D. in northern Mexico and even in some tribes in South America. (Schultes and Hofmann 1992, 162)

From the time of European conquest onward, the mushrooms have been called *god's flesh*, and the Spanish friars equated the ceremonies using them with devil worship. These sacred mushrooms were especially offensive to the European ecclesiastical authorities, who sought to eradicate their use in the religious practices of these indigenous people. In 1656, a guide for missionaries argued against Indian idolatries, including mushroom ingestions, and recommended their extirpation. (Schultes and Hofmann 1992, 156)

Although these mushrooms have been used for many centuries in these cultures, Robert Gordon Wasson, an ethnomycologist, rediscovered this amazing mushroom and brought understanding of it to the Western world. In 1957, *Life* magazine published the account of his sessions with a Mazatec *curandera*, Marina Sabina, who was using this entheogenic fungus in a remote mountain village in the Mexican state of Oaxaca. Wasson was friends with Albert Hofmann, a chemist for Sandoz pharmaceuticals in Switzerland, who in 1938 discovered LSD (lysergic acid diethylamide).

Hofmann then proceeded to chemically identify the psychoactive ingredient of this Mexican *Psilocybe* mushroom; he was able to synthesize its active ingredient, which he named psilocybin, shown to act in a very similar way to LSD.

In the 1960s, with the transformative wave and associated interest in psychedelic-induced altered states of consciousness, thousands of hippies trekked to the mountains of Oaxaca to experience these magic mushrooms. In modern days, the state of intoxication is known as being *bemushroomed* or *beshroomed*. This was much to the dismay of Wasson and Maria Sabina, who felt that the sacred use of Teonanacatl was diluted and desacralized by this onslaught of tourists.

Maria Sabina reverently described the god-given powers of the intoxicating mushrooms passed down through the ages:

> *There is a world beyond ours, a world that is far away, nearby, and invisible. And there is where God lives, where the dead live, the spirits and the saints, a world where everything has already happened and everything is known. That world talks. It has a language of its own. I report what it says. The sacred mushroom takes me by the hand and brings me to a world where everything is known. It is they, the sacred mushrooms, that speak in a way I can understand. I ask them and they answer me. When I return from a trip that I have taken with them, I tell what they have told me and what they have shown me.* (Schultes and Hofmann 1992, 156)
>
> *The more you go inside the world of Teonanacatl, the more things are seen. And you also see our past and our future, which are there together as a single thing already achieved, already happened . . . I saw stolen horses and buried cities, the existence of which was unknown, and they are going to be brought to light. Millions of things I saw and knew. I knew and saw God: an immense clock that ticks, the spheres that go slowly around, and inside the stars, the earth, the entire universe, the day and the night, the cry and the* smile, the happiness and the pain. *He who knows to the end the secret of Teonanacatl can even see that infinite* clockwork. (Schultes and Hofmann 1998, title page)

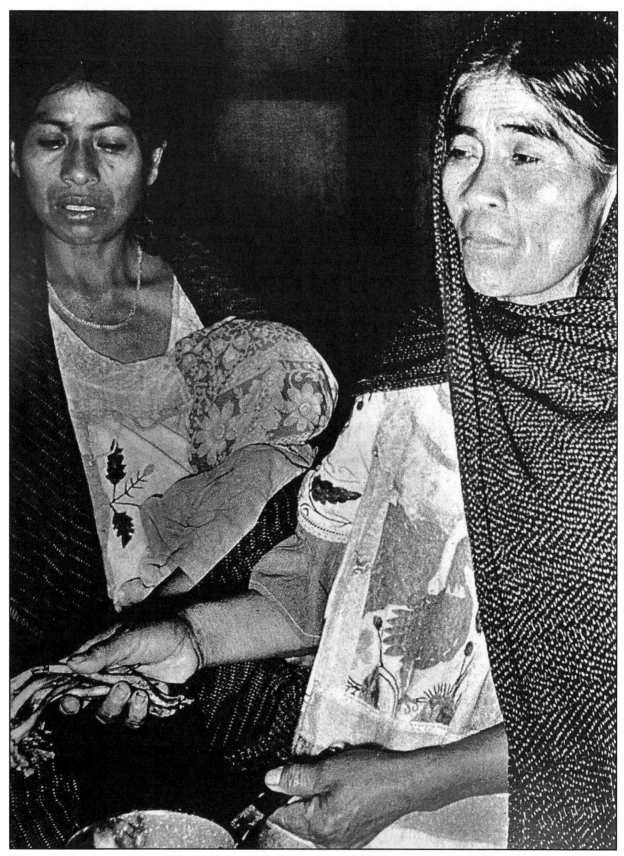

FIGURE 39. Maria Sabina (right) Mazatec Shaman, with daughter (left).

The internal experience of Teonanacatl, or psilocybin mushrooms, tends to be centered in the eye and crown chakras in the head (the Ajna and Sahasrara chakras in the Tantric system). The visionary experience often begins with a very rapid kaleidoscopic phase and then opens into crystalline colorful imagery of various figures, gods and goddess, ancestors, nature deities, and the cosmic awareness of the spirit at work. The medicine also can also travel up and down the Tantric spinal column with imagery of flights of birds or spirits taking one to far off lands for insights into the future. The energy can also be directed lower to the heart space in order for the user to explore relationships and the natural world. There are some accounts of the visionary aspects of these mushrooms in Metzner's book, *Teonanacatl*.

Magic mushrooms (with or without augmentation with Syrian rue) tend to act more on visionary clarity, rather than on a healing visceral spectrum like ayahuasca. Often this medicine is associated with the East, new beginnings, the rising sun, and the inner child within. As a fungus that lives primarily underground with a mycelial network representing a connective and communicative link to the earth and various trees, it contains a tremendous amount of Earth wisdom about the symbiosis of all interconnected species, the health of the environment, and our relationship to the Earth.

Psilocybin is in the chemical class of indole alkaloids that contain dimethyltryptamine (DMT). This hallucinogenic tryptamine is contained in LSD, as well as in some other plant species, such as mimosa and morning glory. It is also found in the ergot fungus growing on grains such as wheat and rye. Psilocybin is rapidly metabolized to psilocin, which is the active hallucinogenic compound. This molecule is found in approximately two hundred species of mushrooms around the world. Because of its prevalence in so many species, it probably evolved for reasons other than serving as an entheogen for human beings with its property of causing an altered state of consciousness. It is possible it may contain other metabolic processes necessary for the survival of these mushrooms and the environment.

It is now thought that the ergot fungus may have been used in ancient Greece as part of the yearly Eleusinian Mysteries celebrated for centuries near ancient Athens; during which its intoxicating effects were collectively used by the followers to obtain visions of Persephone's return in the Spring. This idea is only conjecture, since this ergot can cause poisoning, with symptoms of gangrene in the toes and fingers, vomiting, diarrhea, convulsions, and delirium. In 994 A.D. there was an outbreak of ergot poisoning from infected grains which killed 40,000 people in France. (McKenna 1992, 136)

Terence McKenna extends the possible significance of psilocybin mushrooms in his proposal that they may actually have been the original forbidden fruit creating consciousness, which Biblically is the original sin. He states, "When our remote ancestors moved out of the trees and on to the grasslands, they increasingly encountered hooved beasts who ate vegetation. These beasts became a major source of potential sustenance. Our ancestors also encountered the manure of these wild cattle and the mushrooms that grow in it." (McKenna 1992, 37)

Candidates for these mushrooms include the hallucinogenic species of *Stropharia cubensis*, also called *Psilocybe cubensis*. McKenna postulates further, "I believe that the use of hallucinogenic mushrooms on the grasslands of Africa gave us the model for all religions to follow. And when, after long centuries of slow forgetting, migration, climatic change, the knowledge of the mystery was finally lost, we in our anguish traded partnership for dominance, traded harmony with nature for the rape of nature, traded poetry for the sophistry of science." (McKenna 1992, 39-40)

McKenna considers the chemicals in these mushrooms to be interspecies messengers within nature, allowing communication between plants and animals, thus keeping the natural world in balance. He views nature not as endless warfare among species for the "survival of the fittest," but as a "dance of diplomacy" maximizing cooperation of goals. He continues, "If hallucinogens function as interspecies chemical messengers, then the dynamic of the close relationship between primate and the hallucinogenic plant is one of information transfer from one species to the other . . . in the presence of hallucinogens, a culture is quickly introduced to ever more novel information, sensory input, and behavior and thus is bootstrapped to higher and higher states of self-reflection . . . an encounter with the Transcendent Other." (McKenna 1992, 41)

Terrance McKenna and his brother Dennis proposed the *stoned ape hypothesis* as a theoretical explanation for how humans evolved and developed enhanced consciousness. Briefly stated, early hominids were food scavengers and mushrooms could be easily spotted as a food source.

Psilocybe cubensis was a common species which launched an altered state in hominids. The McKennas offer this explanation for how the early hominid pre-human ancestor came to experience a deity, self-reflection, and a sense of interconnection with nature.

This altered state represented the dawn of human awareness, reminiscent of Stanley Kubrick's film *2001: A Space Odyssey*. The first scene of the movie shows apes encountering a strange monolithic structure and touching it, resulting in a quantum leap of their awareness. The McKennas also believed that the rapid growth in human brains from 500 cc to the present-day 1500 cc in a relatively short period of evolutionary time was spawned by mushroom intelligence infiltrating the human brain. (McKenna 2019, 154)

Andrew Weil, a renowned medical doctor, herbalist, and mycologist, does not endorse this hypothesis. He believes that the perceptual distortions and sensory scrambling typically caused by psychedelics would prove a fatal risk for humans, making them more vulnerable to predation. (Weil 2019, 155) My personal objection to Weil's assessment is that although the mushroom fruit could have disoriented and discombobulated the pre-human ape, thus subjecting it to a higher risk of predation, this aspect of the mushroom would be quickly learned and therefore it would not have been used as a daily food source or remedy. The ape-creature, once intoxicated, would learn wise use of the mushroom in a protected environment for the purpose of experiencing a different reality. Eventually, this state could have brought about self-reflection, a greater awareness of nature, and perhaps a transcendent consciousness. It could have provided the first inkling of a god perhaps infused in nature, similar to that experienced by indigenous peoples. It could have been the same experience of a hallucinogen used in modern times in a sacred and protected setting. Perhaps it was the origin of religion for humans.

In our present time, the use of psilocybin mushrooms remains illegal and their usage suppressed, allowing for the exception of new research in the past several years. As previously discussed, psilocybin (as well as other hallucinogens) is being intensively researched for use in a variety of psychiatric disorders, including depression, anxiety, PTSD, OCD, and addictions, as well as with end-of-life/death concerns. These studies are currently taking place at prestigious universities such as Harvard, New

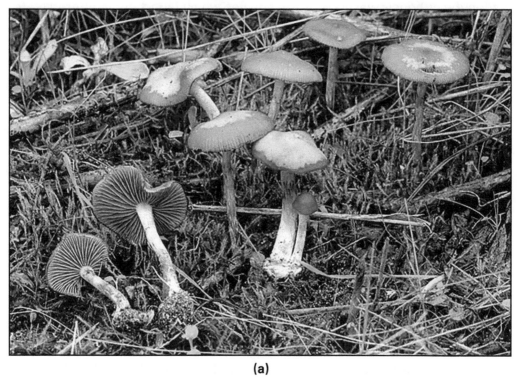

(a)

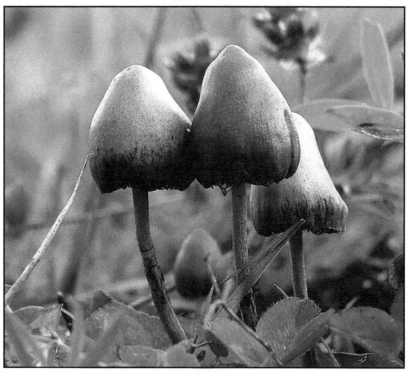

(b)

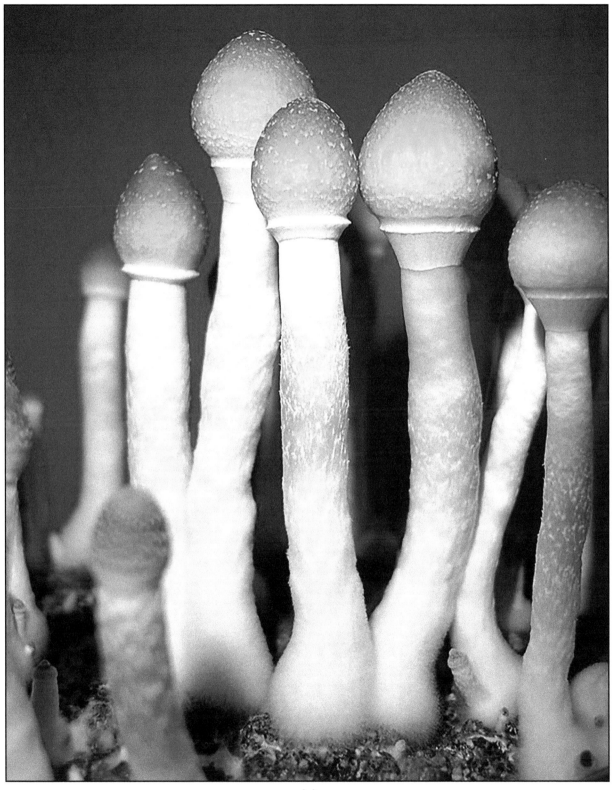

(c)

FIGURES 40 (a, b, c). various *Psilocybe* species.
(photos from Wikimedia commons)

VISIONARY HEALING

York University, Johns Hopkins, UCLA, UCSF, and the University of New Mexico, legitimizing the use of these agents once again. Protocols are being established to ensure the safe, proper use of these medicines and for the specialized training of facilitators.

A beautiful way to end this section is by a quote from Maria Sabina, the Oaxacan shaman who used psilocybin and other sacred plant medicines and expresses to us the essence of healing and the natural world.

> *"Heal yourself with the light of the sun and the rays of the moon. With the sound of the river and the waterfall. With the swaying of the sea and the fluttering of birds. Heal yourself with mint, neem, and eucalyptus. Sweeten with lavender, rosemary, and chamomile. Hug yourself with the cocoa bean and a hint of cinnamon. Put love in tea instead of sugar and drink it looking at the stars, Heal yourself with kisses that the wind gives you and the hugs of the rain. Stand strong with your bare feet on the ground and with everything that comes from it, Be smarter every day by listening to your intuition, looking at the word with your forehead. Jump, dance, sing, so that you live happier. Heal yourself, with beautiful love, and always remember...you are the medicine."*
>
> (inspiringquotes.us/author/2058-maria-sabina)

Chapter 13

A San Pedro Cactus Journey in Joshua Tree

So far, we have been focusing on medicines whose active ingredients include tryptamines. A very different psychedelic alkaloid, mescaline, is the active ingredient in both the San Pedro and peyote cactus. Mescaline activates the norepinephrine neurotransmitter system, which is noradrenergic like amphetamine, although it is a potent hallucinogen.

Intention

My intention for this journey is to explore a part of my psyche which I am aware tends to be critical of myself and others. At times, this is helpful, as when I need to do some critical thinking in medicine and psychiatry regarding my patients. The negative aspect of this function is that it can work overtime when not needed and extend to my observation of friends and loved ones. My evaluation can be perceived as judgmental, lacking patience and tolerance of others, especially when they make mistakes. It can result in stress and discomfort with myself as well, as I become a harsh critic of my imperfections. I have come to believe that there is some type of blockage in my heart center which leads to unrealistic expectations of myself and others. This complex of mine leads to overly negative thinking, which seems to reside within a dark vault in my psyche. My intention for this quest will be to explore this aspect and attempt to remove my "stone shirt" of armor which separates me from others.

115

Preparation

The Joshua Tree desert this spring equinox is beautiful and mild in temperature. I brought my didgeridoo with me and find that I love playing it by myself in the desert. There is a lot of insect life buzzing around and on the ground; I pay attention and try to connect with this realm of the ecosystem. I consider my intention and begin to reflect on all the relationships of which I have a critical view. It concerns me, as I realize how many friends I feel negativity towards. It makes me wonder if they hold such views about me. I decide to try San Pedro, as a medicine to open my heart to insights that I hope will bring about change in my negative thinking and judgement. The heart chakra can be emphasized by the mescaline containing San Pedro or peyote cactus.

Experience

The recipe offered for the evening journey is to take three heaping tablespoons (twelve grams) of ground-up, powdered San Pedro cactus in a tea, as well as a small dose of LSD (100 mcg) to activate the cactus plant. The inner experience of this session emerges gently and colorfully. Early on, some teachings filter through poetically. I hear myself say, "I was once the diamond in your eyes, the ruby flaming in your heart. What have I done?" I then hear an inner voice responding, "I forgive you for all your flaws because I care about you and love you." I end by requesting, "Have mercy on my soul."

I find the visual aspect of San Pedro to be stunningly beautiful, creating a sense of awe. Unlike the kaleidoscopic images of mushrooms, which arise quickly and are rapidly changing, the imagery from the cactus comes on later and is more wavelike, with expansion and contraction similar to breathing. It feels like a slow breath with gradually expanding images of the desert, mountains, and springs, all vividly colorful. Then, like a breath exhaling, these slowly fade away, only for another image to appear of equally intense beauty. The colors and breathing seem one and the same.

My heart feels the wonderment of it all — the love and beauty of existence in which one can let go of judgment and feel the essential core of goodness residing within. My heart is filled with feelings of joy and self-acceptance. The feeling is like a child being born, yet conscious of itself and the profundity of being alive. The message is simply to be quiet, to observe what is going on, and to appreciate. The heart function is about appreciation, gratitude, generosity, and loving all beings and the earth itself.

Later, more of the teachings arise. The central idea is that critical judgment is a necessary discriminating step to help determine whom I care about relationally and of whom I need to let go. Discrimination is a key psychological function at the core of a person. It is based on an ability to trust one's intuition about whether another person is essentially positive, neutral, or negative for one's psyche. This is to help me decide if I'm I able to trust the other person, to enjoy their overall personality, and to take them in. To forgive the other's flaws essentially involves a projection on my part. The other person may not perceive a particular behavior as a flaw, so it is important to reframe it as a shadow projection—my own issue, not theirs. To forgive another's flaws implies letting go of judgment about them and to look at what behaviors disturb me which perhaps exist within myself, of which I am critical about and where my criticism of them stems from.

As I review the stories of my various relationships, I realize that the behaviors in other people that I tend to negatively react to are control issues, lack of playfulness, bragging, a need to preach about their epiphanies, and spiritual superiority. Also, I dislike a person with a lack of communicativeness, excessive passivity, a lack of intimacy and initiative, or unreliability. The bottom line is awareness that I have much to look at within myself regarding these shadow complexes. I realize there is a great deal of work for me to do. I see the blockage as a problem in my heart chakra that needs to heal, first by my being less harsh with myself, then by relaxing and becoming more accepting and patient in life. My own self judgment seems to be the key ingredient requiring work. When I feel judgmental of a person, I first need to put this in my "shadow processor," determine what part of them exists within myself, and then decide whether I need to let go of the other person and move on, or accept them as they are because I care enough about them in my heart.

Another issue that causes me to have negative judgments is my expectations. I seem to have high standards for my own conduct which I place on the behavior of others. It is important to examine these standards, to learn to see each person for where they are, and remember that not everyone has to be a close friend or live up to my expectations. There can be many levels of relationships, and it is up to me to consider each relationship and accept it at the level of closeness or distance that the person presents to me or is willing to offer. I realize that this issue involves my undifferentiated feeling function, described by Jung in his theory of psychological types. As I discriminate/differentiate more wisely, I can choose which "circle of my soul" to which a person belongs.

I also gain the insight that one of my shadow issues is neediness. I seem to primarily desire to befriend a person who likes me and pays attention to me; otherwise, I tend to judge them negatively. Somehow, instead of just shifting my judgment into neutral, a negative cognition tends to occur.

This insight is then followed by an experience of channeling a pre-Neanderthal elder in deep worship in a sacred cave. It is as if the animal instinct in the elder turned inward and began to experience the sacredness of being alive and knowing itself—the beginning of self-reflection. It felt like the first ceremony of a proto-human realizing the *greater other*, the creator and death-taker of existence. I am honored to be part of this ritual in which people were chanting within a cave lit by a central fire. It feels like the first sacred worship ceremony to take place in the cave of the heart. I feel awe and tears of gratitude to be among my primitive ancestors.

I become aware that the plant teachers originate from the ground and bring us awareness of growth and regeneration as well as the importance of a place to be rooted. Also, there are animal teachers who are mobile and teach us the value of mobility through the dynamics of movement, migration, and predator/prey survival.

The image of the chakra system depicts the various centers of consciousness that can be accessed through the use of any sacred medicine, but often San Pedro and peyote center on the heart chakra, as seen in the next two images.

In summary, the insights I gained from the San Pedro are that I need to further meditate on the issues of discrimination, self-judgment with projection, shadow, expectations, neediness, and being neutral. On the positive side, they involve learning to appreciate people more, even with their foibles, and continuing to project my love, gratitude, and goodwill into the world. I need to remember my loving core and allow it to emerge without expectation about how it will be received or returned. Some people will appreciate what I offer and others either will not or will be neutral.

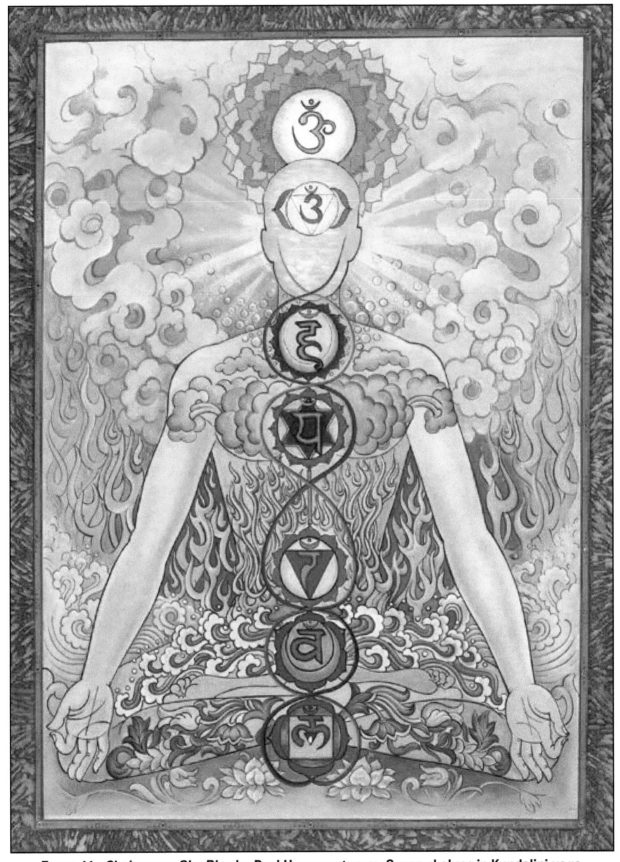

FIGURE 41. *Chakraman Sky Blue* by Paul Heussenstamm. Seven chakras in Kundalini yoga.

119

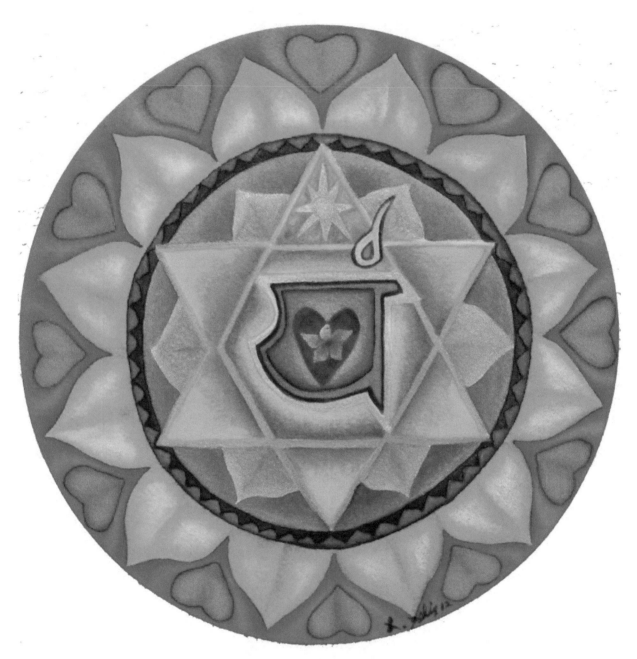

Figure 42. *Anahata* by Lori Felix. A depiction of the heart chakra in the Kundalini/Tantric yoga system of human consciousness, the 4th chakra meditation with this mandala is useful when contemplating the heart center of emotions, feelings, love, trauma, sadness, grief, and judgments.

I am at an age at which I need not care so much what people think of me. At the end of the day, when the curtain comes down and I am with myself, I need to affirm who this person "Alex" is. The above profound teaching is psychological, very simple as far as insights go, yet the cactus experience has impressed it more deeply. I only hope I can make the changes necessary to open up my heart chakra.

Did any real healing around my intention occur? It seemed so, but I realized only time would tell whether this core issue of mine transforms my behavior regarding my relationships. You could say the cactus has spoken to me, but what I do with it is another matter.

Another San Pedro Journey

During one night of our week-long retreat in Ocamura, New Mexico, discussed earlier in the chapter, Ralph shares an induction meditation located in the "Cave of the Heart," where the lineages of father/mother/ancestors, including past life remnants, meet. The medicine for this particular evening is San Pedro cactus extract, six grams, with 125 micrograms LSD augmentation.

My journey starts in a past life of mine that I imagine. I find myself in a Russian peasant village in about the late 1700s-early1800s. I have a wife, a grown son and daughter, and a farm with some cattle and plows. I am also an artist who weaves tapestries. I have some type of chronic lung disease, possibly pneumonia, tuberculosis, or cancer, and am dying. I experience my death, surrounded with the love of my family. I then enter the afterlife space of the chamber of the heart. There is a council of beings deciding upon my reincarnation, since I only lived to about age forty-five to fifty-five and did not complete my karma for that lifetime.

I then gaze into the eyes of the goddess of the South and am transported to a Siberian village in the mountains, the home of my ancestral grandmothers. I meet once again with the grandmothers. They say, "Go plant your seed in this new place (America), and let us dance and sing and love again with the soul and spirit of Mother Russia so we will not perish. We give you our love and bless you, so wake up and eat and be strong." I awaken being nursed, and the grandmothers lift me in the air and, in a circle, start singing a Russian song.

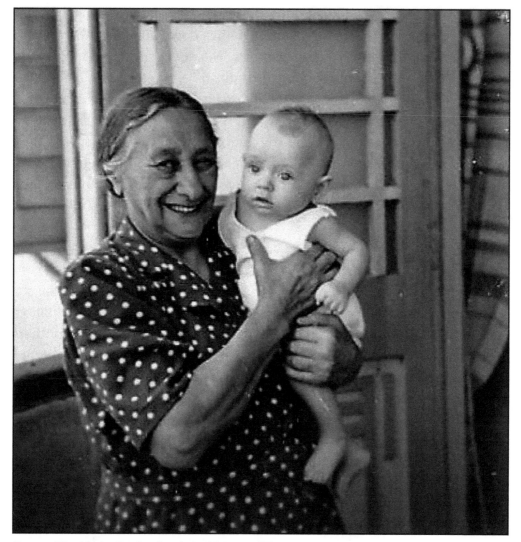

FIGURE **43.** **Little Sasha (me), held by my Russian grandmother, Babala (Sophie), in Bombay, India. Born in Kyiv, moved to Harbin in China then to India, and came with us to America.**

I next go through the actual life experience of my premature birth in Bombay, India, delivered by the doctor, Colonel Waters, as well as my mother's and my near-deaths at that time. I weighed less than four pounds at birth. The doctor tells my mother there is nothing more he can do, and it is now up to God if I survive.

I am then led by my elders toward a place where I meet my present family: my wife Judy, and sons Geoff and Blake, who are the fruits of my seed. I am told by my elders to live life fully, to dance, to sing, and to contribute my gifts as a doctor in this lifetime.

I emerge from this experience with an overwhelming feeling of love and gratitude for my life and with a renewed sense of purpose, not only in my work, but also on behalf of my ancestors. I realize that my Russian ancestral seed migrating to the United States represents my karma in this lifetime.

San Pedro Supplemented by 2C-B

Another journey during this same week utilized San Pedro, with its heart-opening properties, supplemented by the synthesized entheogenic chemical 2C-B. (see chapter 31)

The Wounded Child

My intention for this journey is to transform the wounded child within me into the radiant child through remembering and healing. As a psychiatrist, much attention has gone into this approach of reclaiming the wounded child; many people spend years in therapy in this process. Often, they remain stuck in this complex without much movement. One does not cure the wounded child; since it is always part of the core psyche, it never disappears. However, healing can occur so that this aspect no longer has so much control over a person's behavior and thoughts. One is able to move forward in life and manifest more positively.

The traditional therapy approach for the wounded child is to facilitate mourning the childhood that never fully manifested due to some aspects of negative parenting or trauma. For example, the child was not mirrored accurately to reflect the true nature of the child's self. Instead, the child, in order to gain attention and love, may have adapted to behave in a way that mirrored the mother's and father's needs and expectations and thus created a false self. Faulty mirroring, physical, emotional, or sexual abuse and neglect (absent parenting) — all may traumatize the developing child. Very often, the child grows up feeling responsible for and deserving of the abuse, at the core believing her or himself to be unworthy and unlovable.

In therapy, the patient is encouraged to reparent the inner child by acknowledging the pain, encourage grieving the childhood lost, and providing a more positive cognitive framework, which reinforces the worthiness of the inner child complex. Unfortunately, patients can spend years in therapy, making little progress by looping around the same trauma without healing the inner split. An essential part missing in many therapies is that of helping the patient find the "radiant child" within, the joyful child who has been forgotten. The trauma and its associated false negative beliefs often have suppressed these positive memories. The radiant child is the antidote for the wounded child, is forward-looking, and represents the reclaiming of soul loss. The radiant child may seem like an intellectual concept, but during a medicine journey it becomes a living entity, an experience that can be integrated and brought back to the present. This became an important part of my own journey.

I decided to revisit my inner child, which I believe was primarily wounded by actions of my father. As the pilot of my inner spaceship, I used my intention to head toward the East and, also, using the Janus model, intended to consciously regress to my past memories. Returning to the past in this way would not mean dwelling or indulging in my woundedness; it would allow me to reexamine my memories from an adult perspective and perhaps put the pieces together differently. The purpose for remembering what had been dismembered in my childhood experience is for healing. In this situation that meant coming to terms with the traumas I had endured by remembering them from an observational, adult point of view. Only then could I become unstuck from the traumas lodged in my unconscious that percolate into my behaviors in life. The purpose of poking into pain would be to lance the boil of immobile and stuck trauma and to return with healthy insights into my present predicament of negative attitudes toward work and relationships.

As I centered on my intention, the first memories emerging were of my father's rage episodes, which had often been directed at me, sometimes accompanied by a belt and followed by his abandonment of me, holding back any affection for weeks at a time. I had felt hurt, lonely, and pining for him to love me. I felt responsible for his rages but often could not recall what I had done wrong to incur such a reaction. Since I didn't remember my behaviors, I assumed that there was just something bad at my core. This created a sense of shame and worthlessness about my existence, as well as the belief that I deserved punishment and was inherently unlovable. My father was not a drinker, although some children of alcoholics have similar experiences. It is likely that my father was reenacting his own wounds from childhood with the addition of his Russian temperament. His parents had apparently been angry people who ended up getting divorced; he left home at nineteen for college in Germany, never to return home to see either his parents or his Mother Russia again.

Maternal and Paternal Lineages

The memories continued to come to me; I then remembered Babala, my maternal Russian grandmother. She came to live with us while we were still in India when I was an infant and later emigrated with us to America. She was an unconditionally loving presence for me, doting on my every need as a child. Her support, in addition to my mother's protection, created another aspect of my core being filled with security and love. I also remembered the positive feelings I had as a child about our family outings, as well as experiences with the Russian-American community in Los Angeles that provided a social context for my family.

Following the taproot of my maternal lineage, I realized the creative, artistic, and musical influences my uncles Fima and Jack had on me. Fima became a famous artist of abstract expressionism in Israel and Paris. Jack was a renowned big band leader in Malaya before his untimely death at only forty-four years old. I remembered that my mother had also been reactive, and that she carried distrust of other people as part of her heritage. I recalled the numerous arguments between my parents, which often led to physical violence. As a young teenager, I would often have to intervene to protect my mother from being injured by my father's rages.

The taproot of my paternal lineage was connected more with the scientific and technical interests I cultivated in my life. I developed my critical thinking skills from this side. My father was always supportive of this part of me. My father also had a charming side which endeared many people to him, a personality trait I also developed. He was courageous in his life, traveling from Russia to Germany, then to Malaya, to India, and to the U.S. He was often uprooted from where he lived by circumstances and forced to migrate and to set down new roots. I recognized that although my father had traits that had harmed me, these positive attributes were part of his psychological structure as well.

In reviewing the influences of these two lineages, I found myself wondering how these two lineages came together on the night of my actual conception. Was it out of love, or lust? Either way is fine by me. Somehow, I got here.

These memories of my father's traits then led me to reexamine my connection to my own two sons, the grief I have felt at times when observing their experience of life's travails as well as the regret at times of my angry outbursts with them. After such an event, I remembered I would return quickly to them to reassure them of my love for them, rather than reenact my father's abandonment.

After this thorough review at this stage of the journey, I was able to let all of the negative memories go, to remember that I survived and am still intact, and to begin to experience the other side of the wounded child and to transcend toward my radiant child. I focused on the birth of all the energies within me that represented hope, love, and creativity; and the uncorrupted light I possessed allowing me to carry forth the family lineages and live out a different karma.

The Gift of Life

After this visit to the East, I began to pilot myself toward the other directions. The North was my adult and mature masculine side, and the South represented my adult, mature feminine side. From these adult perspectives, I was able to move my young child from the East toward the West and to reexperience some memories as a teenager, and finally move to my present state of being as a wise elder (or perhaps a wise guy). It seems that the wisdom grew from surviving and integrating these traumas, emerging to the other side with a positive sense of myself and of life in general.

Despite the traumas, I found myself able to thank both of my parents for the *gift of life*. I also came to realize that my personality traits were not all due to my upbringing by my parents, but they represented a longer lineage and the support of ancestors whom I've never known. In healing the inner child, it is important for all to realize that the core of a person is not defined only by the parent's behaviors and DNA, but also by the ancestral remnants which are inherited and can be experienced through memories and journey-work.

This reconciliation with my parents and ancestors left me with a profound feeling of love and connection to the radiant child that inhabits my being. There is a hidden symmetry of love, of giving and receiving, in all relationships that needs to be honored, even if some of the experiences have been interpreted as negative. In the "Cave of the Heart" medtiation, where family, friends, and enemies meet, everyone is given time to express themselves. The enemies and shadow figures all have something to say and to teach. This recognition is fundamental for transcendence of trauma, for wisdom, and for compassion. While not all hurts need to be forgiven for healing, all aspects need time for expression. In the "Cave of the Heart," Ralph's expression of the inward journey to a meeting place residing in the heart chakra, the negative aspects can be overwritten through the support of light-bearing beings. Residual anger can shift into neutral and therefore allow forward motion in life.

The insights and teachings gained from such an experience can be summarized in one word: *profound*. Much can be accomplished with this type of intense inner journey that might have required months or years in traditional therapies. For me, the healing feels deep, cellular. Yet only time will tell how much of this is permanently integrated.

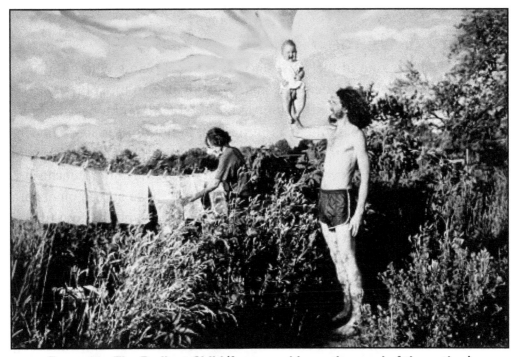

FIGURE 44. *The Radiant Child* (from an old greeting card of the author)

Chapter 14

About San Pedro Cactus (Cachuma) or Cactus of the Four Winds

I sometimes refer to the mescaline-containing cactus San Pedro (*Trichocereus pachanoi*) with a term of endearment, "Uncle Pete." Even though the Catholic priests opposed its usage among the natives, the term San Pedro, or Saint Peter, ironically became the defining name of this cactus. Saint Peter was the guardian at the gates of heaven, an apt reference to the beauty encountered on a mescaline-based journey.

History & Usage

San Pedro is one of the most ancient magical plants where it grows wild in South America, but it also is easily cultivated in most locales. The active main ingredient, found in the skin of the plant, is the psychoactive alkaloid mescaline, the same as is in peyote, although it is less concentrated. San Pedro cactus grows in coastal Peru, in the northern highlands of the Andes (where it is known as Huachuma, or Wachuma in the Quecha language), and in Bolivia (where it is called Achuma). These sacred plants are of the species *Trichocereus pachanoi* and *peruvianus*, and the four-ribbed ones are the rarest, most potent, and thus most sought after. (Schultes and Hofmann 1998, 166-169) It also grows readily in California, as seen in this photo from my garden, and remains legal to grow.

Archaeological evidence has been discovered which depicts this cactus on the stone carvings, vessels, and textiles of the Chavin culture of Peru (1300-600 BCE), and the Nazca culture of Peru (100-400 CE), indicating that they have probably been used by shamans for centuries. As is true of many other entheogenic plants, these plants are seen by indigenous

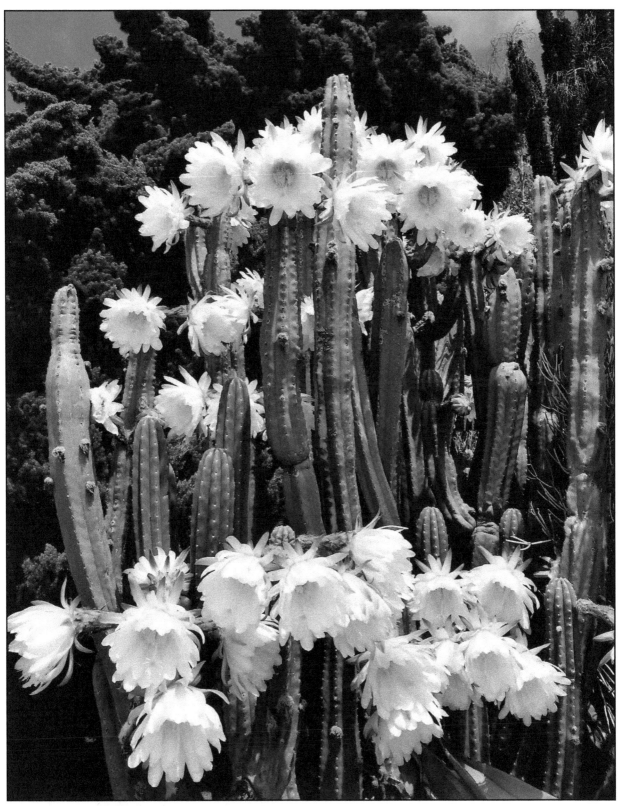

FIGURE 45. San Pedro (*Trichocereus pachanoi*) in bloom in the author's garden. They bloom for three days and are spectacularly beautiful. Photo by Alexander Shester.

people as being given to mankind by the gods to help with the experience of separation of the soul from the body, in a simple fashion and instantaneously. (Schultes and Hofmann 1998, 166-167)

Of course, as with peyote, the Roman Catholic Church fought against its use. "This is the plant with which the devil deceived the Indians . . . in their paganism, using it for their lies and superstitions . . . those who drink lose consciousness and remain as if dead . . . transported by the drink, the Indians dreamed a thousand absurdities and believed them as if they were true." (Schultes and Hofmann 1998, 166-169)

Shamans in contemporary times employ San Pedro, " . . . to cure sickness, including alcoholism and insanity, or divination, to undo love witchcraft; to counter all kinds of sorcery, and to assure success in personal ventures." (Schultes and Hofmann 1998, 166-167) The shaman in his curing ritual aims to make his patient bloom during the night ceremony, to make the subconscious "open like a flower." An ecstatic magical flight is still characteristic of the contemporary San Pedro ceremony.

A shaman describes its effects as follows, " . . . the drug first produces drowsiness or a dreamy state and feeling of lethargy . . . a slight dizziness . . . then a great vision, a clearing of all the faculties . . . It produces a light numbness in the body and afterward a tranquility. And then comes detachment, a type of visual force . . . inclusive of all the senses . . . including the sixth sense, the telepathic sense of transmitting oneself across time and matter . . . like a removal of one's thoughts to a distant dimension . . . participants are set free and engage in flight through cosmic regions." (Schultes and Hofmann 1998, 168-169)

Additives

At times other plants, boiled or powdered, are added as catalysts to activate the San Pedro, and the drink is called Cimora. Some of these additive plants are *Brugmansia* species, the Andean cactus *Neoraimondia macrostibas*, *Pedilanthus tithymalodies*, and *Isotoma longiflora*. Each of these may also possess their own hallucinogenic potential. (Schultes and Hofmann 1998, 166-167)

In the vision quests in which I have participated, I've described other additives which were used to activate the San Pedro experience, such as low doses of psilocybin mushrooms, low-dose LSD, or the synthesized entheogenic chemical 2C-B. To experience effects by itself, large quantities of San Pedro must be eaten and several hours pass for it to have an effect, if at all. These amplifiers activate the effects of the cactus more quickly. Sometimes, people use this medicine in lower doses which, although not psychedelic, brings a sense of increased presence with their surroundings, especially when hiking in nature. There is more acuteness, awareness, and connectedness with the environment.

The essence of the San Pedro experience is heart-centered. The heart is the chakra that is opened up initially, but as with all the described medicines, upper and lower chakra consciousness can be accessed by the participant traveling up and down the Tantric spine through intention. Peyote is also a heart-centered healing medicine.

Chapter 15

Peyote *(Lophophora williamsii)*

The other mescaline-containing desert cactus is peyote (*Lophophora williamsii*), another of nature's gifts to humanity. I will share my personal experiences using this amazing plant under the guidance of Spirit Eagle, a Navajo medicine man. Ralph Metzner never used this medicine as part of his circles, preferring it to be provided only by legitimate Native American Church (NAC) shamans who had been granted permission to take it off the reservation to share with our culture. Even though peyote was consumed as a sacrament at least as far back as the Mayans for more than 1600-2000 years, its modern use by Native Americans of the Native American Church as a practice is only about one hundred and fifty years old. The use of peyote as a sacrament by the NAC was finally legalized in 1978 by President Jimmy Carter in the Native American Freedom Act. Its use outside this church is still illegal; therefore the peyote rituals in which I participated were held in secret.

Spirit Eagle

My experiences with peyote took place during my participation in six sessions led by Spirit Eagle. In these healing circles, he brought knowledge which had been taught to him by his elder peyote shaman, known as Star Man, as practiced on the Shiprock reservation in New Mexico. Spirit Eagle was allowed by his elders to travel to California to teach us about Native American spirituality as practiced through the NAC. It remains essential to remember that when a sacred ceremony leaves its prescribed culture, sensitivity about misappropriating such rituals must observed, and they should be carried out only with the proper permission.

In each peyote ceremony, there were from twelve to twenty participants. These larger circles I found a bit difficult as the rounds became quite extended in length. Each person would share their pain and ask for their specific healing. As they revealed their stories, I eventually became fatigued and overwhelmed and lost my ability to be present. So many participants diluted the experience and I preferred the smaller circles for their greater impact on me. Here is a quote about creating a mindset for approaching this powerful medicine, "You must come to peyote as truth, in an attitude of worship. (Hammerschlag, 58) "... peyote's gift really depended on how you came to it. If you were a skeptic and approached it with fear, peyote would not reveal itself." (Hammerschlag, 60) The same could be said regarding any of the medicines previously discussed; it is a reminder that the experience is influenced by set (mindset) and setting.

The leader of the ceremony, Spirit Eagle, was called the Road Man. We would surround an altar he had made in the center with a prayer rug, which had a pan of hot coals brought from the fireplace as well as other ceremonial symbols he had brought, such as a fan made of eagle feathers, dried sage, and sacred tobacco. He would have certain participants carry on the several roles of the Fire Man or Woman, who tended the central fire or hot coals in the circle, as well as a Cedar Man or Woman, who sprinkled cedar on the coals to add fragrance. Often during the prayers and blessing, sage was lit and spread around by an eagle fan. Sage is considered by the peyote people to be the first plant God gave the Earth Mother. (Hammerschlag 1989, 66) The Drum Man or Woman would entrain us all by a rapid rhythmic beating (approximately five beats per second) of a water drum, which by itself would put us all in a trancelike state. Spirit Eagle usually led the drumming, but at times he would hand the drum over to another person. Over the various circles, I occasionally had the honor of beating the drum, as well as taking on the roles of Fire Man and Cedar Man while under the guidance of the peyote medicine man.

Often during the ritual, Spirit Eagle would chant and sing songs in his native Diné (Navajo) language. At times we would chant along with him using his vocalizations and syncopations, even though we did not understand the language. This created a sense of community, which was an important element of the ceremony. There was less time for individual meditation, but listening to the various stories triggered many associations and memories with similar themes which were specific to each of us.

Spirit Eagle would provide the peyote to each of us with a blessing at the beginning of each circle. The doses he gave us were generally small so that we could function as a community. He provided more peyote to the experienced participants, but the effects depended more on mindset than on the actual dose. Some people experienced little or no effect, while others were deeply affected by the medicine. The effects generally lasted about four to five hours unless more was taken during the night.

Peyote Journeys

My characterization of peyote is that it is heart-centered and heart-opening, similar to San Pedro, but more concentrated, likely because the main chemical ingredient is also mescaline. My experiences are mirrored by this description, ". . . only the body is grounded . . . the spirit soars and tears speak . . . It has taught me how to feel small, to appreciate specialness in things ordinary, to be less serious about knowing . . . An overwhelming sense of well-being came over me as I stared at Father Peyote. The colors were incredibly vivid, the songs were unbelievably melodic; and the coals formed a sparkling, volcanic mosaic." (Hammerschlag 1989, 67)

The medicine assists one to go deeply into the core of being and to suspend negative cognitions regarding past traumatic experiences. It helps to untangle the knots of psychological trauma embedded in the psyche. Forgiveness of oneself and others occurs, which allows the flow of positive energy to emerge once again. Transformation in a heart-felt way can then occur, freeing the psyche and bringing appreciation of the deeper indwelling spirit in ourselves. Such an experience can leads to the Navajo path called "The Beauty Way."

Carlos Castaneda in *The Teachings of Don Juan* talked about the path of the heart, and his words serve as a reminder for how important it is to clear heart/emotional blockages. "Does this path have heart? If it does, the path is good; if it doesn't, it is of no use. Both paths lead nowhere; but one has a heart, the other doesn't. One makes for a joyful journey; as long as you follow it, you are one with it. The other will make you curse your life. One makes you strong; the other weakens you." (Castaneda 1968)

In one particular circle, I experienced an incredibly beautiful vision. From the beating drum emerged cupped hands from which fire with many vivid colors sprung forth. The pair of hands was holding a red rose in full

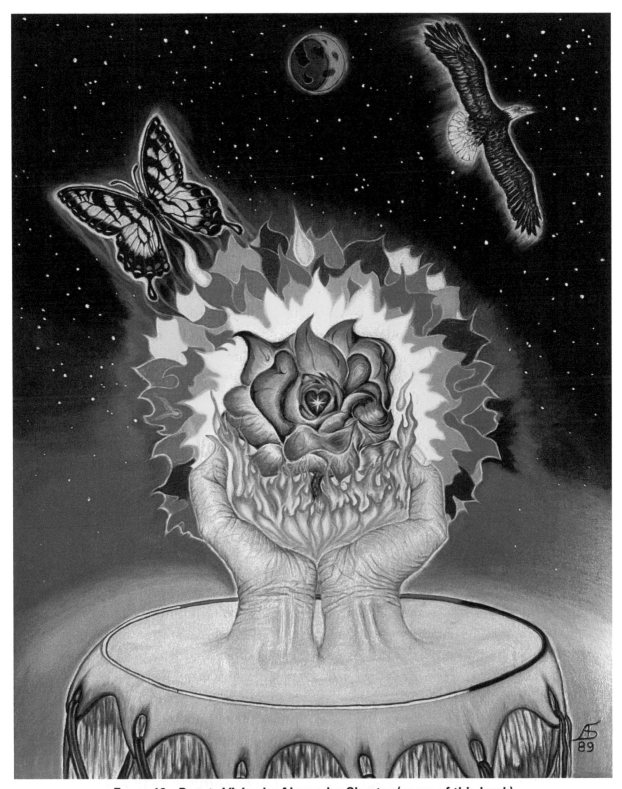

FIGURE 46. *Peyote Vision* by Alexander Shester (cover of this book)

bloom, highly scented. As I went deeper into the vision, a heart appeared. I was overwhelmed with sadness for all the pain in the world and within myself, and tears began to flow. They turned into tears of joy as I felt myself going deeper to meet my soul. At the center of my vision was a brightly lit star emanating tremendous energy outward toward me. As I immersed myself in this light, I felt I was in the presence of the Creator, lit up like flickering fire, with the face of an old man with a benevolent smile gazing at me. I again found myself totally naked in front of this force; I bent down and prostrated myself in total humility, honored to be with this presence. Forgiveness for all my shortcomings was felt, and a blessing was offered for my life.

From this fire sprang forth an eagle which soared up into the dark sky full of stars. Then a swallowtail butterfly slowly emerged, accompanied by the feeling that my soul was set free of its burdens for a time as it soared upward. I now understood and incorporated the feeling of grace as I witnessed all this vision with a sense of awe. The beautiful colors accompanying these images seemed to come from within myself, fueled by the beating of the drum by Spirit Eagle, the hot coals in the central fire, and the incense of cedar and sage in the room. All was one, a unity from which sprung forth the manifested world. I knew I must create some form of art to symbolize this vision in order for me to always remember this experience. Thus the cover of this book was born from that work.

The Native American Church Intervenes

Unfortunately, as a few years and more circles passed, Spirit Eagle became psychologically corrupted. He seemed to have become inflated by his position as a shaman and the money it brought him. While on the reservation, he lived a humble existence, but when he started earning a significant amount through fees he charged, some animosity grew on the part of the members of his tribe who were still living at a poverty level. The elders of his peyote church began to feel that he was diluting the potency of the sacredness of peyote by using it primarily with the privileged white participants who were not part of the Native culture. Some participants noted that he seemed to show preference to some of the females in the circles. The elders sensed Spirit Eagle becoming corrupted and withdrew

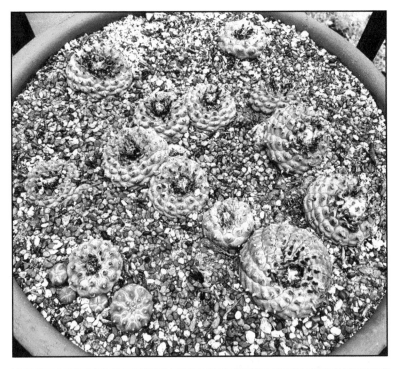

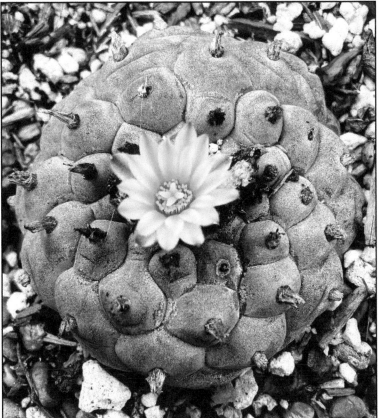

FIGURE 47. Father Peyote (*Lophophora williamsii*)
(photo by permission of an anonymous colleague)

permission to share the Diné Way outside of the tribe. He was eventually censured by his tribal elders and forbidden to carry out further peyote ceremonies outside the reservation. Despite these failings, he did teach me and others much about sacred space and healing. I benefited both personally and professionally from the insights I gained through these circles.

In later years, I visited him on occasion at his home on the reservation in Shiprock, New Mexico. He taught me how to make and beat a water drum, but I never took peyote with him again. His life ended in an early death secondary to pneumonia. I often wondered if the power of the peyote finally humbled his existence and contributed to causing his illness due to his having drifted from the sacred path. Barbara Myerhoff in *The Peyote Hunt* quotes a Huichol *mara'akame* (shaman), Ramon Medina Silva, "Peyote can 'read one's thoughts' and can punish one for being false or evil. The peyote rewards or punishes a man according to his inner state, his moral deserts. The sanction is immediate, just, and certain, an effective regulator of behavior in a small, well-integrated society."

Chapter 16

About Peyote as Medicine

Peyote is a very interesting cactus in that it has no spines and is relatively flat rather than columnar, like San Pedro. It is very slow-growing and thrives in the deserts of Northern Mexico and Texas. The active ingredient of peyote was identified at the beginning of the 20th century as a crystalline alkaloid substance extracted from a dried cactus called Mescal Buttons (*Lophophora williamsii*) and is therefore known as mescaline. As noted, this is also the active hallucinogenic ingredient of the San Pedro cactus (*Trichocereus pachanoi*).

The chemical name for mescaline is 3,4,5-trimethoxy-phenylethylamine, which is similar to the brain neurotransmitter norepinephrine. Therefore, it is different from the tryptamine-based entheogens, which primarily affect the serotonin neurotransmitter system. Both brain pathways can lead to the gateway opening up the mind, a retuning of it to an ability to experience the transpersonal realm. Interestingly, these two systems, when not functioning properly, are implicated in various psychiatric disorders such as depression, bipolar disorder, anxiety, and psychosis. Different medications target these disorders through modulation of serotonin, norepinephrine, and dopamine.

History of Use

As mentioned, the sacramental use of peyote dates back at least 2000 years in various indigenous Mesoamerican Indian tribes, such as the Chichimeca, Toltec, and Tarahumara. It eventually spread to the Cora and Huichol tribes of Mexico. In the early 1900s, its use spread from northern Mexico to North American Indian tribes such as the Navajo, Apache, Kiowa, and Comanche, as well as about forty other tribes.

The Native American Church was formed in 1885 for the sacramental use of peyote, primarily due to opposition from the Catholic Church and local governments. Peyote was considered a divine messenger enabling individuals to communicate directly with God without the medium of an intervening priest. Between 1885 and 1922, the NAC had 13,300 members. It is presently thought to be a pan-Indian religion with more than 300,000 participants nationwide. (Schultes and Hofmann 1998, 152) NAC members are universalists, regarding all religions as basically good, and variations on the same theme. They stress humility, faith, and love toward all beings along with the belief that a man or woman trying to function alone outside of community is weak. Peyote offers the communicant a method of establishing contact with the Creator. Observers have considered the ritual use of peyote to be the single most effective program dealing with the problem of Indian alcoholism. (Hammerschlag 1989)

It is thought that peyote first came to the Oklahoma territory over a century ago through a Comanche Indian leader, Quanah Parker. Carl Hammerschlag in The *Dancing Healers* (1989) tells the story as follows, " . . . while living with his white mother's family in Texas, Quanah fell ill. When the doctors could not help him, the family called an Indian healer; she cured Quanah with the help of songs and a bitter tea. When Quanah recovered, the woman told him that the magical tea must never be taken for its own sake. It must be taken as a sacrament, with ceremony and respect."

"The medicine, peyote, came from the buttons that grow on the mescal cactus, and it was to be used for prayer, understanding, and healing – it was a sacred thing... When Quanah returned to Oklahoma, it was a time of seething Indian discontent...Quanah brought the beads and sash worn by the Peyote Chief, called the Road Man. He brought the elements of the peyote ceremony: fire and cedar incense, the water drum, the peyote fans, the staff, the gourd, the rattle, and the smoking of sweet tobacco, and peyote." (Hammerschlag 1989)

The ceremony among the Cora, Huichol, and Tarahumara Indians of Mexico has probably changed little in content over the centuries; it still exists, in great part, of dancing and singing (Schultes and Hoffman 1998). A description of such a ceremony of the Cora tribe was published in the 17th century by a Spanish missionary, "Close to the musician was seated the leader of the singing, whose business it was to mark time . . . Nearby was placed a tray filled with Peyote, which is a diabolical root that is ground up

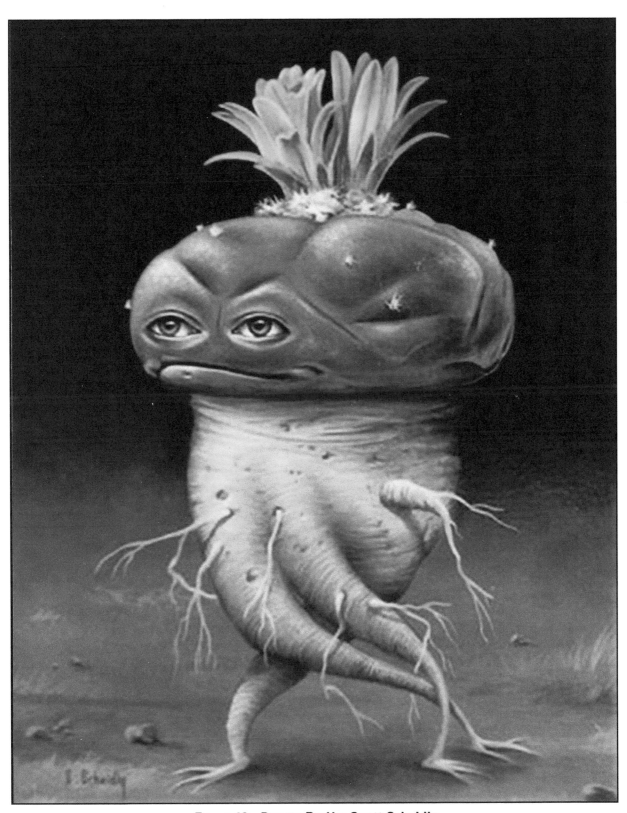

FIGURE 48. *Peyote Bud* by Scott Scheidly.

and drunk by them so that they may not become weakened by the exhausting effects of so long a function, which they begin by forming as large a circle of men and women as could occupy the space. One after the other, they went dancing in a ring or marking time with their feet . . . They would dance all night from 5 o'clock in the evening to 7 o'clock in the morning, without stopping nor leaving the circle . . .for the majority . . . were unable to utilize their legs." (Schultes and Hofmann 1998, 144-155)

The Huichol – Peyote Hunt

The modern Huichol Peyote ritual is closest to the pre-Colonial Mexican ceremonies, as described by a Spanish priest, Sahagun (1499-1590), among the Chichimeca and Toltec Indians. The Huichol Indians, a lesser-known tribe of Mexico whose population is about 9000, reside in the Sierra Madre mountains throughout the states of Durango, Jalisco, Nayarit, and Zacatecas. To this day, they gather for the *peyote hunt* about three hundred miles northeast of their homeland in the mythical sacred mountain called Wirikúta.

The purpose of the yearly peyote hunt in the birthplace of the gods in Wirikúta is to return to paradise. The ritual pilgrims temporarily suspend their human condition in order to become their divine counterparts. The late anthropologist Mircea Eliade states, "The Myth of the Eternal Return" is the universal longing for paradise; to return to an original place and time." (Myerhoff 1974, 245) It is equated with a state of wholeness, an absence of differentiation between man, god, animals, or male and female. It is the cosmic wholeness before creation, before consciousness, before the separation between dark and light.

At the time there was found abundant peyote on the ground to be collected; they sang all night and all day and wept exceedingly. (Schultes 1998) In present times peyote is considered scarce from over-harvesting. The Huichol Indians consider peyote to be above any of the other psychotropic plants, such as the sacred mushrooms, morning glory (containing lysergic acid), and Datura, all of which they consign to the realm of sorcerers. (Schultes and Hofmann 1998, 144-155) The pilgrimage to the sacred grounds of Wirikúta was only opened to outside anthropologists in the 1960s, and is now led by an experienced *mara'akame* (shaman). This *mara'akame* is in touch with the oldest Huichol god, Tatewarí (our

Grandfather-fire), also known as Hikuri, the peyote god. Therefore, peyote is also sometimes called Hikuri. (Schultes and Hofmann 1998)

The peyote hunt is described in great detail in the book *Peyote Hunt: The Sacred Journey of the Huichol Indians* by Barbara Myerhoff (1976). She reports a peyote experience described by Ramon Medina Silva, a Huichol mara'akame:

> The first time one puts the peyote into one's mouth, one feels it going down into the stomach. It feels very cold, like ice. And the inside of one's mouth becomes dry, very dry. And then it becomes wet, very wet. One has much saliva then. And then, a while later one feels as if one were fainting. The body begins to feel weak, it begins to feel faint. And one begins to yawn, to feel very tired. And after a while one feels very light. The whole body begins to feel light, without sleep, without anything.
>
> And then, when one takes enough of this, one looks upward and what does one see? One sees darkness. Only darkness. It is very dark, very black. And one feels drunk with the peyote. And when one looks up again it is total darkness except for a little bit of light, a tiny bit of light, brilliant yellow. It comes there, a brilliant yellow. And one looks into the fire . . . One sees the fire in colors, very many colors, five colors, different colors. The flames divide—it is all brilliant, very brilliant and very beautiful. The beauty is very great, very great. It is a beauty such as one never sees without the peyote. The flames come up, they shoot up, and each flame divides into those colors and each color is multicolored— blue, green, yellow, all those colors. The yellow appears on the tip of the flames as the flame shoots upward. And on the tips you can see little sparks in many colors coming out. And the smoke which rises from the fire, it also looks more and more yellow, more and more brilliant. Then one sees the fire, very bright, one sees the offerings there, many arrows with feathers and they are full of color, shimmering, shimmering. That is what one sees. (Myerhoff 1974, 219)

Although this description is repetitive, I am sharing it in its authentic narrative form as told by the shaman, rather than by a Catholic priest. He does not describe any of the sacred teachings that came from the session with the medicine. Peyote is often construed as a private experience, and the individual visions and teachings are not shared outside of the group, which keeps it confidential. (This is also true of modern psychotherapy and dreams, which are held in confidence.) It is believed that the energy must be contained to help in transformation; otherwise, it could become diluted if it were indiscriminately shared with another person.

It is interesting to compare and to note the similarities of these described visual effects with my own peyote experiences, which I had many years before reading this book about the Peyote Hunt. I have chosen to share some of my personal experiences in this writing because many years have passed, and I have integrated what is necessary. There will always be some aspects that remain respectfully sealed in my personal inner vault.

Among the Huichol, there is a belief in a holy trinity making up a unity, consisting of the *Deer*, the *Maize*, and the *Peyote* complex. The deer (animal) is associated with the period of Huichol history marked by masculine dominance, hunting, independence, adventure, and freedom. The maize or corn (vegetal) represents the period of cultivation and partnership between the male and female. It symbolizes sustenance within the community, food, regularity, sharing between the sexes, family, labor, and diligence. It is the daily life of the community necessary for survival, but like "all work and no play", it can become burdensome. There is a need for periodical transcendence and spiritual sustenance. Peyote, like the holy spirit, is the source unifying the needs of the community for survival and the needs of the individual for the restoration of the soul and spirit. The peyote brings something precious and beautiful, with no utilitarian purpose, to Huichol life and makes the daily struggles of life meaningful.

"This combination of deer, maize and peyote represents remarkable completeness. When the Huichol juxtapose them and consider each to be an aspect of the other, they are stating that man cannot live without a sense of the past, working for his living, or finding moments of solitary beauty." (Myerhoff 1974, 227)

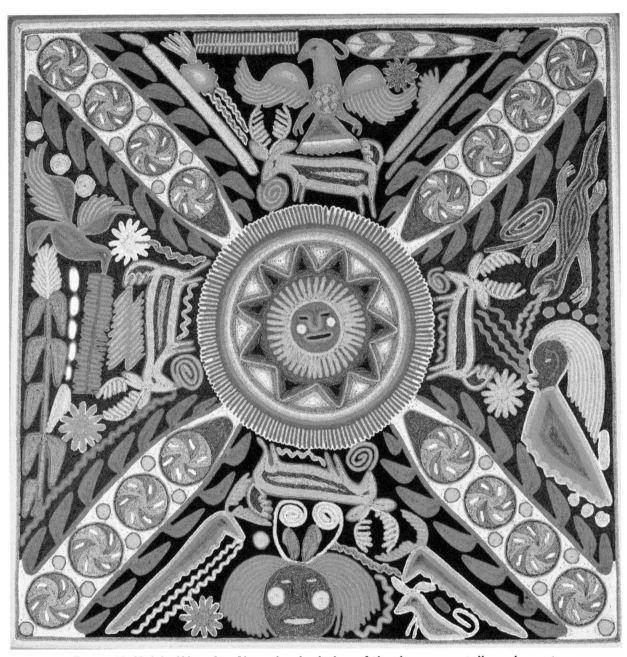

FIGURE 49. Huichol Yarn Art. Note the depiction of the deer, corn stalk, and peyote.
(Collection of the author)

Archetypal Visions

This archetypal, mythic longing to return consciously to our origin is exemplified by the oft quoted segment from the end of T.S. Eliot's *Four Quartets.*

"We shall not cease from exploration
And the end of all our exploring
Will be to arrive where we started
And know the place for the first time."
(Eliot 1971, 145)

Entering paradise has its dangers in that everyone desires to stay in a perpetual state of ecstasy: to live without the responsibilities, routines, and stress of daily living. This desire for transcendence is a powerful dynamic behind addictions. The addict initially uses a substance to seek the pleasure of a high or to avoid emotional pain. This phase of an addict's experience is replaced with the compulsive need to escape stress and pain, only to be enslaved by the drug itself. The harsh reality of being separated from a paradisial state (the mother's womb) leads one to the painful knowledge of human loneliness, impotence, pettiness, and deficiency.

Jung would call this entranced state of paradise (the Huichol Wirikuta) and the refusal to leave it *uroboric incest* (the snake eating its own tail). This signifies the individual's refusal to enter the world, to encounter the universal principle of the opposites, to come to terms with the inner and outer worlds, and thus to avoid the essential tasks of human and individual development (Myerhoff 1974, 250). Jungian psychology holds that it is important to differentiate between the mother complex, which incestuously embeds a person into infantile fantasies and dependencies, and the Great Mother archetype, which is regenerative and life-enhancing to the psyche. Wirikúta, for the Huichol, is the mythical space where the Great Mother dwells. Staying in this space too long blocks individual development (individuation) toward becoming a mature person. In this state, one remains infantile, needy, and in the worst case, becomes delusional or psychotic.

Briefly, the archetype of the positive mother is a universal experience of nurturance, fertility, and protection, which is life-promoting and comforting for an individual. Examples occur in mythology and stories of the goddesses, mother nature, queen of the rainforest, and the fairy godmother.

As with all archetypes, there are positive and negative, light and dark aspects. The darker side of the mother archetype may manifest as the maleficent witch, intent on controlling, poisoning, or holding back the development of a child; abusing and or preventing separation of mother and child. Examples in fairy tales include Baba Yaga of the forest in Russian tales, or the European tales of the witch who poisons Snow White or the evil stepmother in Cinderella. Therefore, the mother archetype contains the potential for both the creative and the destructive energies of life and death. In fairy tales, often one must embrace and humble oneself to the dark mother and do a number of tasks for her before she will transform to the positive form. One must first earn her respect and work for her before she becomes an ally.

Archetypes manifest themselves by descending to the personal plane and becoming expressed in certain qualities in the individual. Depending on a person's experience with parents, the personal mother mirrors degrees of positive and negative mothering to her offspring with the hope that there is "good-enough" child-rearing to enhance growth and trust in the world. Too much abuse or neglect, as with narcissistic parenting, leads to psychopathology later in life. A female then may not experience her power and nurturing qualities as an adult and may become developmentally fixated with immature traits. A male may not be able to separate adequately from the maternal matrix and will have a lifelong need to be taken care of by others, rather than become self-sufficient with a strong identity.

Once paradise is experienced, the difficult task for the participant is to leave this blissful state and return to ordinary existence. Barbara Myerhoff best expresses the importance of leaving paradise and coming back to home:

> On the sociological level, the temptation to remain in Paradise is due to man's desire to dwell in a permanent state of ecstasy, forever outside of social obligation and responsibility. In Wirikúta, the hirkuritámete are in a state of intense communion with each other, where the social self is shed and men [and women] stand beside each other as totalities,

in spontaneous, joyous vulnerability, without the protection or requirements of social structure. This state of fusion of the individual with the group is antithetical to everyday life and its requirements . . . This concern cannot be suspended for long. Thus, the experience of ecstatic communion with another—something outside of the self, whether god, the cosmos, or fellow mortals—is as fleeting as it is universally sought . . . at one pole, mundane needs met through social structure and at the other, the ecstasy of communion, which [Victor] Turner calls communitas. To attempt to make either of these opposed states the whole of life is perilous. Without communitas—which must be periodic and short-lived— mundane considerations are overwhelming—tedious, trivial business, mere survival. The spirit starves. Without social structure, the body starves. (Myerhoff 1974, 247)

During the annual pilgrimage of the Huichol to the land of Wirikúta, the participants approach slowly, with intention and patience. They enter with their empty baskets to collect the sacred cactus. The tracks of the deer lead them to where the peyote grows. Once collected, they participate with the lead *mara'akame* in the sacred ceremony and meet the Creator in ecstatic visions. Once the ceremony concluded, they would hustle quickly but respectfully out of Wirikúta with their baskets full of peyote, back to their regular life, so as not to be seduced into staying there. It was known that sacred energy can turn destructive to the human if one tries to capture and possess this state of consciousness. The above warning about paradise also applies to anyone who journeys to the altered state of the transcendent realm, whether using a psychoactive medicine or not.

As a final description of the ceremonial use of peyote, following is a Huichol myth of the journey to Wirikúta as described in Joan Halifax's *The Fruitful Darkness*:

According to Huichol mythology, in ancient times after the world had been put in order by Our Grandfather Fire, Grandmother Growth, and the Divine Deer Person Kauyumari, Our Grandfather Fire called the gods into council. All of the gods were suffering from various illnesses, and they assembled so that Grandfather Fire [Tatewarí], the first shaman, could cure them. In Council, Grandfather divined that the gods had not followed the traditions, had not made the pilgrimage to the Sacred Land of Peyote. Only by doing so would they 'find their life.' So, the gods prepared themselves for this difficult journey by fasting, abstaining from sex and salt, taking ritual ablutions, and making votive arrows and gourds. The gods prepared themselves for the pilgrimage as Huichols still prepare themselves today.

The gods then left the comfort of their village and went on the sacred journey. After many days of traveling and near death, the Ancient Ones arrived at the edge of a spring-fed lake. From a nearby rancho, Huichol women emerged bearing gourds of sacred water and tortillas. These were Our Mothers, owners of the rain and all terrestrial waters.

After drinking the sacred water and washing their heads, after being nourished by the holy corn, the gods, being of one heart, traveled into Wirikúta. The Great Shaman, Tatewarí, saw Elder Brother Deer on the first altar far in the distance, and though Our Elder Brother transformed himself and tried to escape to the second altar, he was not able to do so. Setting up snares, The Old Ones ran him down, and they saw that where he left his footprints peyote grew.

As Our Elder Brother Deer laying dying, they caught the radiant energy streaming from his head and were strengthened by it. In fact, Elder Brother Deer did not die, but was peyote. They ground up his antlers and drank of this, and this was also peyote. His hooves were peyote, his flesh and bones, all were peyote.

After singing and dancing and seeing many beautiful things in the desert, they climbed the sacred mountain and made an offering to the place where Our Father Sun was born. Wearing the skin of the holy deer, they returned to their village by way of many holy places. They brought with them the sacred water from the springs of Our Mothers and the wonderful gift of peyote. In that way they returned to where they started, but now they were fully healed, as Tatewarí had told them. (Halifax 1993, 37)

Conclusion About Peyote

In combining my personal experiences with the historical ones presented above, I conclude that peyote is a primarily a heart chakra experience of intense beauty and radiance in which one is in the presence of a benevolent Creator. It recharges the spiritual side of the human and heals the sufferings accumulated by the daily travails of living in the world. As with all of the medicines discussed thus far, partaking of peyote reorients our connection to the earth; it reminds us that humans are part of nature. It reinforces the notion that the plant and fungi realms know more about us than we do about ourselves and can serve as powerful assets to transpersonal consciousness. They are available to help us thrive on this planet if we allow them to do so. The key is respecting nature and understanding our role as servant-stewards of our planet, as we are all interconnected in this extraordinary ecosystem we call Mother Earth. We are reminded of the connection of the earth to the universe, as well as what a great privilege it is to be incarnated, able to manifest creation in this beautiful island in space and time.

Peyote may not create as rambunctious visual displays as the other entheogens but is a very physical and beautiful emotional encounter with the Creator. The peyote experience creates magnificent and colorful visions. It has inspired the Huichols to make yarn paintings and very detailed beadwork of these visions, which often incorporate the peyote cactus, the deer, and the maize. The book *Huichol Indian Sacred Rituals* by Mariano Valadez is a valuable resource for those interested; it is filled with pictures of their complex yarn paintings, which can provide a sense of how peyote inspires creativity through its psychedelic, mind-manifesting effects. It also describes the rituals and mythology of the tribe. (Valadez and Valadez, 1992)

As mentioned, the hallucinogenic chemical isolated in peyote is mescaline, which is also the active component of San Pedro cactus, although in lower concentrations. In his famous book, *The Doors of Perception*

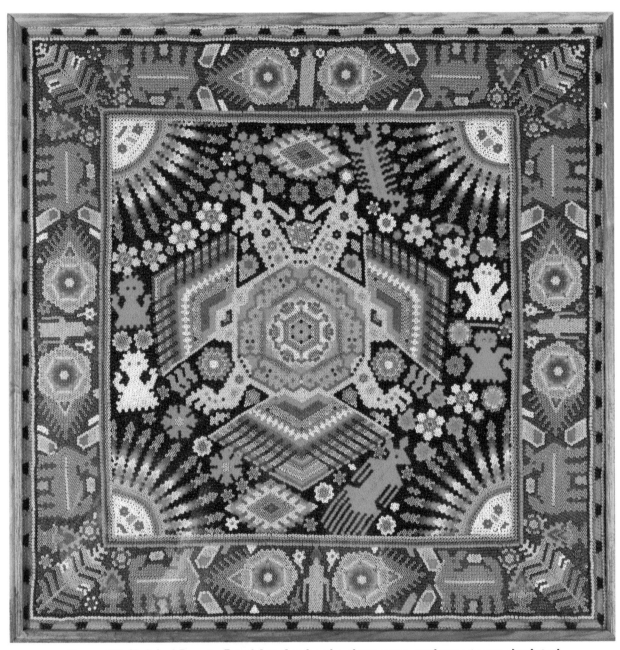

FIGURE 50. Huichol Peyote Bead Art. Again, the deer, corn, and peyote are depicted.
(collection of the author)

151

(written in 1954), Aldous Huxley discusses mescaline as the extraordinary compound that generates the above-described heart-centered journey to the godhead.

Since my forays participating in peyote ceremonies, there has been a backlash from the Native American Church and community about the misappropriation of this substance and their cultural sacrament and rituals by white people and other Westerners. The harvesting of peyote in Mexico and southern Texas has led to a shortage of this cactus with the potential for its extinction. Real estate development and farming have also contributed to the destruction of its habitat. The Native communities have requested outside cultures to avoid harvesting and exploiting peyote for personal use and to exclude it from being decriminalized even if other substances such as psilocybin and MDMA become legally available. Alternatively, Native Americans suggest using synthetic mescaline or San Pedro cactus as an alternative. San Pedro cactus grows readily in many climates and is not endangered. They are not against the chemical but are trying to protect the peyote plant and its habitats. It is why Ralph Metzner never brought this cactus to any of his circles. It was out of respect for the Native American concerns.

I am now aware of the peyote's plight and would like to apologize for using it in the past, even though a Native American peyote medicine man led the ceremony. Although enticing, I do not recommend using the peyote cactus but suggest seeking alternatives. Respect is one way of demonstrating reciprocity.

Chapter 17

Earth Vision Circle at Joshua Tree: Iboga Experience

We gather again at the Joshua Tree retreat house in the early evening under a full moon, with an arctic blast of cold reminding us of the seasons and the elemental forces of nature. This will be my sixth circle. So much has opened up for me over the past year and a half. I have met some wonderful people and have begun to speak at several workshops and seminars on the topics of Jung and Shamanism. I desire to learn about different forms of love and how to differentiate the personal and transpersonal, romantic and relational: *eros*, *agape*, and *philia*. According to my friend and fellow Jungian Analyst, Robert Johnson, there are ninety-three different words in Sanskrit texts describing all the many forms of love. The English language lacks this detailed vocabulary to describe all types of love, which leads to many misunderstandings of this experience.

Gathering Ritual

We open with a shamanic drumming exercise. Ralph asks us to choose to go either to the underworld, middle world, or upper world. For an underworld imaginal journey, we are to find an opening in the earth and descend; for the middle world, to enter through a gate, as between two trees; and for the upper world, to climb a tree and perhaps catch a flight on the back of a bird.

I choose a middle world meditation. I am met first by a leopard in the dark whom I follow deep into an African jungle. I arrive at a village where there are dark, leopard-skinned natives with faces that look like wild boars and with stiff, spiked hair brushed back. One native throws a spear, which

I follow in flight, and it lands in front of some Spanish conquistadors with metal helmets, shields, and spears. The natives and Spaniards then engage in conflict with the Africans on the left and the metal people on my right.

The scene changes, and there is no more conflict. There are now only wandering spotted giraffes with long necks eating from the treetops. I ride on the back of one and we gallop through the savannah. Now there is a cauldron containing a bluish iridescent brew from which I drink. On the other side appears a beautiful woman with blond-grayish hair, seated cross-legged, greeting me with a serene smile. I place a drum between us. The rhythm of the drums synchronizes to our heartbeats, and we are thus joined as one. As Ralph ends the drumming, I again rejoin the circle. This entire vision has taken place without the use of any medicine.

Earth Walk: Saturday

It is very cold in the desert, yesterday an Arctic storm blew through, dumping rain. The Sun-Fire energy I remember from spring is absent, but there are still trickling brooks running over rocks making a soothing noise. The desert is unusually moist, and I have to walk to stay warm. I occasionally rest in small nooks I find in the boulders. There are two ravens squawking and flying above, messengers of the upper world region. There is very little life on the desert floor other than a few rabbits peering out. I contemplate what medicine I will choose to take that evening. Initially, I was planning to take some psilocybin mushrooms or San Pedro cactus for its heart-centered effects. But I learn that Ralph has also brought some iboga, from Africa, which is difficult to procure, so I volunteer with one other adventurer to try it that evening. This medicine would correspond to the meditation on Africa I had the evening before. I am told that iboga (*Tabernanthe iboga*), with the active chemical ibogaine, facilitates ancestral communion, which sounds interesting, although my initial intention was to explore the many realms of love.

Evening Medicine Circle

We gather again in the familiar Joshua Tree home as the Velada (a term used by Mazatec curanderos for late-night or all-night healing rituals) begins at around five in the evening. There will be some taking ayahuasca, some choose to take Teonanacatl (psilocybin mushrooms), and a few will take the San Pedro cactus with an initial booster of a small dose of LSD for activation. It is confirmed that just one other experienced traveler and I decide to experiment with iboga.

We begin with an appetizer of desiccated Toad Slime (5-MEO-DMT) to open up the gateways of our brains. This time Ralph mixes the desiccated Toad with other herbs, including some crushed *Amanita* mushrooms, *Damiana*, *Datura*, and cannabis. I inhale two puffs, and within a few seconds, my ego-body dissolves and I am transported into a geode with crystalline edges, which breaks apart to open up a hole leading out into space. I float into a dark, gentle universe. This time there is no anxiety; I am propelled to a place of energetic calm. As I quickly return, I breathe to circulate the energy to parts of my body, particularly my head region. As we all return, we each begin to take our medicines for the prolonged nighttime adventure of mind-expanding consciousness.

My dose is one tablespoon of the iboga tincture mixed in ethanol, which has an astringent taste but not unpleasant like that of ayahuasca. Ralph recommends also taking a small dose of LSD (65 micrograms) to synergize and to activate the ibogaine derivative, in order to bring on its visions more fully. Otherwise, he tells us the experience would consist more of memory thought-forms, rather than visual ones.

The induction is with some music "Dolphin Dreams," which takes me underwater. After an hour or so, only a few visuals of animals appear, so when the booster time arrives, I ask my body wisdom whether I can handle more medicine and receive an affirmative answer. I lie back with my eyeshade on, and soon the visuals begin with full-scale intensity of iridescent, luminescent, and neon-like psychedelia. They are unlike the kaleidoscopic and fractal patterns of mushrooms or LSD, but more static patterns which slowly change and are highly detailed like great works of baroque art. The visions are driven by the music, first of ayahuasca icaros (songs), field recordings from the jungles of the Amazon, and later by the music of Ladysmith Black Mambazo, an African vocal group with amazing harmonies.

The mellow introduction soon begins to intensify to a very stimulated and high, electrical-like state. My lower chakras are activated, experienced as an urge to urinate as the serpent awakens at my base. I try to breathe through this to raise this Kundalini energy upward through the chakras until I start feeling ecstatic and stimulated with a very warm feeling in my head. At times the ecstasy is so intense that I feel I may explode, disintegrate, and be unable to contain it. Disintegration is a form of death, so I experience some anxiety as to whether or not I will return intact. I realize in an instant that there is more difficulty in experiencing such ecstasy in the psyche than dealing with the darkness and depressed thoughts more common to humans.

The Kundalini experience is the tremendous energy that can be likened to the serpent power of instinct rising up the spinal column as it is awakened through forms of ecstatic Tantric meditation or yoga. For the unprepared and uninitiated psyche, it can become dangerous, leading to panic anxiety or a disintegrative psychosis. It is why practitioners of this type of Kundalini yoga must develop, over years, the ability to withstand, appreciate, and integrate this spiritual ecstasy. When an entheogen does this quickly, it can be discombobulating, disorienting, and frightening. Stanislav and Christina Grof describe this type of encounter as a *spiritual emergency*.

Ralph calls us all for the first round of songs, and I utter sounds I feel coming from deep down in my soul. Although I do not remember my vocalizations, later in the night after the circle ends, I am told that my songs were beautiful. I think of my body as a musical instrument changing my sounds through what I am feeling; I experiment by going up and down my chakras and vocalizing from each of them. I let the energy flow from my throat through my nasal sinus passages and the hollow regions of my skull, and then down through the center of my heart, lungs, abdomen, and pelvis. I make air sounds, water sounds, clicking noises, animal growls, lullabies, intense to calm melodies, masculine and feminine vocalizations, all without words. It all seems so sensual yet natural as I further explore the feelings of sadness, ecstasy, and areas of blockage. It is an experience of letting go of all performance anxiety, which is part of my intention, as I plan to give workshops in the future.

After this round, Ralph tells us a metaphorical story about the seed, which contains the memory of the entire life cycle of a tree as it grows and branches. Birds come and alight on the branches, like positive or negative thoughts, and eventually fly off, but the tree remains. Negative thought forms do not have to make a permanent nest in the psyche. Ralph then continues to speak that at the base of the tree is a serpent-like life force which winds up the trunk and spirals into the branches, like Shakti awakening at the base of the spine and climbing up the chakras. I realize that this is a Kundalini experience of ecstasy, which can be dangerous to an unprepared mind. I am thankful that by my preparation, I am prepared. The sap brings nutrients from the earth and, with the sun, nourishes every cell of the tree. It is like the soul of the tree, similar to the blood and oxygen, which nourish life in animals. The tree is a metaphor for our life's growth. The wind, rain, and sun shape the branches, much as our experiences shape us during our growth from childhood to maturity and on to death. (see figure 14, pg. 41)

The Eternal Feminine: Queen of the Rainforest

As I return to my journey, the music intensifies with the music of Reinhardt Flatischler's *Schinore* carrying a rhythmic beat. It feels like every neuron in my body is cranked up to 100 percent stimulation as my ecstasy continues. My brain is lit up and on fire. It is then that the main image of the Goddess appears to me in all her bounty. She is the mother of all things, giving and nurturing, a supportive, positive ground. She is also the great lover, sensual, giving pleasure, and also desiring to be loved by us humans. She carries a seed in her mouth, bends down to kiss me, and transfers this seed into my mouth. She tells me to take this seed and all of her bounty, to carry it, plant it, and then care for it as it grows. She says she will feel loved by me if I become a potent servant of her. All things will regenerate if I do this and continue to set this as a primary goal of my life. She says, "Use your gifts and dreams for good." It requires potent masculinity to join with potent femininity to allow nature to continue to thrive. We become her guardians. She is a goddess of the Amazonian rainforest but does not want to enslave us to her. She is the feminine soul and spirit who motivates a man (and all humans) by giving her love to us rather than demanding service. Stewardship needs to be voluntary, a way of giving back what we take.

The face of the lover appears, and I realize that this is not personal, but an image of the lover through all time for me: past, present, and future, over many lifetimes and dimensions. I have envisioned that same face in

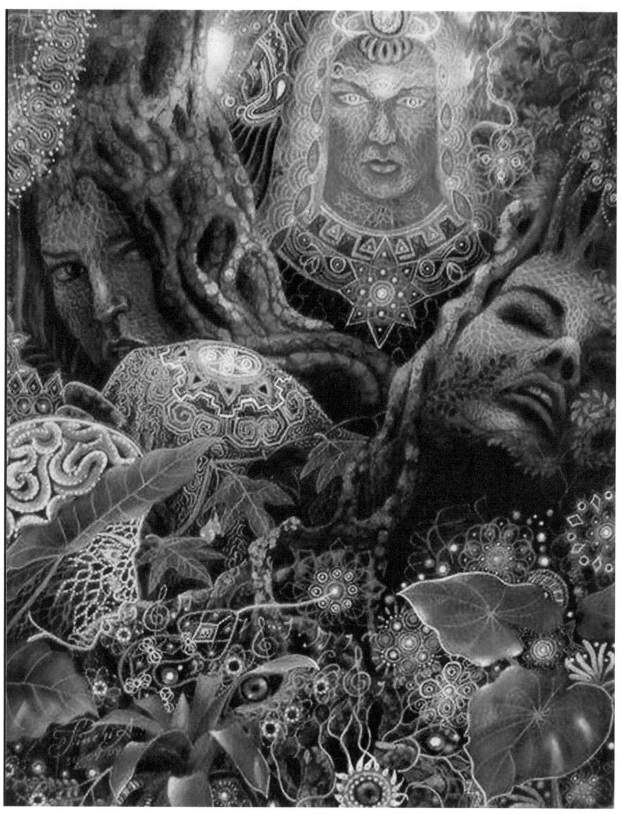

FIGURE 51. *Sueno* by Felix Pinchi Aguirre.

goddesses in Africa and other cultures over time. There is no sin or shame with her as a lover as long as she is respected and cherished in the heart and mind. As a goddess, she is not a destroyer (negative mother), but she will depart from a person who does not understand her gift of bounty. No person can be separated from her who understands life, love, earth, and creativity.

I feel the need to sing to her. I realize that it is easy to project the lover archetype in its erotic aspect onto another person. The key is to remember where you live, who is at home waiting and has taken care of you, and then to take that eros energy back where it may find expression in the body of the partner at home.

The energy then shifts to my ancestors in Russia. I experience Mother Russia with all her earthiness, peasant demeanor, saltiness, and survival ability. I find myself in a marketplace with a number of old, heavyset women who seem physically strong. They are buying and trading fruits and food. The food is abundant in the market, and the women are arguing and laughing with each other. I realize this is a women's culture, but I am a part of it, witnessing the grief, the laughter, and the passion of the collective Russian woman's soul.

The next image is of a group of pigs (sows and boars). They are all snorting in a pile of food, driven compulsively in an erotic frenzy, trying to penetrate the wet food and eat. Erotic images of large buttocks, hips, and openings are all mixed in with this fertile muck, the undifferentiated prima materia, with the sows groveling in the garbage. (*Prima materia* is an alchemical term referring to the formless base of all matter.) The pig is my guide animal at present, mediating between the interface of the earth and the animal consciousness of survival, the need to eat. The sow seems to be the primal mother, the unabated Russian passion. I can relate to this pig-passion, at times seeking immediate gratification without reflection on the needs of my partner. The pig nature pushes, shoves, and grunts—the peasant of the culture, impatient, needy, but also representing merriment, spontaneity, food, and love. It is also the wild boar in its masculine manifestation.

I relate this part of my ancestral nature to my relationship with my wife, whose ancestors are Irish and English, representing the refinement and reserve of the Protestant/East Coast culture. I realize the difference in each of our souls and in the way we were raised. It is the meeting of the Russian boar with the faerie energy of Britain, the pig passion of Russia with the refined eloquence of the country-dwelling Irish ancestors. With this awareness, I am able to see the benefit of refining my "pig" nature in order to delay gratification and be more sensitive to my wife's needs. My coarse nature could be refined into a Russian-style charm with my faerie queen. I could meet with her sensibilities and thus develop a more mature relationship through deeper mutual acceptance—in the place where the pig and the faerie meet. My wife represents balance for me, and I need to further appreciate her quiet, introverted, yet solid demeanor. I realize the lusciousness and eros of my wife, a true beauty, appealing in every way. Without awareness, my piggishness could lead to infidelity, and I realize I must cultivate absolute integrity in the way I express my erotic nature.

The Ancestors

I next see Russian men singing in spiritual communion with each other, like Volga boatmen drinking vodka and bemoaning their harsh lives. The face of my grandmother, Babala, appears as the embodiment of the strength that allows survival in Russia, as well as the passion expressed for all things high and low. It is not the type of rarefied, crystalline, pure spirituality that is imbued with angels but a mixture of body, work, and joy transcending all the suffering of the Russian community.

This is my maternal ancestry at its core. I am sitting around a campfire in the countryside, seemingly in the 1700s, with all my Russian grandmother ancestors praising my birth and singing lullabies to little "Sashinka" (baby Sasha—me), while looking over me with pride. I am feeling such acceptance and ecstatic love from them. They display their caring for my life, then reveal that my path and the ultimate meaning for my life is to transplant the life force of my Russian heritage to the New World in America. There I can transform the suffering and suppression of their lives into freedom and fruitfulness. This is my main *raison d'être*, and everything else will be frosting on the cake of my life. This scene then leads me to other memories.

I then think of my father in his heroic attributes. He was born and raised in Odessa, now Ukraine, when the communists arrived. Luckily, his family survived. He left Russia and his parents at the age of nineteen, never to see them again. He wandered through Germany to get his college education in engineering, only to encounter the growing power of the anti-Semitic Nazi regime. He was fortunately evacuated by his uncle Anatole (from whom I get my middle name) in time to avoid disaster. Anatole enabled him to travel to Malaya, a British colony, where he worked as an engineer and met and married my mother. Then, Malaya was invaded by the Japanese during WWII. He and my mother emigrated as refugees, first to Ceylon and then to India, which was also a British colony at the time. In Bombay, my sister and I were born, and my father worked there for eight years.

When Gandhi came into power during the Indian independence movement in 1947, the country was undergoing significant unrest. In 1949, our family emigrated to the United States. We crossed the Pacific Ocean by freighter, the Mano Oran. My father brought us to this country to plant the seeds of his Russian heritage in American soil, where we then thrived amidst freedom and bounty. I realized more fully that his capacity to deal with life circumstances, with many starts and stops, took a great amount of confidence and energy.

My mother was also a strong and practical person, born in a Russian-Jewish enclave in Harbin, China (Manchuria). She migrated with her family to Malaya, where she met and married my father and then moved with him to India. Unfortunately it seemed she never experienced the adoration of love within her marriage, but she passed on to me her genetics, strength of character, and artistic inclinations. In a vision of my mother and father in their youthfulness, I was able to see them dancing together, full of passion and love. It was good to see them happy.

I realized that my purpose in life was to take this heritage, transplant this seed, grow it in this country, and then pass it on to my progeny. This basis represented a strong building block in my life toward my pursuits of becoming a doctor, a healer, a teacher, and a father. More importantly, this journey allowed me to perceive my father from a different perspective. His path took a lot of courage: leaving his parents at an early age, escaping the Nazis and then the Japanese invasion of Malaya, leaving India due to its independence movement, moving to the United States and finding employment, starting his own successful engineering company, and raising us children.

My previous image of my father had been that of an abusive person, who had both emotionally and physically injured me deeply. The medicine enabled me to heal from this one-sided perception of him and to develop gratitude for all he was able to accomplish, as well as awe for his heroic adventure, considering all his trials and tribulations. Also, I felt a renewed love for my mother, who I realized had protected me as best she could from my father's abuses. I could now mourn my loss of them with a sense of peace and closure. I grieved and cried profusely as I mourned them both again.

Ancestry, however, goes beyond my Russian heritage, as seen during my iboga journey. I recall that in other journeys I had met black African ancestors and the Black Queen, Isis, further back in time. Also, during prior ayahuasca journeys, I encountered indigenous Indians of South America in the Amazon rainforests. While on psilocybin mushrooms and San Pedro cactus, I also met up with Australian Aborigines as ancestors. Additionally I have met some Biblical Jewish ancestors, including Abraham, Isaac, and Jacob, with whom a reciprocal relationship was formed. They have all "been through it before me," and I have been grateful for all of their valuable insights into the vagaries of my dilemmas.

I came to appreciate the way in which a person's connection with ancestors may come about through forming a mutually respectful relationship with ongoing memory and sharing. If I could love my ancestors, I realized I also could love and care about my descendants, even those yet unborn. The past, present, and future are all possible in the transpersonal realm in which time and space dissolve. This is a concept promoted by quantum physics theory, where time and space are artifacts created by human consciousness. It is also a tenet of the philosophy of biocentrism, in which human biology creates the reality that is observed. (Lanza 2009, 1-2)

Eternity is the absence of time, and infinity is the absence of space. Ancestors are from the past, descendants are in the future, and our present life is the melting pot that can experience both. These teachings emerged more like thought-forms when the visual part started to diminish. These thoughts came very quickly and intuitively, rather than through a logical progression.

Those of us in the circle end the evening session with some very exquisite music sung by the Irish Noirin Ni Riain, which furthers my ecstatic trance of the feminine. During our closing round, I learned that my fellow iboga traveler had quite a different experience. Instead of ecstasy, he felt depressed in seeing images of his cold Scottish ancestors who were withholding and distant. He felt isolated, then had images of Africa which displayed only suffering and famine, as in Somalia. He witnessed the degradation of humanity in a world that had gone barren, lacking any bounty from the Goddess or Mother Earth.

These two experiences exemplify how different the forms of the visions can take from person to person, even with the same medicine. The truth of the medicine seems to lie in the reality that we receive the vision we need to see. His vision is certainly an aspect of truth, albeit from the shadow side of life. I remember that I had experienced that type of vision in the past.

As we end the circle and break our fast, I am still feeling very stimulated, while the people who have taken other medicines seem to have come down and are calmer. I do eat some soup and crackers and then a small orange. I peel the skin and suck on sections of the fruit. As the juice flows, I kiss the fruit lubricating my mouth and throat with this sweet, citrus nectar. It feels like the Goddess is feeding me and then a seed enters my mouth. I realize this is the same as in my vision, in that I am to take this seed and plant it so that regeneration will occur. I realize that I, Alex, Sasha, am a potent servant of the Goddess of Nature. The deforestation of Earth will continue unless I replant her life-giving seed. Otherwise, the unhindered masculine energy will continue to plunder Earth and to dominate her destiny, with the result that the human race will not survive. This outcome would not be dissimilar from my fellow iboga partner's experience during the circle.

Aftermath and Summary

The most significant aspect I took from this journey was the importance of maintaining a memory of the messages from the Goddess of the Rainforest and the experiences of my own ancestors. The primary piece of wisdom was that the aspect of love, in all its fertility and eros, is transpersonal but incarnated in each of us. We need to choose to peel back the veil of daily realities and step outside them to experience this understanding. The second teaching was to form reciprocity with the Goddess and the ancestors to clarify the purpose of each of our lives. One must replant the seeds of one's heritage in daily life and become a potent servant of stewardship of our planet, families, and love life. The third was to realize that the face of the lover (the lover archetype), which exists through all times and all cultures, needs to be discerned. Otherwise, it will be projected onto real individuals, which will lead to discord in a marriage or relationship. The face of the lover throughout all times is recognized but is not to be confused with erotic love. One must bring eros back home and live it more fully with an ongoing partner, thus replanting and cultivating it.

While time and age separate us from multiple lovers in our practical daily relationships, time does not separate us from the transcendent archetypal lover. The face of the lover can be seen in many people throughout a lifetime, in those who are older as well as younger than oneself. It can be easy to confuse the face of the lover with an individual of a different generation and it is important to remember that the other person may not perceive you in the same way. An example would be that of an older man who misperceives his attraction to a younger woman and acts upon the urge. Very likely he will be rebuffed, viewed as having come across as creepy, and there is nothing more pathetic than a dirty old man, desperate to find love with someone not kin to his soul. In modern times, this errant sexuality is one factor that has led to the #MeToo Movement, secondary to the real or perceived abuses of a man's power needs in the disguise of sexuality.

The final takeaway from the journey is that ecstasy can be more difficult to contain than depression, which is counter-intuitive. I had always thought the opposite; that joy and pleasure are more desirable, possibly because these positive energies are often more fleeting, while negativity can become stuck in the psyche. It is reminiscent of a quote by one of my mentors, Michael Meade, from my time working in the Mythopoetic Men's Movement. He called this the Samba Prayer:

> *"It is better to be happy than sad*
> *Happiness is the best thing there is*
> *A Samba is a form of prayer*
> *But to make it more beautiful*
> *One has to remember the sorrows of the world*
> *It is like this to the light of the heart"*

From Michael Meade I also learned the drum rhythm for the dance the Samba, which has been called the "Morse code for happiness."

I found that indeed, it is a difficult task to carry out the insights gleaned by such a journey as the travails of life, routine, and daily demands intervene. Over time, it is easy to forget these enlightened visions and their associated insights, which, as I have emphasized, need to be integrated for any lasting behavioral transformations. As I have suggested, some possible aids for maintaining insights include meditation, journaling, and sharing with other like-minded people who understand the terrain of journey work.

It is difficult, if not impossible, to put into words the visionary experience of a mind-manifesting medicine. It is such a visceral experience that those who have not been on such a journey may have difficulty understanding the depths of wisdom gleaned. Over-proselytizing about the experience generally tends to alienate people, who may interpret it as a drug-induced false fantasy. It is easy to become inflated after visionary journeys and come across as "holier than thou" or superior to other people and their belief systems.

From my experiences, I offer the suggestion that a person contain these insights and only discuss them after others first show interest. The wisest stance for one returning from a journey is to remain humble, expressing the value of the insights through actual positive behaviors. An additional insight is that wisdom seekers and carriers may continue to have psychological problems that have not as yet been integrated. We can have degrees of wisdom and still be rather "screwed up" at times.

When someone tells me that they have seen the Godhead, I have on occasion thought to myself: How has that changed you for the better? How do you treat your friends and family differently? How has your transpersonal encounter become translated into something practical? It reminds me of the old saying, "What's the use of going to the mountaintop and getting your hair parted by a light beam if you are not kind to your family below?" It suggests that when you look for wisdom, also look for humility.

Chapter 18
About Iboga

Chemically, iboga, also called eboka, is a psychoactive indole alkaloid whose main ingredient is ibogaine, which has a strong stimulating effect on the nervous system. It comes from a shrub, the *Tabernanthe iboga* (from the family *Apocynaceae*), which can attain a height of four to six feet. The active part is the yellowish root or bark of the plant that is rasped and eaten directly, in powdered form, or drunk as an infusion.

Over the last few years, ibogaine has been researched for the treatment of various forms of end-stage drug addiction. The experience was described by one ex-cocaine addict after ibogaine therapy in a research article (Da Silva 1995, 24-26): "It's arduous. Ibogaine is not a drug you take to get high." This research has been taking place in the Netherlands, in Mexico, as well as places like the University of Florida and, more recently, Johns Hopkins, NYU, UCLA, and UCSF. Ibogaine is now showing promise in dealing with addictions of all sorts, including heroin, cocaine, alcohol, and tobacco. It is not yet fully understood whether the positive results are due to a direct chemical effect on the brain or from the profound psychological effects.

The mechanism behind the medicine is thought that it tends to reset the neuroreceptors in the brain and associated entrenched neural addiction pathways, thus untangling the root causes of addiction. Published studies demonstrate that 75 percent of end-stage addicts give up their drug use after one or two sessions. (Da Silva 1995, 26) Another positive result is that it seems to help modulate, or in some cases actually to eliminate, withdrawal symptoms suffered by heroin addicts.

However, Mexico has presently stopped ibogaine research because it caused the drug lords to have concern that a cure for addiction would result in a loss of its trade and affect the drug-based economy. The FDA and DEA also may be complicit in suppressing trials of ibogaine due to its potential dampening effect on other pharmaceuticals being researched by Big Pharma.

The Bwiti Cult

Iboga is utilized by the Fang Cult of Bwiti and other secret societies in Gabon and the Congo in West Africa. It is used to initiate members into the Bwiti culture by breaking open the head to have contact with the ancestors through collapse and hallucinations. Sorcerers use iboga to seek information from the spirit world and their cultural ancestors. During intoxication, the shadow (soul) is believed to leave the body to wander with the ancestors in the land of the dead. As a powerful stimulant, iboga enables the partaker to maintain extraordinary physical exertion without fatigue over a long period. Warriors and hunters have used it to stay awake during night watches.

The Bwiti culture has been growing in number and social strength over the past half-century, and it appears that iboga helps these indigenous-based societies resist the loss of identity due to the encroachment of Western civilization and the conversion efforts of Christianity and Islam. The iboga cults exist as an alternative belief to Christian dogma, whereby its members are able to maintain a connection with their ancestors and thus to preserve a direct relationship with their indigenous cultural origins. One member expresses the common view, "Catholicism and Protestantism is not our religion. I am not happy with mission churches." (Schultes, Hofmann, 1992, 115)

A Myth of Eboka

It is also said that eboka was brought to more developed West African tribes by the more primitive Pygmies of the jungles of the Congo. There would be an exchange of the plant for various tools and utensils. A myth regarding eboka is recounted as follows, "Zame ye Mebege (the last of the creator gods) gave us Eboka [iboga]. One day. . . he saw. . . the Pygmy Bitamu, high in the Atanga tree, gathering its fruit. He made him fall. He died, and Zame brought his spirit to him. Zame cut off the little fingers and the little toes of the cadaver of the Pygmy and planted them in various parts of the forest. They grew into the Eboka bush." (Schultes and Hofmann, 1992, 112)

Another story, from Ndong Asseko of Gabon, states, "When I ate Eboka, I found myself taken by it up a long road in a deep forest until I came to a barrier of black iron. At that barrier, unable to pass, I saw a crowd

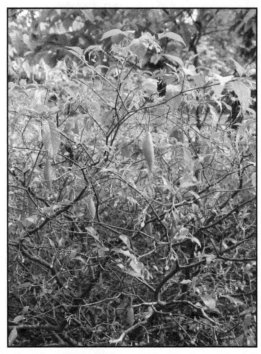

FIGURE 52. Marco Schmidt – Iboga plant – Limbe Botanical Garden, Cameroon.

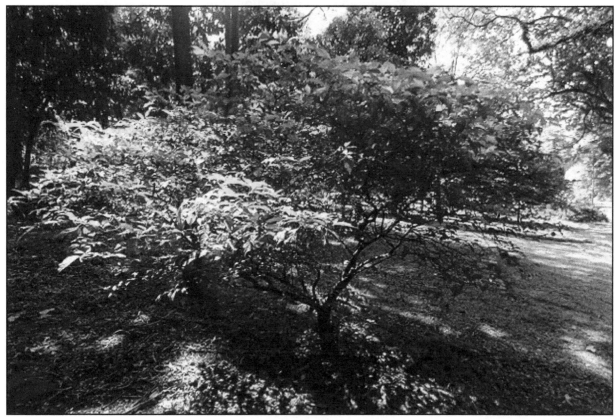

FIGURE 53. *Tabernanthe iboga* shrub, from which ibogaine is extracted.

(photo – Wikimedia commons)

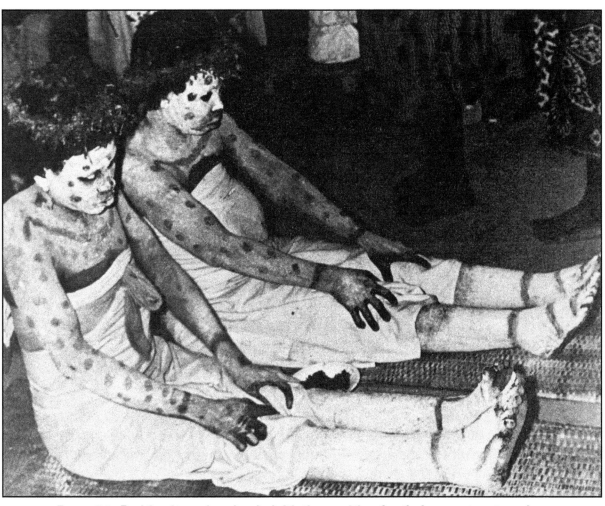

FIGURE 54. Bwiti cult novices begin initiation waiting for their ancestors to arrive.
(Schultes, Hofmann, 1992, pg. 115)

of black persons also unable to pass. In the distance beyond the barrier it was very bright. I could see many colors in the air . . . Suddenly my father descended from above in the form of a bird. He gave me then my Eboka name, Onwan Misengue, and enabled me to fly up after him over the barrier of iron." (Schultes and Hofmann 1992, 114)

Afterthoughts on Iboga

Although this medicine can produce great insights, I found that, after trying it three times over a ten-year period, it is not my favorite plant for journeying. For me, it is too powerful a stimulant and too long-lasting compared with the other medicine choices. The effects can last several days, rather than several hours, and put a strain on the body and brain. Deaths have been reported, albeit rarely. When they have occurred, it is unclear whether the cause was a concomitant medical condition or an interaction with another drug. As a potent stimulant, it may induce an arrhythmia or a seizure in a vulnerable person.

In my personal experience, it felt like my brain was overwhelmed with energy, as though I was in a manic state. Despite these drawbacks, I do conclude that I learned a great deal from my journeys with iboga. The experiences assisted me in untangling my ancestral roots and provided me with a sense of purpose, which is ultimately artistic and creative. In addition, it helped me overcome my performance-anxiety issues which were based on my compromised self-esteem. My renewed interest in so called roots music, including Mississippi Delta blues, and Old Time Appalachian mountain music, is possibly an outcome of these far-reaching psychedelic events. This type of music provides the rhythm and voice for the American soul. It is all in the roots, like the life-giving roots of a tree, or the instinctual roots (chakras) of the body and soul.

In considering these medicines, one might ask what the difference is between iboga and cocaine or methamphetamine, since they are all potent stimulants of the central nervous system. One distinction is that since iboga is mind-manifesting or expanding (making it a psychedelic) with the potential to heal wounds and to provide deep insights, as well as to counteract and help those with addictions, it is better classified as a medicine. Amphetamines and cocaine are not mind-enhancing and only convey physical prowess, energy, alertness, and focus. Amphetamines can be useful in treating ADHD and thereby be useful as a medication for some who suffer from this disorder.

Other differences are that these amphetamine drugs do not provide teachings of any transpersonal lessons to the soul. Their use can cause abuse and addiction through aiding a person either seeking a pleasure-high, or in avoiding the conflicts and pain of reality. All drugs of abuse, including opiates and alcohol, are able to temporarily relieve psychic tension and to distract from the difficulties of life. The high is not an ecstatic release infused with insights, but a temporary feeling of well-being or euphoria by alleviating pain, both physical and psychological.

In contrast, iboga and other hallucinogens do not promote addiction or euphoria through avoidance. Their positive effect is allowing the partaker to confront the roots of the pain and to unravel the knots which bind the person in an unhealthy prison. The psychedelics may in fact be anti-addiction remedies. The medicine may be viewed as a teacher, transformer, and healer. It is considered a "truth serum."

From my perspective, this concept is the real difference between a medicine and a drug. Medicines heal, whereas drugs carry the connotation of abuse. A drug has a greater tendency to congeal neurotic or unhealthy patterns, but a medicine is expansive; it can break down dysfunctional neural pathways and lead to spiritual experiences and healing. A hallucinogen can promote *karma* whereas a drug of abuse solidifies *dogma* and old negative patterns. *Karma* is a spiritual concept, but *dogma* is a rigid religious or psychological belief system. One frees the mind, while the other controls and imprisons the psyche.

Lastly, it is important to distinguish the highly stimulated state of the central nervous system of the psychedelic experience of iboga from the mania one sees in bipolar disorder. In bipolar mania, one jumps from subject to subject (known as "flight of ideas") without any central connection of thoughts, and is thus a very rambling, distractible state of consciousness. It is possible to have transcendental experiences while manic, but these usually appear as delusional (false belief) states typified by hyper-religiosity. They do not persist once the person is well. The insights gained on iboga and other hallucinogens are more organized, rooted in the deep psyche, and are remembered and hopefully integrated as a lasting, life-changing spiritual or mystical experience.

Ibogaine remains illegal in the United States, classified as a Schedule I drug in 1970 by the government, along with other psychedelics. This declaration states that there is no legitimate medical use and a high potential for abuse with these drugs. However, a recent article in *Time Magazine* (April 12-19, 2021), describes a new interest in researching ibogaine for opioid addiction and withdrawal, as well as for end-stage alcohol addiction. Human clinical trials are underway in Spain and soon will be in São Paulo, Brazil. Interestingly, in France, ibogaine was sold and prescribed as an antidepressant and stimulant for more than thirty years before it was outlawed in the 1960s. Its anti-addictive benefits were not well known until 1962, when researcher Howard Lotsof successfully experimented with it in New York for heroin addiction, from which he himself suffered.

This led to the opening of underground ibogaine clinics in other countries, including Mexico, where addicts flock and pay high fees for treatment. These patients have failed numerous rehabs or medication attempts with methadone or buprenorphine to treat their opioid addiction. Instead of just treating symptom reduction using a substitute opiate, ibogaine seems to work at a deeper level where the patient reexperiences the roots of their addiction and psychological trauma. The success rates vary at these clinics, which differ greatly in the amount of supervision and competency of the providers.

At this time there have not been any completed controlled trials of ibogaine, so the results are still anecdotal and observational. For those who benefit, many do not return to drug use, and so they feel that the benefits to chronic end-stage opiate addiction outweigh the risks of possible death. The main issue regarding ibogaine is that some people have died or had heart attacks due its arrythmia-causing potential. MindMed, a pharmaceutical company in the U.S., is developing a synthetic analog of ibogaine called 18-MC for opioid addiction and withdrawal that has less cardiac side effects. (*Time* April 12-19, 2021, 82-87)

As with psilocybin and MDMA, ibogaine appears to be a promising drug to treat various psychiatric disorders such as addictions, PTSD, depression, and anxiety. Other than the symptom reduction that traditional psychotropic medications accomplish, these drugs are like psychoanalytic medicines. The medicines cause the patients to go deep into the roots of their life experiences and meet with helpful entities and ancestors that untie the knots that keep them stuck in their chronic pathology patterns. These entheogens appear to enhance the neuroplasticity and neurogenesis of the pathways in the brain and unjam the chronic dysfunctional neural networks that reinforce psychopathology. People feel and think differently about themselves after the experience, and often these changes persist.

The Medicine Wheel

A few remarks before we conclude this survey of the major psychedelics. One of the teachings in shamanism is that of the four directions as an orientation to place. The four directions in the horizontal plane always are North, East, South, and West. The teaching can be expanded to the vertical dimension of up, down, and middle. These four directions are associated with different animal spirits, elemental qualities, and colors depending on the culture and its geography.

With the four major medicines under discussion, a four-fold way can be visualized by making a cross of a horizontal and vertical axis. For the direction of the North, one can place the medicine iboga as it relates to ancestral exploration. For the East, the medicine Teonanacatl can be placed, as it relates to upper chakra visions. The West can be symbolized by ayahuasca, referring to its healing aspects. In the South resides the San Pedro medicine, which is heart-centered. Following is a medicine wheel diagram depicting these four directions:

WHEEL OF THE FOUR MEDICINES

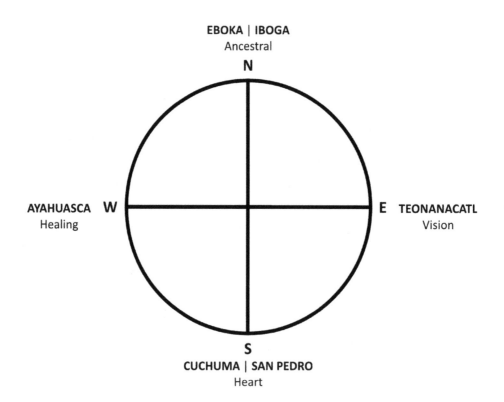

EBOKA | IBOGA
Ancestral

N

AYAHUASCA **W**
Healing

E **TEONANACATL**
Vision

S

CUCHUMA | SAN PEDRO
Heart

FIGURE 55. **Wheel of the Four Medicines**
(As shared by Ralph Metzner)

Chapter 19

A Week-Long Vision Circle at Ocamura, New Mexico

Some of my psychedelic vision quests followed the weekend format I have described in previous sections, others occurred during weeklong retreats. I participated in a weeklong vision workshop with Ralph Metzner called "The Web of Life." The workshop was located in Ocamura in the mountains between Las Vegas, New Mexico, and Taos. The retreat center was an isolated place amidst nature that had some cabins, tent camping, and a mess hall where organic food was prepared for our sustenance. I chose to tent camp on the open grounds for the week. I drove there from Carlsbad, California on my trusty BMW motorcycle with a tent and sleeping bag packed on the back of my bike. This made for a great road trip adventure on each side of the quest.

There were about fifteen participants in the workshop, all veteran psychonautical explorers who had worked with Ralph in the past. The workshop was to involve a series of shamanic teaching seminars during the day, followed by a medicine journey at night. Each evening, a different medicine or combination of entheogens was to be used to augment the daily teachings, for personal healing and envisioning. My primary concern was how anyone could handle nightly medicines for a week and maintain physical and mental health, sleep, and not be overwhelmed by the powerful insights of journey work. As it turned out, it went well for all of us, providing an opportunity to integrate the sessions with each other over a period of time. What we all learned was to use the insights of one session to help explore the dark recesses and yet unexplored areas in another session.

Since I have shared in detail some of my previous visionary experiences as examples, I will foreshorten the nightly sessions to give a hint of the journeys, and also present some of Ralph's shamanic teaching. The workshop represents a hybrid of the psychological, shamanic, and the religious-celebratory realms. Each session calls for an invocation of the spirits, allies, animals, plants, ancestors, teachers, gods and goddesses, as well as for place, time, and the four directions (see appendix 2). The basic assumption is that all of us live in a world of multiple realities, in that the world is both material and transpersonal, and inhabited by other spirit beings. The visionary experiences that I share in this section contain additional psychological material regarding my personal healing. I share this vulnerable information to demonstrate the power of healing rituals within the context of a vision circle as well as the previously described ways sacred medicines can reach deeply into the psyche in a brief period of time. One teaching from Monday night is described below. I share this to introduce you to Bert Hellinger, whom I had never heard of in my professional education.

After we all experienced the jaguar (the 5MeO-DMT rich slimy venom of the Colorado River Toad), the rest of the first evening was spent doing the Hindu chant, Om Shiva, followed by a presentation of Bert Hellinger's video *Coping With Survival*. I learned that Bert Hellinger is considered as one of the most influential and provocative psychotherapists in Germany doing family and group work. He initially worked as a priest and missionary with the South African Zulus; he then converted his spiritual orientation to a psychological approach. He studied various psychological disciplines, including psychoanalysis, primal therapy, Gestalt therapy, hypnotherapy, transactional analysis, and family systems therapy. He became known as a "caretaker of souls" (*Seelsorger* in German), working with a patient's deepest spiritual questions and difficulties. He is not well known among my contemporaries in the U.S.

His unique approach was assisting families in looking at their ancestral entanglements in order that they might achieve a more harmonious family life. (Hellinger 2002) His blending of the spiritual and psychological domains is reminiscent of Jung's transpersonal approach, as well as Ralph's. There are videos available of Hellinger's teaching methods, in which the participants of a family act as mediums to the ancestors and where there is release of deep grief that was previously unconscious in the members.

This presentation was highly moving for all of us; viewing it brought up many insights into our dead relatives. A deeper visit to Hellinger is warranted for all psychotherapists who work with families wishing to explore ancestral roots as part of their dynamics.

Orientation

When describing journey-work, I likened it to being a psychonaut sitting in the center of a globe-like space ship holding a joy stick. The globe surrounds the perimeters of the four horizontal directions and the two vertical directions. Once oriented to the six directions of space, right/left, forward/backward, and up/down, the pilot becomes oriented to space and time. From there the participant can venture in any desired direction or time to follow the path of their pre-determined intention.

Once settled into this orientation capsule, after setting an intention and after the medicine is imbibed, the participant may lie down with the other people in the circle, usually with the head facing a central altar and the feet at the outer perimeter. The leader of the group leads a meditative invocation. After the invocation, some music is usually played at a light volume so as not to be intrusive, acting as a vehicle of transfer or flow as the journey progresses. The musical themes are varied but usually involve instrumental trance music, indigenous music, or electronic music, some with vocalizations but not lyrics. Some music features rhythm through shamanic drumming, flutes, or pipes. Both slow and rapid tempos can be employed by the lead shaman depending on what phase of the journey the group is in. The music acts like synesthesia, driving the visionary experience to the various senses and to other places—underwater, outer space, the jungle, etc.

Week in Review

Here is a summary of the week at Ocamura:

Saturday night — Gathering with shamanic drumming and dance of the bees giving us direction.

Sunday — Empathogen journey with 2C-B and San Pedro to the East with the childhood themes with mother and father.

Monday — Jaguar session with evening singing of Hindu chants; presentation video of Bert Hellinger.

Tuesday — Journeying using LSD and San Pedro to the South to meet the feminine and the goddess.

Wednesday — Walk to the surrounding mountains using Salvia divinorum.

Thursday — Journey with Jurema to the North to meet the masculine and the gods.

Friday — Using mushrooms with Syrian rue to explore the West region of the elders and ancestors.

Saturday morning — Final integration session outdoors, then dispersal.

Typically, at the end of each night's session, we would send a thanksgiving prayer to the four directions. As the week proceeded, the experience coalesced into a four-directions mandala, with each medicine becoming identified with a different point on the circle.

MEDICINE WHEEL OF LIFE CYCLE

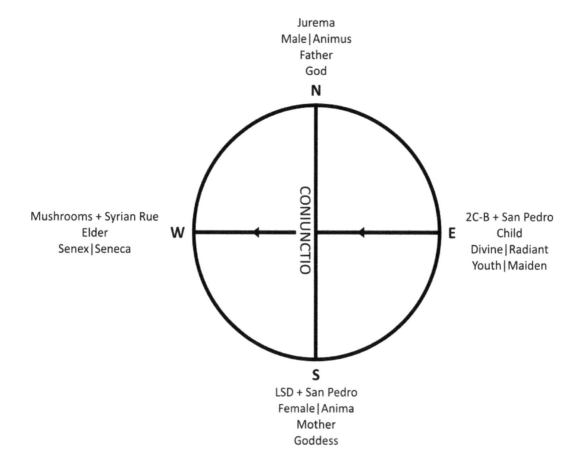

FIGURE 56. Medicine Wheel of Life Cycle.
(As shared by Ralph Metzner)

178

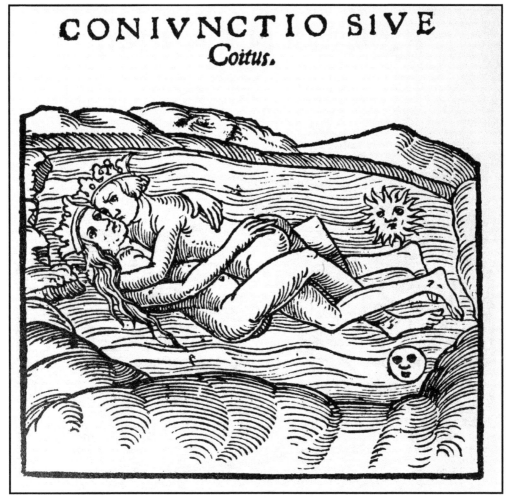

FIGURE 57. Coniunctio from the *Rosarium Philosophorum*.
(Jung CW 12 1968, pg. 330)

Note that in Figure 56, there is movement of the life pathway from the East (birth and the child) toward the West (the elder and death). On the vertical axis are the male and female components representing a union of opposites called *coniunctio*.

Coniunctio is a Latin word meaning conjunction of the opposites, the uniting of differences, often symbolically expressed as the union of the male and female having intercourse. It is also often used in alchemy to describe the end process of the work (opus) from which new creation springs forth. A premature union can lead to the creation of a monstrosity, whereas a union, after proper discrimination and differentiation into the

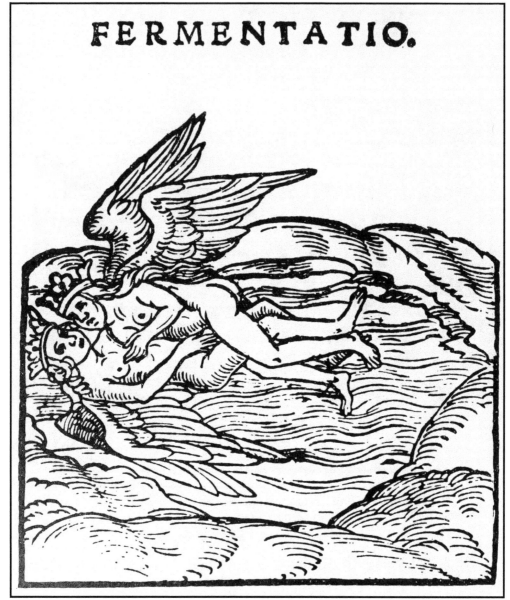

FERMENTATIO.

FIGURE **58.** **Fermentatio from the *Rosarium Philosophorum*.**
(Jung CW 12 1968, pg. 478)

opposites, generates a tension that eventually resolves with the creation of new insight or manifestation.

Two alchemical images of the coniunctio from the *Rosarium Philosophorum* text are shown on the preceeding page and above.

Week's End

At the end of this weeklong excursion to other worlds and within, I was tired physically yet psychologically energized, feeling clear and clean in my mind and body. After all the goodbyes, I fired up my BMW motorcycle and decided to take a dirt road through a mountain passage to go to Taos to meet up with my wife and her sister who lives there. I was met with an unexpected, intense rainstorm that made the dirt road rutted, muddy, and slippery — quite a challenge for my motorcycling skills. I was alone on the road and fatigued, but with focus I persisted without crashing. Once over the summit and some miles further on, I again rejoined a smooth and paved road to take me the rest of the way to Taos. I was greeted whole-heartedly but wondered: how would I ever begin to describe this powerful journey to someone who did not experience it? So, for the time being I just contained it and kept quiet and felt the comfort of the present reality and love of family. Eventually, I rode home from Taos to end this journey of nearly two weeks duration.

In the next chapter, I will share my experience doing a weeklong vision quest without any sacred medicine augmentation. Not everyone is suited for or willing to take entheogens, but a potent healing experience can still occur without them, with proper preparation and mindset.

Chapter 20

Vision Quest Experience: A Week in Temagami, Ontario, Canada Without Medicines

A vision quest has become a popular experience of our times, yet it has also become somewhat cultish. Traditionally, it is most associated with Native American tribes but also takes place in the initiation rites of certain other indigenous cultures. It is important to remember that the term "vision quest" has been appropriated from native cultures and is being incorporated into modern Western healing practices. Credit must be given to these societies, and the respectful usage of their rituals must be led by wise experienced leaders. The integration of multicultural stories and ceremonies may help our present dominant civilization to value the natural world and the spirit realm.

In native cultures sacred medicines are rarely used to augment initiation rites of passage; however as noted previously, the Bwiti cult in West Africa uses iboga for the experience. Typically, other shamanic techniques involving fasting, water restriction, isolation from the community, and sleep deprivation are employed to induce an altered state of consciousness. A vision will hopefully occur which will guide the initiate in the transition from childhood and adolescence into adulthood with all of its responsibilities. A vision may also be sought with an intention to heal an illness or become clearer about a future path. Implied in such a quest is a voluntary submission to a ritual death and rebirth, and often a new name is given to the person once the vision manifests and the initiate completes the quest.

Facing death of the body is possible because it is a strenuous ordeal physically. Usually the experience of the death/rebirth experience is more emotional and spiritual, but still can be a harrowing trial. Therefore, preparation is of the essence and an experienced leader is necessary to minimize the inherent risks.

As previously forewarned, there are many charlatan shamans leading such quests who exploit this collective interest. We have all read about those who have actually perished, rather than experienced the ritual of ego death, during such quests and sweat lodge ceremonies. The same preparation of intention and proper set and setting as described for sacred medicine sessions is necessary. Most often, these quests take place in a natural setting. Preparation may also include drumming, chanting, meditation, dream work, and movement exercises.

The Setting

I had the opportunity to participate in a very powerful weeklong vision quest at Temagami Lake, at Ontario, Canada in 1993, sponsored by an organization called Journey to Wholeness, which led these experiences for many years. I learned about Temagami through sending my two sons to wilderness canoeing camps there during many summers when they were in high school and college. These experiences taught them to become experienced wilderness guides and develop self-reliance and a love of nature. The vision quests for adults were held after these summer camps.

To get to the island on Temagami Lake required flying to Toronto, then taking a bus, then a train 250 miles straight north to the town of Temagami, and finally a float plane to land us at the base camp island on the lake. When I landed there, I walked to the dining hall of the lodge and the first thing I saw was this framed quote from the famous Seth Speaks material, "You are not here to cry about the miseries of the human condition, but to change them when you find them not to your liking, through joy, strength, and the vitality that is within you." I immediately recognized how much complaining I was in the habit of doing in my life based on my comfort needs not being fulfilled, with the expectation that I should be taken care of by someone else. This was a quick reorientation for my intention of the upcoming journey.

The preparation prior to the vision quest included dream work groups outdoors on the island, sweat lodge ceremonies, and some predator/prey game-playing, all of which put the participants in contact with the region's natural elements and ecosystem. What follows is my personal experience, intended only to inform about the transformative power of undergoing such an ordeal and without the aid of psychedelic medicine. As you read this account, remember that I paid to do this for my summer vacation. It was not exactly like going to Cabo San Lucas and relaxing with margaritas under a cabana and listening to Jimmy Buffet.

First, the sweat lodge was too hot, and the rainy weather was too cold, and when I was in one setting, I wished for the other. I told myself it was time to stop complaining and being dissatisfied with my present situation, but just to accept it. From my human standpoint, I felt miserable, but from the standpoint of the Earth, the hot fire was energizing and the rain brought fertility. So, I became determined to fit in with the needs of the Earth—not from sitting in the center of comfort, but from the edges, knowing that the opposites can turn into each other, from death and misery, to life and grace.

The Solo

After several days of preparation, each of the participants set out in their own canoe and paddled across the lake from the island to the mainland wilderness. I took no food or water with me for the three-day quest. If I became dehydrated, there was always the lake to drink from, but both fasting from food or water as well as isolation help promote an altered state. Once on land, I found my private sacred spot among the trees, far from anyone else. I carved out a seven-foot diameter circle within which to experience the entire quest. I only left this circle to attend to my bodily needs.

I marked each of the four directions by a tree. The tree of the South was the largest and my main support to lean on. I then invoked the seven orienting directions with trees also to the North, East, and West, as well as up, down and the center point on the ground level where I sat. As I had previously learned, I sought to clarify my intentions, and to review and honor my relationships, including my family and ancestors. I invoked the spirit of this place, the rocks, vegetation, the four and two-legged creatures of the earth and sky. I then sat in reverence and waited for the sun to ebb. I experienced a light drizzle which blessed this place. I was aware of how different this ecosystem was from my desert excursions in the past.

The Ordeal

Soon enough, I saw lightning and heard distant thunder, a beautiful display of light and sound that shimmered like a strobe light behind the trees of the forest. I was unprepared for how quickly the storm moved in to where I was sitting, drenching me with a cold and powerful rain and wind. It was too late to change out of the clothes I was wearing, which got wet, so I shed everything and placed it into a waterproof garbage bag. It felt like a dismemberment of my bones. I had a poncho but, after ten minutes, it started to leak, and I was left naked facing the full brunt of the storm. The cold climes of the northeast were something I was not accustomed to. I huddled into a fetal position to preserve warmth as the darkness, cold, mud, and fear took over. I began to uncontrollably shiver from the cold and probably also from fear. I quivered down to my bones, not just from fear of the storm but from all the fears, anxieties, and depressions that had lodged in my body and mind during my life. I said over and over, "I can't believe I'm here and paid for this misery." I realized that the weather was scripting this vision quest with a synchronistic cooperation.

I told myself, "This is the real experience of dismemberment of the psyche in the form of a physical ordeal." It was presenting me with a survival course. I was being pelted and worn down, not by something evil but by the divinity in nature. Memories of my traumas came to me—my losses, hurts, fears, and disappointments—so I reiterated a curse that I believed followed my life: "Nothing works out for me." I was filled with self-pity: "Poor me, wah, wah, wah!" I wondered, were all my accomplishments for naught?

Never mind the weather, I was being victimized by my own belief system and negative interpretations. Could I get past all of this, take responsibility, and proceed more positively? Could I accept all this as a baseline and see this situation as the earth needing rain to flourish? The energy of the Sky World was speaking, discharging from the heavens to meet the earth. This image was very grounding for me. I reiterated that I didn't care anymore if I died or was struck by the lightning surrounding me. I had done a lot in my life and what a way to go if need be. Deep down, I knew I would survive this within the sacred space I had created. All storms pass and I had to ride this one out. I told myself to hold fast and to calm down.

The mud, wetness, and pine needles were now in my buttocks. My knees, back, and legs were stiff from sitting, and every bone was crying out its aches and pains. I realized that my body had absorbed much physical and psychological trauma over the years and that I was aging. My work at home is sedentary, and I had become softened. I realized the storm is like a forge to toughen my body and soul and make me less thin-skinned. So, before any vision, I am to strengthen myself and be more flexible and less brittle. I must strengthen myself to the changing reality of what lies ahead in my profession. The invasion of corporate medicine and managed care are challenging to my core values of what it means to be a healer. Like the earth, I need a storm, a divine catastrophe, to help me to adapt to these collective changes. Comfort and success will not bring me the answers. I asked Mother Earth to give me support as she replenishes her fertility. I become aware there is a great difference between the *Great Mother* (archetypal) and being stuck in the *mother-complex* (personal, which is comfort, safety, dependency, laziness, and passivity). This storm, with its cold, rain, harsh wind, as well as darkness, sleep deprivation, and nakedness, are exactly what I needed at this time of life. It is the correspondence between nature and my human weaknesses that will contribute to my healing.

I realized that I have abandoned my heritage, diminished my intellectual abilities, become disillusioned with Judaism and Jungian work, and lost faith in my abilities to be a teacher and to deepen my inner wisdom. Being burned out at work has been partly due to my over-emphasizing the material aspect of it, which I equated to being successful. I lost my way in order to gain recognition through having more patients, making more money, and being a better provider for my family. I thought more money would lessen my anxiety. This desperation led to a feeling of failure and depression.

The mother-complex had embedded me in the negative aspect of the *Lover* archetype, which desires comfort and appreciation. I need to reactivate the "warrior within" to continue to manifest my destiny and toughen up a bit. On the other hand, the Great Mother gives life and can take life. While the nurturing mother, Gaia, gives life and sustenance, the death crone mother, the witch, (e.g. Baba Yaga of Russian folklore), takes back life and forces a trial to prove worthiness to continue to live.

The poison of the negative mother is like the storm, requiring tasks to be performed in order to show reverence and humble respect for Mother Nature. This storm completely dismembered my ego, humbled me to the ground, and destroyed the burned-out concepts that I held to be true, but were actually just my arrogance and narcissism. It was the correspondence between nature and my human woes that contributed to my eventual healing, as well as my realization that my vulnerability was my strength. I needed to develop respect and empathy for myself first of all. I needed to self-nurture instead of expecting all to come from some outer source. "God helps those who help themselves." Simple and true. Time to take more accountability and responsibility for my lot in life.

Thoughts of nature emerged next. As I felt personally beaten down, I wondered about all the animals that must endure the elements of nature, especially in its raw fury. What about the worms, birds, and all creatures that become drenched and need to seek cover? What about the Native Americans who used to live here, as well as indigenous people around the world, where storms, droughts, and disasters are frequent occurrences? The reptile and primitive nervous systems are all geared for survival, the life force in action. I then pondered disabled, chronically ill humans and those dying of terminal diseases. My personal plight at the time was put into perspective by awareness of these adversities within humanity, and my heart became filled with empathy for all unfortunate beings.

A Vision

I found that the night and its darkness last forever when a person attempts to stay awake. It amazed me how much time we usually sleep in everyday life. The dark and empty forest seemed like death with nary a sound or any light. It forced me to turn inward, and soon the visions began. First, I saw an underground cavern with no life or vegetation, with breast-like stalactites hanging down and dripping a nourishing, milky substance. Then a large snakelike boa penetrated this realm. Next, I saw a lotus flower embedded in my third eye, which was slowly opening. It was reminiscent of a mild psychedelic experience but, due to the intense outdoor setting, I was actually glad I was not taking any hallucinogens. What I was spontaneously envisioning was amazing.

I then realized that, slowly it was beginning to get light, and the surrounding trees emerged in silhouettes. The dawn was finally returning but the rain continued on and off, and the winds picked up, creating more chill. I was still soaking wet, but at least my poncho helped to break the wind. I remembered that the camp leader, David, said that even the thinnest person would not develop hypothermia in this weather, but I wondered. However, I learned that it was better to be naked and pelted with rain then to continue to wear wet clothes. I also learned that it is important to keep your clothes as dry as possible because they can quickly warm you up. As the day broke, there was no sun, just intermittent rain and wind. I wondered whether I could endure another night of this and how the other participants were faring, especially those who were older and frailer.

As the day drew on, the weather continued overcast with sporadic rain, and I remained cold. Amazingly, I was tired but not hungry or particularly thirsty. My senses, especially hearing, became hyperacute. I found myself dozing off and having fragments of dreams with images of trees, boats, and people by their cabins on the shore. These were perhaps minor hallucinations, because the reality was pure wilderness with only light flickering among the trees. When awake, I heard music in the forest that sounded like Native American chants. I soon started singing along with the melody and rhythm and found it exhilarating. But in actual reality, no one was there except for me.

The day wore on very slowly and by late afternoon, the sun came out and the rain abated. I was able to hang my wet clothes out on the tree branches where they slowly dried. I could now track the sun, which seemed holy. My wet clothes became a metaphor for my dismembered bones. I started to dress again once they were dry and "put Humpty Dumpty together again." I was recollecting my parts, remembering the Egyptian story of Isis reconstituting the dismembered body of Osiris. The feeling of warmth was such grace; such a small and common everyday thing as dressing filled me with incredible joy. The storm had passed and I pondered, now what?

Slowly twilight came, and now the forest was no longer foreboding, taking on great beauty and tranquility. What a difference a day can make in the psyche! As the day darkened, I sat in prayer, asking to receive a vision and more teaching, as I felt I could integrate these now that my physical survival was no longer of primary concern. I then saw an old man with gray hair and beard emerge from the water of the lake to greet me. When I asked, "Who are you?" he told me he was known as "Old Man River." He said he comes from the river and is very old, yet ageless. "I have come to help you, to respond to your requests, needs, and laments. You may ask of me whatever you want, I am your friend."

Old Man River

Here is my dialogue with Old Man River (OMR), which represents an altered state combined with active imagination:

Alex (A): My worries and blocks are with my work, my vocation. I can't keep going on in its present form. I am having trouble envisioning and manifesting my next steps. I am feeling contracted. Gaining help with this issue is my intention.

OMR: Speak more simply and directly. Shorter questions will bring more answers. You talk too much. That is the first step.

A: You are honest and clear. Thank you.

OMR: Yes, and now you can better hear me. You are unhappy and have conditioned yourself to put that into work.

A: That is a starting place. Say more.

OMR: In your history, you never enjoyed school or work very much. It's the mother complex. You are lazy and always want more comfort. You procrastinate when you are moody.

A: Is that it?

OMR: There is that part that wants to be cared for and thinks that will happen of itself. You expect it to just come to you.

A: Do I have early Alzheimer's?

OMR: Not organically, but you have forgotten what is important, and your mind has become dull.

A: I've wasted a lot of time worrying, too.

OMR: You want a great vision, but you need to take smaller steps and focus.

A: What about living a life of heart?

OMR: You live enough of that, but your fine mind has devolved; you've become lazy and scattered and have lost focus on your priorities. You have lost touch with the stream of your unconscious process. Take it all more seriously—that's what you have spent your life studying and doing.

A: Yes, I know you are right. I have been resisting my heritage and legacy and yet still expect it to all go well.

OMR: Focus on the task at hand—your next workshop on the Lover. Pick your stories and work on the details with the other presenters. Do this before you spend more time reading about your current interest in shamanism.

A: What stories should I tell?

OMR: Start with "Sir Gawain and the Loathly Damsel" and "The First Sons and Daughters," the Native American story about how men and women got together. Consider presenting "The Love Flute." Pick a story like "Tristan and Iseult", and perhaps the story of "Isis and Osiris."

A: Good suggestions, and I can present them while I drum.

OMR: Prepare for one event at a time. This will reduce your performance anxiety. Take notes on what you read. For instance, outline the book *Power and Love* by Angeles Arrien.

A: Why will all this help manifest a more positive future for me?

OMR: This you must trust like the movie *Field of Dreams*. Do your homework and "they will come." More opportunities will open up.

A: How can I trust that advice?

OMR: Trust is a big issue for you, but Old Man River knows. Feel your resistance to do the work and to write. You have to struggle with your mother-complex, otherwise it will immobilize you and lead to more depression. After this workshop, you can again tackle your "Plants and Shamanism" lecture. There is plenty of time for that. For now, maintain your focus and priorities, and learn to be more direct.

A: I like what you say.

OMR: I'm cool like you but not holier than thou. Do a little preparation each early evening.

A: Yes, but I'm so tired after work.

OMR: Stop with the "yes, but" phrase. It is only an excuse. You can work even if you are tired. Start with spending a few minutes with this task each morning or evening. You will still have plenty of time to rest and play. Get more disciplined.

A: It seems like everything I pick to do is not popular, for example Jung or shamanism.

OMR: It's your soul, man, so you have to live it out no matter what. You are too old and wise to continue to win popularity contests.

A: Yes, but what about making a living to support my family?

OMR: You are doing already what you must. You are making changes and adapting slowly to the onslaught of corporate medicine and managed care. I must remind you that you have chosen this solo path, not signing up with a group practice that would dictate to you how to work. You would lose your independence in being the healer you wish to be. This success and money obsession distracts you back to your core neurosis. Stay with your interests and the work will follow to support your body and soul. Like this storm, be patient for the new day.

A: Is this the great vision of this quest?

OMR: You are always looking for something bigger and better and not accepting what is given to you. I am giving you this vision, and it is what you have to do as a start to reorganize your life.

A: What about love and my upcoming workshop on the subject that I will be doing with J.?

OMR: Your task is to work with her. Let your respect and loving feelings for each other fuel your work but keep it separate. Her professional interest is focused on love. Do not try and live this out with her. Remember that you're in a good marriage and family where the hearth burns for you. Bring the eros home with you.

A: I've had enough for now. I'm tired, but is there more I should know?

OMR: There is always more, but you've done well for this journey. Take a rest. It's OK if you sleep a little. I'll wake you up when needed.

A: Thank you, Old Man River. You are firm yet I do not feel criticized or judged. I seem to be able to listen to you without being defensive.

OMR: Remember, I am you but from a deeper perspective. It is because you are ready and need to hear some answers, or should I say suggestions, to move onward.

A: Again, I thank you and am grateful you exist within me.

(See Fig. 81, page 330.)

After this message, I drifted off to sleep a bit in some mild nighttime weather. I awakened in the early glow of light before the sunrise. I was overwhelmed by a feeling of grace: awe, beauty, and security. All the indescribable pain, coldness, suffering, abandonment, abasement, fear, and trembling were gone. This was death and rebirth, the main function of a vision quest initiation. All was still in the environment. I heard birds again. All seemed well. I survived and received what I needed. I said, "I'm alive—still alive. Why worry?" This is what I would call a "violent adventure" that turned out well.

As the morning wore on, I heard the sound of the motorboat from the island, meaning it was time to return. I went down to the shoreline where I got into my canoe. I slowly paddled the distance back to the island with a feeling of joy in accomplishing the quest. It didn't seem necessary to spend more days questing alone. I was ready to rejoin the group, carry out some integration of the experience, and hear from the others.

Once ashore, I headed to the large teepee where everyone congregated, first hydrating with water. We all then entered the teepee for a sweat lodge ceremony where blessings were dispensed. Ritual has a way of making the mundane holy. When I left the sweat lodge, I felt dizzy from the lack of nourishment and dehydration. I was helped by some of the staff, resting by a rock to regain my equilibrium. I then proceeded to take the short hike back to the lodge where all of us were greeted with cheers by the staff as if we were heroes returning from the battlefield. All of the staff in the past had completed similar vision quests and thoroughly understood its meaning. A feast was awaiting us in the dining hall as we sat down to what tasted like the best meal ever.

The next few days were spent in small groups integrating the experience. Everyone had important things to share. A few of the participants returned the morning after the storm, but there was never any judgment or failure implied. Everyone bore what they could and learned a great deal from their time. At the end of the week, we exchanged goodbyes and well-wishes. I realized I had gown very close to several people during this week at Temagami. We flew back on the float plane to the railway station in town. Most of us sat in silence on this ride back. Finally, from Toronto I flew home to my family for whom I had even more deep feelings of love.

Afterthoughts

The above portrayal is intended to reveal the power that vision quests can manifest. It is my hope that it demonstrates how a life-altering peak experience can provide insight for change. As time passed, I found that the intensity of the memories diminished, but the key to integration is to remember the lessons and do something with them. When I compare this journey to the vision quests I have carried out using sacred medicines, I see that the same results are possible. The above quest was definitely more physically demanding, but it accomplished the process of altering my consciousness, allowing me to perceive, think, and feel extraordinary ideas, and again reoriented my psyche to the natural world. Living out these insights in my daily work and routines remained the challenge.

Now that years have passed since this experience, I did create a successful career, living out my destiny as a healer. I earned a good living but realize I no longer focused on making money. I continued to trust my inner wisdom, and the rest just followed. There were difficult times and recurring doubts, but remembering my experiences helped me cope more effectively with new obstacles that arose. I will always remember that "perseverance furthers," that storms and crises pass, and new opportunities return. There is rebirth after death. My philosophy of life can be summarized by these simple quotes, "Keep on truckin'," "bop till you drop," and "don't die until you're dead."

Section Three

More Shamanic Lore: Other Sacred Medicines

The following chapters are included for informational purposes rather than the sharing of my visionary memoirs. I found these stories of the ways various sacred plants and chemicals were used in the past to be fascinating and deserving of attention, especially for those with curiosity regarding consciousness. However, it is important to realize the difficulty in distinguishing speculation from facts, and fantasy from truth. Historical interpretations are subject to the opinions and biases of the researcher, so as a reader, please take what follows with a grain of salt. At the very least, the stories make for good conversation.

Solanaceae: Witches, Brews, Love Potions, Werewolves, and Headhunters

A family of plants (the *Solanaceae*) exist that are hallucinogenic, widespread, and of great importance in the Old and New World. This order of plants is related to the potato, the tomato, chili peppers, and tobacco. A discussion of solanaceous herbs is essential to an inquiry into entheogens, since they have been used extensively in shamanic rituals, witchcraft, and vision quests in Europe, Asia, Africa, South America, and among Native American tribes since ancient times. (Harner 1973, 125-150) I do not advocate using these plants for present-day shamanic journey work because of danger from their toxicity.

These plant hallucinogens include the deadly nightshade, belladonna (*atropa*), henbane (*hyoscyamus*), mandrake (*mandragora*), and hemlock. Also in this class are the *Datura* species, sometimes referred to as Jimson weed, devil's apple, thorn apple, and mad apple, and the *Brugmansia* species, Gabriel's trumpet or Angel's trumpet. The common active ingredients are atropine and the tropane alkaloids hyoscyamine and scopolamine (used for seasickness). These plants are all potentially hallucinogenic but can be extremely dangerous, in that their therapeutic range is adjacent to the toxic dose. They can be both physically and mentally harmful and can sometimes cause death.

Michael Harner (1929-2018), a present-day anthropologist of shamanism, discusses the usage of solanaceous plants and postulates the following in his book, *Hallucinogens and Shamanism*:

In ancient witchcraft, these plants were made into ointments and unguents, and were rubbed into the skin and mucous membranes. They were often called flying ointments or witches' salve. "A staff or a broom served as an applicator for the atropine-containing plant to the sensitive vaginal membranes [see illustrations]." (Harner 1973, 131) This possibly accounts for the image of a witch flying on a broomstick. "The witch then indeed took a 'trip': the witch on a broomstick is a representation of that imagined aerial journey to rendezvous with spirits or demons, which was called a *Sabbat*." (Harner 1973, 129)

All women, young and old, could thus participate in the joys of these ecstatic experiences, and sensual pleasure was open to all. These fantasies occurred while the women were motionless, asleep, or unconscious.

However, current research does not support the notion of these witch's sabbats as wild gatherings of women intent on erotic gratification or a wild hunt. It may be a male fantasy to speculate that these women, the so-called witches, would concoct a potion that allowed them to have erotic, ecstatic, sensual experiences on a Saturday night (Sabbat). Perhaps they were no more than a "girls' night out" allowing some participants a respite from men and their domination.

Historic reports of erotic themes frequently dominate the hallucinatory images attributed to the solanaceous herbs; modern-day users who have tried these concoctions report similar results. Images of flight commonly occur, despite the partaker remaining motionless or unconscious on the floor. These excursions can be considered "flights of fancy or fancy flights." Erich Hesse writes about the effects of these admixtures of witches' brews and love potions: "The hallucinations are frequently dominated by the erotic moment . . . In those days, in order to experience these sensations, young and old women would rub their bodies with the 'witches' salve.'" (Hesse 1946, 103) Again, this is a conjecture.

The Inquisition, during which hundreds of thousands of supposed and real witches were tortured and executed, has supplied the bulk of data on hallucinogenic plants in late medieval Europe. (Harner, 1973, 129) An account by the Catholic priest of the Dominican order, Bartolommeo Spina (1523), describes the witches' flight: "She finally confessed that she had been carried on the journey; from which it is manifestly clear that they (witches) are deluded not bodily, but mentally or in dreams, in such a way that they imagine they are carried a long distance while they remain immobile at home." (Harner 1973, 133) Nevertheless, I have included two artistic depictions of the application of erotic, solanaceous ointments for these sabbats (see Fig. 59, 60).

It is crucial to note that Spina lived during the Inquisition, and that the confessions occurred while these women were tortured by priests. The veracity of these sabbat experiences was coerced, and they probably did not occur. Instead, the confessions served to rationalize and justify the church patriarchy's misogyny and domination of women. The male-dominated Catholic clergy of the Middle Ages were threatened by any form of sexuality, eroticism, or pleasure. They perhaps felt controlled by female sensuality, in which they could not participate. They suppressed these sabbats according to the mandates of their patriarchal dogma. This display of feminine ecstasy could only be controlled by demonizing such women and burning them at the stake. Hence the term "witch" became synonymous with consorting with the devil and evil. Present thinking is attempting to redefine the witch with a more positive connotation.

The projection by men onto these women of evildoing was a way of blaming a woman when something went wrong that could not be explained, such as a cow mysteriously dying, someone getting ill, or something being stolen. The men would say a magic spell was cast by these women that caused this misfortune. Throughout history, the human psyche has had a need to blame someone rather than take personal accountability. In a male-dominated society, this takes the form of blaming a female or some shadow figure. Hate, anger, and jealousy are notorious emotions that are commonly projected onto the other.

Some witches were healers, herbalists, midwives, and also ordinary women. The term "pagan," often used to describe these women, means "country dweller." Also used to describe them is "heathen," which means living on the heath (open, uncultivated land). They tended to have nature-loving, polytheistic views of God and Earth spirits that contrasted with the patriarchal Church's monotheistic viewpoint. Witches and polytheism had existed long before Christianity emerged. Their polytheism was another reason to suppress and stamp out witches, and along with it, sexuality and pleasure, all in the name of God.

It is also essential to note that not all witches were good. Like any humans, there were some women who were maleficent, having intent to harm others to gain power or revenge. It is also crucial to know that the term witch did not only apply to females. Approximately one-third were males, but the torture and sacrifices were mostly visited on women.

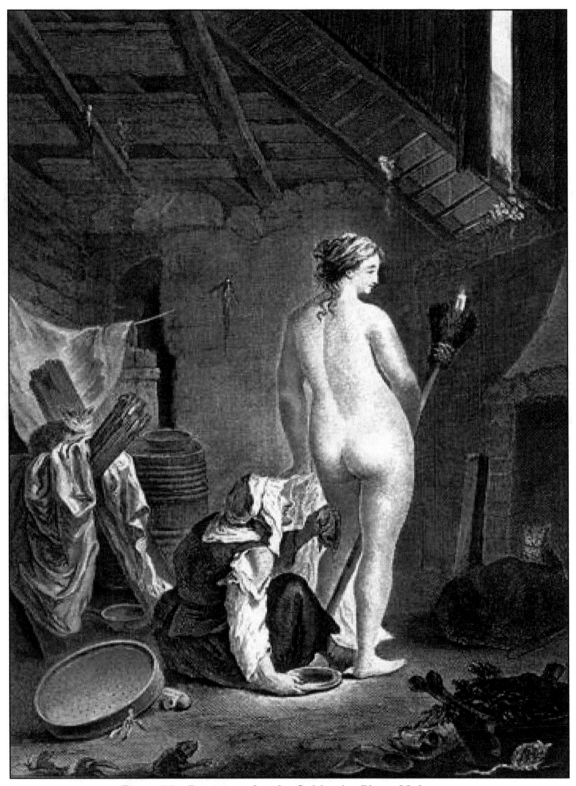

FIGURE 59. *Departure for the Sabbat* by Pierre Maleuvre.
Witch applying the ointment with a broomstick preparing for the sabbat.
(Pierre Maleuvre, Public domain, via Wikimedia Commons)

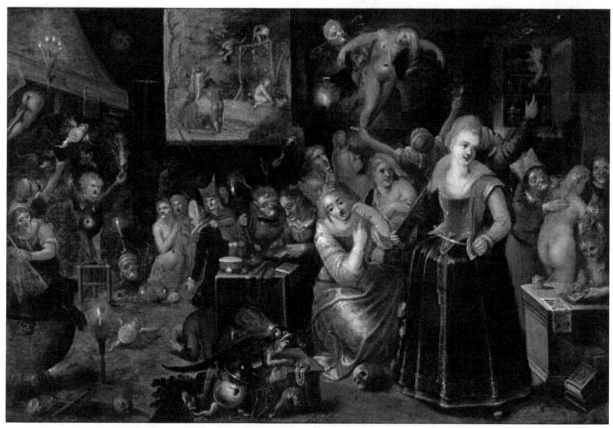

FIGURE 60. *The Witches' Kitchen* by Hieronymus Francken II.
Being rubbed down with the ointment.
(Public domain, via Wikimedia Commons)

In the 20th century, re-creations of the above-described flying oint-ments included belladonna, henbane, aconite, opium, hashish, and *Datura*, which were based on 17th century formulas. Professor Will-Erich Peukert (1966) describes such a modern journey: "[He] rubbed it on his forehead and armpits and had colleagues do the same. They fell into a twenty-four-hour sleep in which they dreamed of the wild rides, frenzied dancing, and other weird adventures of the type connected with medieval orgies." (Krieg 1966) Another recent German scholar, Gustav Schenk, describes his exper-iments with henbane, including this, ". . .the crazy sensation that my feet were growing lighter, expanding and breaking loose from my body . . . Each part of my body seemed to be going off on its own . . . At the same time I experienced an intoxicating sensation of flying." (Schenk 1955, 139-140) The sensation of gradual body dissolution has been reported as a side

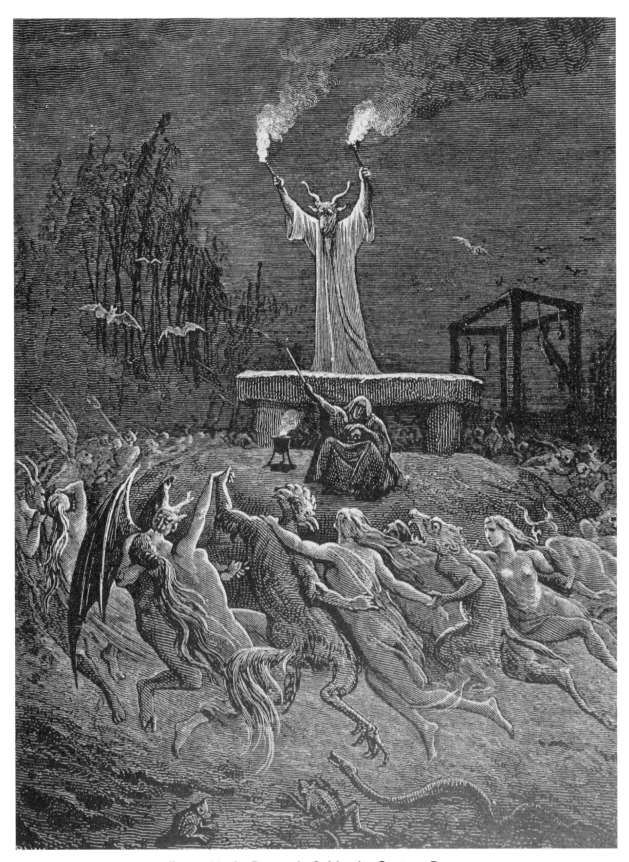

FIGURE **61.** *La Danse du Sabbat* by Gustave Dore.
(Émile Bayard, Public domain, via Wikimedia Commons)

effect of henbane poisoning.

Carlos Castaneda described the use of the solanaceous Datura plant as a visionary agent in the book *The Teachings of Don Juan*: "The motion of my body was slow and shaky . . . The momentum carried me forward one more step, which was even more elastic and longer than the preceding one. And from there I soared . . . I saw the dark sky above me, and the clouds going by me . . . My speed was extraordinary . . . I enjoyed such freedom and swiftness as I had never known before." (Castaneda 1968, 140) It is essential to note that despite Castaneda's descriptions as an anthropologist from UCLA, Don Juan was a fictional character throughout his series of books. His writings, though interesting, must be viewed with a grain of salt, and should not be considered accurate anthropological research.

The noted cultural anthropologist and recognized authority on the use of sacred plants, Christian Rätsch, in a private conversation at the 1994 International Transpersonal Conference in Killarney, Ireland, relayed that henbane and other solanaceous herbs are currently being used in some circles to promote erotic experiences. Often these herbs are mixed in a mead-like drink. With a skilled practitioner of these plants, as well as with a safe set and setting, the correct non-toxic dosage of solanaceous compounds may indeed provide a heightened erotic and pleasant journey for those wishing to explore this realm.

Werewolves

It is speculated that solanaceous plant ointments were not only used in sabbats to experience the witches' flight, but also for metamorphosis into wolves. *Lycanthropy* is an ancient belief that humans can change themselves into wolves or similar predatory animals. The use of solanaceous hallucinogens possibly fueled this metamorphosis.

An account by Paulus Aegineta, a 7th -century Greek physician, describes the disease of lycanthropy: "Those labouring under lycanthropia go out during the night imitating wolves in all things and lingering about sepulchres until morning. You may recognize such persons by these marks: they are pale, their vision feeble, their eyes dry, their tongue very dry, and the flow of saliva stopped; but they are thirsty, and their legs have incurable ulcerations from frequent falls. Such are the marks of the disease."

(Adams 1884, 1:389-390). Here is another description by Pierre Bourgot in 1521: When "...rubbed on the body, [the ointment] was to change them into wolves for one to two hours, and that in this state they physically attacked a number of persons, biting them with their teeth, killing them and even eating parts of their bodies." (Wier 1885 [orig. 1660]) These above quotes may indeed be the basis of fear of werewolves prowling at night under a full moon as depicted in horror movies.

These symptoms resemble the clinical (anticholinergic) effects of atropine, specifically, dryness of the throat and mouth, difficulty swallowing, thirst, impaired vision, staggering gait, and delirium with hallucinations and delusions. As we know, humans will use any drug to get high or to experience an altered state, despite side effects. Erich Hesse notes: "A characteristic feature of solanaceae psychosis is . . . the intoxicated person imagines himself to be changed into some animal, and the hallucinosis is completed by the sensation of the growing of feathers and hair." (Hesse 1946, 103-104) While these experiences may serve as the origin of werewolf beliefs, it is unclear whether people purposefully tried to become wolf-like with the intent to harm others or to become aggressive.

Headhunters: The Jivaro of the Amazon

These plants were also used in Jivaro (hee-va-ro) shamanism. The Jivaro are an indigenous tribe of the Western Amazon in Peru and Ecuador, sometimes known as headhunters and head-shrinkers. They were a tribe known for their fierceness and independence, strengths enabling them to thwart and drive off the Spanish conquerors. In his book *The Jivaro: People of the Sacred Waterfalls*, Michael Harner, the anthropologist and Western shaman, shares the results of his studies of this tribe and their strange sociocultural ideology. They used hallucinogens to produce visionary trance states to stem the onslaught of progress and outside civilizations, allowing them to maintain their cultural integrity. Their warrior nature was fueled by hallucinogens. They considered daily, ordinary living as relatively unimportant and viewed killing as a highly desirable activity. Their belief system rationalized killing to acquire a new soul, which provided the individual with immunity from death. "The Jivaro believe that the true determinants of life and death are normally invisible forces which can be

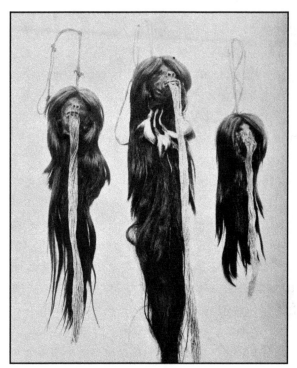

FIGURE **62. Shrunken head (Tsantsa) trophies.**
(Harner 1972, 138, fig. 21)

seen and utilized only with the aid of hallucinogenic drugs. The normal waking life is explicitly viewed as "false or a lie." (Harner 1972, 135) What our culture deems as violence and murder, for the Jivaro was considered normal. The plants would be used to encounter the supernatural and the shamans would use the trance states for their rituals and warrior activities.

Their warlike reputation spread in the late 19th and early 20th centuries, when Jivaro shrunken head trophies called *tsantsa* made their way to the markets of exotica collectors in the Western World. (Harner 1972, 1) This perhaps is the origin of the word "headshrinker" or "shrink" for modern day psychiatrists. Presumably, the psychiatrist would shrink the grandiose ego-beliefs of their patients and realign them with a humbler reality.

It is known that the Jivaro used *Datura arborea*, called *maikua*, with its high content of the solanaceous compounds, hyoscyamine, atropine, and scopolamine. (Harner 1972, 137) They also used *Banisteriopsis* vines to make a drink called *natema*, better known as ayahuasca, to induce trance states.

This Jivaro practice was in contrast to this plant's usage in European witchcraft. The witches did not use these solanaceous compounds to acquire an altered state for healing ceremonies, considering them too powerful to simultaneously navigate both worlds. They were used primarily for their sabbatical adventures.

In Western medicine, the pharmacologic effect of solanaceous substances is known as anticholinergic. These drugs block the action of the neurotransmitter *acetylcholine* (Ach), at the synapses of the central and peripheral nervous system. They are used today to treat a variety of conditions, including vertigo and motion-sickness (scopolamine). They are also used to decrease bowel spasms and pain in gastrointestinal disorders, including ulcers, ulcerative colitis, and vomiting. Additionally, they can treat genitourinary problems such as cystitis and prostatitis that cause urinary frequency and incontinence.

Certain of these drugs are used as antidotes to organophosphate nerve agent poisonings, such as from VX, sarin, tabun, and soman, as well as pesticide exposure. In psychiatry, these anticholinergics are used to treat the extrapyramidal side effects and abnormal movements caused by antipsychotic drugs. The side effects of these medications can cause delirium, hallucinations, delusions (especially in the elderly), fever (hyperthermia), constipation, tachycardia, urinary retention, pupil dilation (mydriasis), and anhidrosis (dry skin and mucous membranes). Some psychiatric patients request these medications for purposes of getting high. In therapeutic doses, these drug analogs can be helpful, but the toxic dose is adjacent to the therapeutic range and can be deadly. There are many safer alternatives for the psychedelic experience, and the general recommendation is to avoid these solanaceous compounds unless properly guided and with a proper intention.

Personally, the only time I have tried such a solanaceous herb was in a journey using an admixture of *Brugmansia*, Damiana (a non-psychoactive, presumably aphrodisiac herb), and cannabis, smoked in equal parts. (The *Damiana* flower has been used since prehistoric times in North America and the Mayan region as both a medicine and a love potion. The Catholic Church decried its use among the clerics of the 11th century, known for their loose morals.) I smoked this combination in a joint and did not experience anything extraordinary or erotic. Perhaps it was more stimulating than cannabis alone, but I experienced more irritability. My conclusion was, "Why bother?" It was not a fantasy enhancer, teacher, or guide for me.

Chapter 22
Salvia Divinorum: Herb of the Shepherdess

This plant is being included for discussion since it is considered sacred and has come into prevalent use (and abuse) during the new wave of psychedelic experimentation. *Salvia divinorum* is a psychoactive plant, sometimes called seer's sage, sage of the diviners, and *yerba de la pastora* (herb of the shepherdess). It rarely seeds, so it is usually propagated through cuttings. The natural environment is in the Sierra Mazatec mountains and ravines, in a relatively cool and mild climate, with temperatures ranging between 60 and 70 degrees. (Sociedad para la Preservation de los Plantas del Misterio 1998, 29)

Mazatec shamans in the state of Oaxaca, Mexico, have used this plant to facilitate visionary states of consciousness for spiritual healing sessions. It is also used to find lost objects and to clear up thefts. The Mazatecs use its leaves when they are unable to obtain magic mushrooms. They consider the plant to be the incarnation of the Virgin Mary. María Sabina, the famous Mazatec shaman, remarked, "When I am in the time (the off-season) that there are no mushrooms and want to heal someone who is sick, then I must fall back on the leaves of pastora." The ritual usually takes place at night in complete darkness and stillness. (Schultes, Hofmann, and Rätsch 1992, 164-165)

Salvia divinorum was known only to the Mazatec Indians of Mexico until the latter half of the 20th century. Later, knowledge of it filtered down to anthropologists and botanists, first documented in 1939 by Jean Basset Johnson. In October of 1962, it finally came into the hands of R. Gordon Wasson and Dr. Albert Hofmann (of LSD fame). (Sociedad para la Preservation de los Plantas de los Misterio 1998, 8) They also postulated that this salvia plant could be the mythological *pipilzintzintli*, the Noble

Prince, used by the Aztecs. This is the only species among nearly a thousand other plants in the *Salvia* genus with hallucinogenic properties. The more familiar white sage, *Salvia apiana*, is often burned as incense for smudging, purifying, and blessing ceremonies, but is otherwise not psychoactive. (Rätsch 1992, 53-154)

Salvia does not appear to be toxic. Most commonly, about thirteen pairs of leaves and stems are rolled up into a cigar and chewed. The juice is absorbed through the mucous membranes rather than being swallowed. The Mazatecs would often wash it down with a swig of tequila because it is very bitter. Sometimes it is smoked (with two to three leaves), made into a tea, or juiced. The effects may vary depending on the method of ingestion, and whether one meets the ally on the *Path of Leaves* (chewing), or the *Bridge of Smoke* (smoking). (Pendell 1995, 158) The psychoactive effects of Salvia are short-lived, lasting from about forty-five to ninety minutes.

This plant is in the chemical class *neocerodan-diterpenes*, also known as divinorum A and divinorum B, which are potent opioid agonists. It is not considered an alkaloid (that is, it does not contain nitrogen) as are other hallucinogens, which usually act on the brain's serotonin 5HT2A receptor. The term alkaloid refers to a diverse group of some five thousand molecular compounds that contain nitrogen, carbon, oxygen, and hydrogen. They are mostly of plant origin, and they are all alkaline, hence their name, and are usually bitter to the taste. (Schultes 1976, 17) There exist some older references for the possible use of *Salvia divinorum* for divination.

Descriptions of Effects

Subtlety, darkness, quietness, and patience are necessary to tease out this plant's shy ally. Some claim the experience to be like yoga, meditation, or trance. As a spirit ally, "She may not appear for a while until she gets to know you." (Pendell 1995, 156) Some users say that the power of the leaves slowly builds up after successive use. Others have described it as a "root energy network, or that it is about becoming a plant" and that "it is plants that have consciousness. Animals get consciousness by eating plants." (Pendell 1995. 158-159) Another assertion is: "The ally loves darkness. Light can interrupt and suspend even wildly cosmic and disembodied states, seamlessly returning the petitioner to the mundane . . . What is amazing is how immediately the interdimensional space reasserts itself when the lights are again put out." (Pendell 1995, 168)

Variable descriptions about the effects it may have on a particular individual have been reported. The bottom line is that it is dependent on set and setting. Some additional descriptions by Pendell of its effects include these:

"The most 'Zen' of any plant ally excepting rice." (Pendell 1995, 168)

"Staggering. Lurching. But not the drunkenness: the mind is completely clear. The effect is reminiscent of kava." (Pendell 1995, 168)

"It's like heavy zazen, like after a long period of sitting." (Pendell 1995, 169)

"There is something very pagan about it . . . Sex is fantastic. It sensitizes the skin." (Pendell 1995, 169)

Some describe it as a mirror. "It just gives you where you are. Wherever you are, that is what you get. If you are in darkness, you fly through darkness . . . If you are with your lover, the plant is an aphrodisiac." (Pendell 1995, 171)

"It helps me with some of my business dealings: like it told me how to talk to the producers . . . We call it 'the balancer.'" (Pendell 1995, 170)

"Sometimes the sage whispers, sometimes it shouts. Sometimes it tells you to sing, sometimes it takes your voice, walks off, leaving your rooted, eyeless, and with the kind of voice a plant has." (Pendell 1995, 175)

I have personally experienced *Salvia divinorum* several times through direct ingestion of chewing the folded leaves. In one journey, I was inside a gothic church with vaulted ceilings of immense proportions. Inside, it was very dark and quiet, but the feeling was sacred. There were several hooded monks about in dark cloaks, faceless. It felt like being in a holy sepulcher, with monks presiding over the dead and the ancestors with reverence. No one spoke.

I found the visions to be short-lived, and the experience was over within one hour. After this period of calm meditation, I felt more irritable. There were no profound teachings to be integrated or even a pleasurable high, although I noted the plant's sacred quality. I must say that the visionary aspect of it underwhelmed me, thus it is not a visionary medicine of choice for me. Perhaps with repeated use, the ally would become more apparent and guide me further.

As previously stated, each individual will respond to the spirits within each plant medicine differently. Often trial and error are required to find which plant spirits are allies and which ones are unhelpful. I would like to include a firsthand experience of a colleague and friend who felt a tremendous benefit from Salvia.

> *From my experience, Salvia divinorum is in a class of its own as far as psychedelics and dissociative medicines go. Unlike LSD, peyote, ayahuasca, and mushrooms, Salvia takes me completely out of my body to a place 100% removed from what is happening around me. Each time I have smoked the leaves, everything around me disappears as I am drawn toward a complexly beautiful and powerful rectangular vortex moving in a curve downward, pulling me into it as it progresses. There is a slight fear of going with this throbbing entity, but I always surrender. I'm in a ribbed tube that is actually a mass of enlightened beings that connect with me, not through words but through energy and some type of deep joining. Too soon, the medicine wears off, and I feel a deep sadness at not wanting to leave.*

> *After each journey, I return feeling like I have reset my perspective on life. I try to keep the vision of the vortex clear in my mind to get a better understanding of what really matters. Salvia divinorum is the most intense reset button I have ever pushed. Unlike other psychedelic medicines, Salvia does not rob me of energy the next day. For me, it is a gift, although one I use only once in a while because of its intense power. Oddly enough, it is still legal to buy at shops in California.*

This example shows how there are "different strokes for different folks." Sometimes, the plant chooses a particular individual to express itself fully. An experienced shaman and a proper, safe setting can also make all the difference. It is important to note that Salvia has potential to be abused. For some, it has become an alternative for marijuana to get high or is often blended with cannabis as a smoke. It has been made illegal in many countries; it is illegal in at least thirteen states in the United States. Lawsuits have been filed from adverse effects attributable to this sage. I conclude that with the current availability of other plant medicines, it is probably best to seek wisdom elsewhere.

Chapter 23

Amanita Muscaria: Santa Claus as Shaman

A type of magical mushroom called the *fly agaric*, better known as *Amanita muscaria*, is a red-capped mushroom with white dots that has become the image common in many illustrations in children's and Christmas books. It is the foremost hallucinogenic mushroom used by most Nordic shamans. Its use can be traced to the Laplanders and various Siberian nomadic people, such as the Samojeden, Ostjaken, Tungusen, Jakuten, Koryak, Chukchi, Yukagir, Yakut, Ostyak, Samoyed, and Kamchadal tribes. Some North American Indians also utilized it. Its use was clearly widespread. (Rätsch and Mueller-Ebling 2003, 45)

Throughout the world, shamans, magicians, and healers viewed this mushroom as a magical plant, while ordinary people feared it as a poison. In antiquity, it was used by Taoist alchemists as an additive in a variety of elixirs of immortality. It was called Raven's Bread by the Egyptians. In Greece, it became associated with Dionysian festivals for its ability to bestow enormous physical power, erotic potency, visions, and the gift of prophecy. The ancient Germans associated this mushroom with Wotan/Odin, the all-seeing god of ecstasy, and the discoverer of magical runes. One author even suggested that Christianity began as a fly agaric cult. (Rätsch 1992, 83)

"The name 'fly agaric' is probably derived from the fly's reputation as a magical animal or the mushroom's ability to enable a person to fly." (Rätsch 1992, 83) Others have said that when mixed with milk, it is a poison to flies.

The shamans of the Chuj Indians of Central America sometimes use the fly-agaric and smoke it with tobacco. For them, it induces a clairvoyant trance in which they can detect the causes of diseases and unleash special healing powers. They associate the consumption of fly-agaric with the god

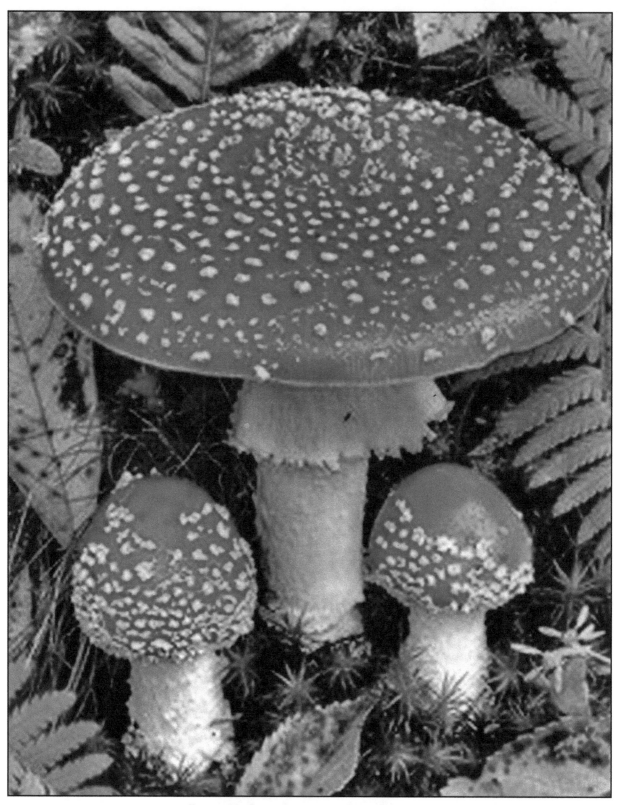

FIGURE 63. Amanita muscaria mushroom
(photo – Wikimedia commons)

212

of lightning and thunder. (Rätsch 1992, 83)

It was also used in ancient India, where this magical plant was called Soma. It was both a god and a plant dating to 2000 B.C. among the warrior Aryan tribal religions, which swept down into present-day Afghanistan and the Valley of the Indus. Soma was the sacred plant in the Rig Veda of ancient India. R. Gordon Wasson advances the notion: "In a word, my belief is that Soma is the Divine Mushroom of Immortality. My candidate for the identity of Soma is Amanita muscaria, in English, the fly agaric..." (Wasson 1972, 9-10)

A good description of *Amanita's* effects is given by Michael Harner, who quotes Jochelson as follows:

> The alkaloid of "...fly-agaric produces intoxication, hallucinations, and delirium. Light forms of intoxication are accompanied by a certain degree of animation and spontaneity of movements. Many shamans, previous to their seances, eat fly-agaric in order to get into ecstatic states . . . Under strong intoxication, the senses become deranged; surrounding objects appear either very large or very small, hallucinations set in, spontaneous movements, and convulsions. So far as I could observe, attacks of great animation alternate with periods of deep depression. The person intoxicated by fly-agaric sits quietly rocking from side to side, even taking part in conversations with his family. Suddenly his eyes dilate, he begins to gesticulate convulsively, converses with person whom he imagines he sees, sings, and dances. Then an interval of rest sets in again. However, to keep up the intoxication additional doses of fungi are necessary . . . There is reason to think that the effect of fly-agaric would be stronger were not its alkaloid quickly taken out of the organism with the urine. The Koryak knows this by experience, and the urine of the person intoxicated with fly-agaric is not wasted. The drunkard himself drinks it to prolong his hallucinations, or he offers it to others as a treat. (Harner 1973, xii-xiv)

There is some speculation whether the book by Lewis Carroll, *Alice's Adventures in Wonderland*, was a children's novel based on the psychedelic effects of the *Amanita* mushroom. A blue hookah-smoking caterpillar advises Alice to eat from different sides of a mushroom to make herself big or small for her adventures. It is an interesting conjecture, but there is no evidence that Carroll ever used plant substances for this inventive book, but he may have read descriptions about its effects.

The psychoactive compounds in this mushroom contain ibotenic acid and muscimol, which are cholinergic agents (activates the acetyl choline, ACh, receptor) and are located in the mushroom's cap. They intoxicate the brain and cause both the hallucinogenic and side effects. Cholinergic agents usually cause pupils to contract (miosis). The side effects include delirium and ironically mydriasis (pupil dilation). This dilation is probably due to other anticholinergic constituents in the Amanita mushroom such as atropine and muscarine. Muscimol is also a potent GABA-A agonist, like benzodiazepines, which accounts for its sedative effects and the pupillary dilation rather than contraction. These are different constituents than are found in the magic mushroom psilocybin, whose active ingredient is psilocin, a tryptamine-based serotonin agonist.

Amanita is prolific in multiple cultures throughout antiquity, used by shamans around the world. Some fascinating history of this plant involves the Nordic cultures' use of this mushroom and how it pertains to creating the stories about Santa Claus as a shaman during the Winter Solstice period and Christmas time.

The legends of the modern American Santa Claus evolved through Europe in the 19th and 20th centuries. He originated from Saint Nicholas (Nicklaus), who was born in Greece around 280 A.D. and who eventually became a bishop in a small town on the northeastern shores of Asia Minor, what today is modern Turkey. He defended Christianity during the Great Persecution in 303 C.E. by the Romans, who at the time executed those in that faith. Nicholas died in 343 C.E. and was made a saint because of his association with many miracles. The name Santa Claus comes from the Dutch, Sinterklass, and is a nickname for the early Christian Saint Nicholas. St. Nicholas Day is celebrated by Catholics on December 6th. He was revered as a protector of children, orphans, sailors, and prisoners. (Handwerk 2018)

In one tale, three young girls were saved from a life of prostitution when the young Bishop Nicholas secretly delivered three bags of gold to their indebted father to pay off their dowries. Later, the custom of the gift of oranges replaced gold as a less expensive alternative. St. Nicholas was then considered the patron saint of gift-giving, especially to children.

He is not only the patron saint of children, but also of sailors, travelers, and many other professions. As the patron saint of sailors, Nicholas probably accounts for why the modern Santa Claus's home is located at the North Pole, right under the North Star, Polaris; this star is the most stable point in the heavens and does not move as the Earth rotates. The Pole star guides sailors on their sea journeys around the world. It is the most important star in the sky: "Since if you ever get lost, it will help you find your way and orient you." (Carus 2002, 1-3)

St. Nicholas Day fell out of favor in the 1500s after the Protestant Reformation. The gift-giving shifted to the celebration of the birth of Jesus on Christmas. (Handwerk 2018) In early America, the holiday was shunned in New England, but elsewhere it became associated with celebrations of alcohol-fueled, rowdy blowouts, not with gift-giving. Saint Nicholas was revived only in the 19th century through the works of a series of writers. The pipe-smoking Nicholas soaring over rooftops in a flying wagon, delivering gifts, was first portrayed in Washington Irving's 1809 book, Knickerbocker's *History of New York. Later*, in 1821, in an anonymous poem entitled "The Children's Friend," the appearance of St. Nicholas, dressed in furs in a wagon pulled by a single reindeer, was the progenitor of the modern-looking Santa Claus.

In 1822, Clement Clarke Moore wrote for his six children, *A Visit From St. Nicholas*, better known as *The Night before Christmas*. Here the description of the jolly and plump Santa figure, riding a sleigh pulled by eight reindeer, first emerged. The grandfatherly face of a chubby Santa, created by Thomas Nast, a political cartoonist, also added to the modern image of the generous gift-giver.

In his portrayals in America and European countries, Santa Claus usually symbolizes a mythical, magical father figure for young children, the bringer of gifts for the good and punishment for those who are bad. Adults hoped this served as a means of social control over children's behavior throughout the year. As mentioned, for Catholics, the eve of December 6 was called Nicholas Day. Saint Nicholas was often fully dressed in a red bishop's cap (miter), reminiscent of the *Amanita* cap, accompanied by his helper *Ruprecht*, who carried a sack and a rod. His visitations bring all sorts of fruits, nuts, and homemade toys for those children who have been good, and the rod for children with bad behavior. (Rätsch and Mueller-Ebeling 2003, 33-36) The rod was considered the rod of punishment for the bad children during the Christmas season. In the Alpine regions, Ruprecht is known by the more familiar name, *Krampus*. (Rätsch and Mueller-Ebeling 2003, 32-36) Santa Claus is sometimes called Father Christmas and Mr. Winter. In Germany, he is referred to as Sunnerklass, and in Switzerland is known as Samichlaus, as well as by various names in other countries.

Some Christians object to the story of Santa Claus, believing that it dilutes the true meaning of Christmas, which is to honor Christ's birth, and insisting that it fills the heads of children with false, superficial notions. In recent times, many decry the over-commercialization of Christmas and the increase in buying expensive gifts, which has made the holiday more material than spiritual or religious. In days of old, the presents of Santa Claus were usually apples, nuts, almonds, dried fruits, chocolates, candy, toffees, spices, biscuits, winter greens, and homemade toys. As a gift, the hazelnut was holy to Donar, the old Germanic name for Thor, the god of marital and animal fertility.

Santa Claus:
The Shaman and Father Christmas

The pagan, pre-Christian origin of Christmas can be surmised from the usage of *Amanita* muscaria. The fly-agaric mushroom was widely used by Nordic shamans, especially during the winter solstice, and can be traced to the Lapps, the Siberian nomadic people. The red and white mushroom caps are associated with the colors of Christmas, and Santa's pointed red hat and clothing. These north Siberian shamans ritually ingest these mushrooms to make soul flights to communicate with the souls of their ancestors or to make contact with the spirits for divination and to heal the sick. (Rätsch and Mueller-Ebeling 2003, 47)

"According to many researchers, the wonderful voyage of Father Christmas in his reindeer sleigh through the midwinter sky is another surprising remnant of the shamanic flight of the soul . . . of [the] reindeer

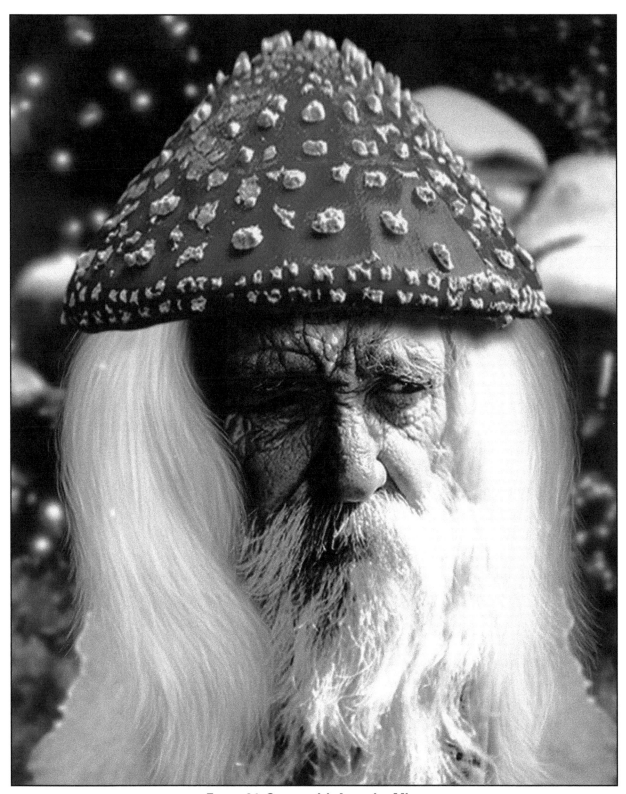

FIGURE **64. Santa with Amanita Miter**
(photo – educateinspirechange.org)

217

breeding tribes of arctic Europe and Siberia. These people experienced their soul flight with the help of the hallucinogenic fly agaric mushroom ... Even Homer considered mushrooms a connection between heaven and Earth." (Rätsch and Mueller-Ebeling 2003, 46-47)

Siberian mythology describes the shaman riding on a reindeer sleigh through the air. Probably it was just one reindeer, since the idea of eight reindeer came about in the 19th century, as noted previously. The goal was to reach the top of the *World Tree*, where the reindeer lived. The association between reindeer and shamanism is ancient. Paintings of reindeer have been discovered on the walls in caves of Ardèche, France, which are approximately thirty thousand years old. (Rätsch and Mueller-Ebeling 2003, 47)

"It has been observed that reindeer appear to get high on the agaric mushroom and they are seen searching for them in the snow. Reindeer are keen for the urine of people who have taken the fly agaric. Likewise, the reindeer who eat the *Amanita* are able to detoxify its poisonous component and to excrete it in their urine. The urine can then be safely consumed by the shaman and retain its full hallucinogenic effects without toxicity. "Among the Siberian peoples, it was a common custom to collect the urine of those who got high on the fly agarics and drink it in order to achieve yet another state of mind —one said to be even more intense than caused by the fly agaric itself." (Rätsch and Mueller-Ebeling 2003, 50)

Another story recounts that these mushrooms, usually found at the base of trees such as ash or fir in the Nordic environment, would be eaten by the reindeer; the urine would then be collected by the shaman and imbibed. In the cold and darkness of a dead winter night, the partaker would return to his cabin, light up the Yule log for heat, and enjoy the spirits of the forest and visions of dancing fairies and wights (ghosts).

The inside of the lodge would appear to be lit with flittering scintillas, and the shaman could experience himself in flight with his reindeer. What better way to celebrate the isolation of wintertime, whether it be for a shamanic ritual or entertainment? Bringing light into the home during peak darkness on the shortest day and longest night is an aspect of the solstice. It symbolizes the rebirth of light, which was appropriated much later by superimposing Christmas (the birth of Christ) onto the solstice celebrated by pagans. It represents the meaning of generosity and hope during this

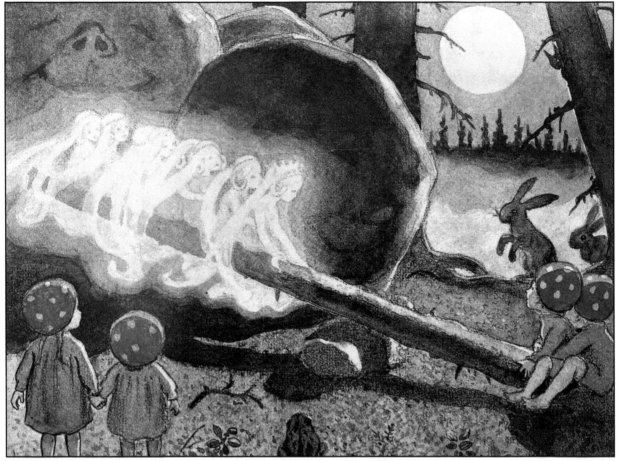

FIGURE 65. *De Sma Skovnisser* by Eska Beskow.
(Rätsch and Mueller-Ebeling 2003, 10)

bleak time of year.

The abilities of Santa to shape-shift, slide down chimneys, and to time-travel to deliver a nearly infinite number of gifts to everyone in one night are also typical features of the visions of shamanic hallucinations. Flying around the world on a reindeer-driven sleigh delivering gifts is a vision of fly-agaric mushroom intoxication and represents the spirit of generosity, hope, and giving at this dark season.

Another Nordic winter ritual is the burning of the Yule log in the fireplace. The log was often from the ash tree, honoring the World Tree, Yggdrasil, in Nordic mythology. This log is burned along with herbs and resins, and the resulting ash was retained for healing and considered holy.

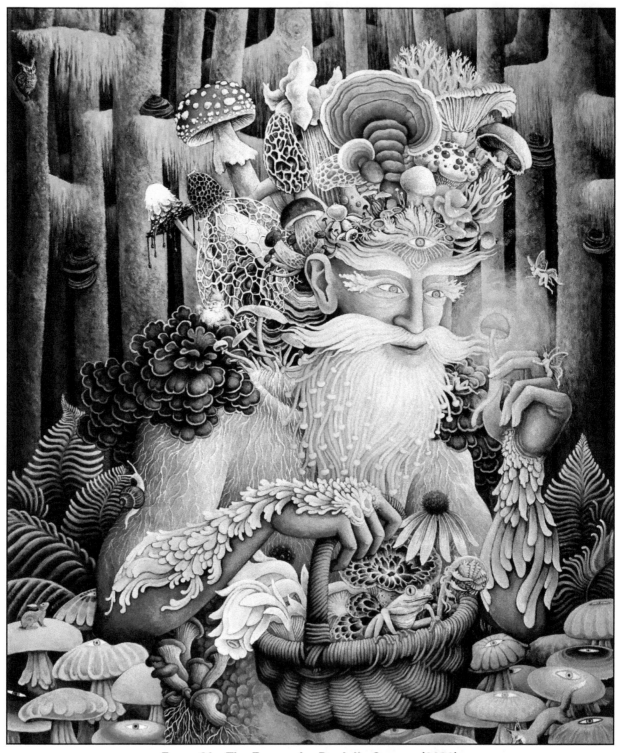

FIGURE **66.** *The Forager* by Danielle Caners. (2020)
(daniellecaners.com)

The ashes were also thought to bring about outward and inward wealth.

From the ashes, the rebirth of life occurs, reminiscent of the Egyptian Phoenix myth. It also represents the ritual of Christ's birth and his return each year. (Rätsch and Mueller-Ebeling 2003, 116) Bringing the Christmas tree into the home and decorating it is presumably a German invention. The earliest written description was in 1419. Others claim the first illuminated tree dates to 1604. Usually, the tree was a Northman fir or the noble spruce and again honored as the World Tree. (Rätsch and Mueller-Ebeling 2003, 21) As recounted in previous chapters, the tree symbolizes an entryway to the lower and upper world in shamanistic practice. It represents the *axis mundi* or world navel, the center-point of culture and the soul. It is a starting point for the shaman's journey.

It is not too far-fetched to theorize the shamanic origins of Santa Claus as the visionary lore filtered down through history from the Nordic regions to Western Europe, and later to the Americas, and melded with the stories of Saint Nicholas. This may be the origin of Santa Claus, the supreme shaman of Christmastime, powered by a mushroom-based hallucinogen perhaps found in reindeer urine. At the very least, this radical speculation makes for interesting conversation around the campfire. Short of being Santa Claus, it's best to steer clear of the *Amanita* species for doing visionary work, due to its tricky toxicity, unless you would enjoy a drink of reindeer urine.

Chapter 24

Snuff Stuff: Yopo and Cebil

As previously described, the hallucinogen DMT (dimethyltryptamine), in its various forms, is found in the skin secretions of the Colorado River toad, *Bufo (Incilius) alvarius* (5-Meo-DMT). As stated, it is an indole alkaloid tryptamine compound sometimes called bufotenine after the namesake toad. This same compound is found in the hallucinogenic snuffs from certain plant beans found in South America. *Yopo*, sometimes called *Cohoba*, has been used as a powdered snuff by tribes in Colombia and Venezuela along the Orinoco River basin. Its scientific name is *Anadenanthera peregrina*, also known in the literature as *Piptadenia peregrina*. It similarly grows in the open grasslands, or *campos*, of the northern Amazon of Brazil. It is used as a snuff, which is finely ground leaves that are inhaled into the nasal cavity. Artifacts utilized with snuff have also been discovered in archaeological digs in the Caribbean, Haiti, and Costa Rica.

One story describing its effects is as follows, "In the beginning, the Sun created various beings to serve as intermediaries between Him and Earth. He created hallucinogenic snuff powder so that man could contact supernatural beings. The Sun had kept this powder in His navel, but the Daughter of the Sun found it. Thus, it became available to man—a vegetal product acquired directly from the gods." (Schultes, Hofmann, and Rätsch 1998, 116-123)

It is commonly used as a daily stimulant, and by the shamans (called *payés*) to induce trances to communicate with their Hekula spirits. The snuff is forcefully blown through a blowpipe into the nostrils of the *payé*. It acts rapidly, causing a profuse flow of mucous, a quivering of the muscles, gesticulating, prancing, and shrieking. The *payé* then collapses into a trance-like stupor, during which visions are experienced. It lasts for thirty to sixty minutes. While in a trance, the shaman would confer with the Hekula

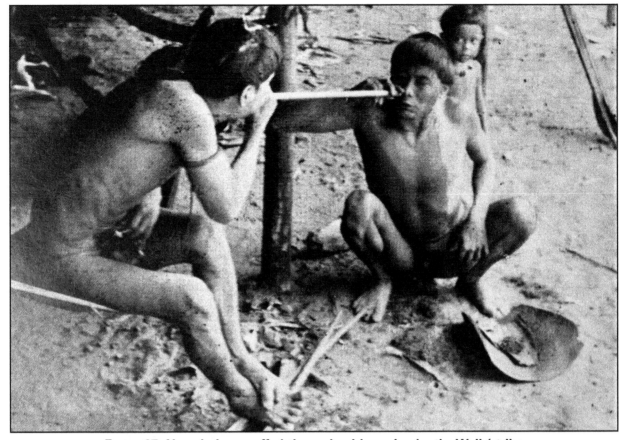

**FIGURE 67. Yopo being snuffed through a blow pipe by the Waiká tribe
in the Venezuela Amazon region.**
(Schultes, Hofmann, and Rätsch 1998, 118)

spirits "to prophesy or divine; to protect the tribe against epidemics of
sickness; to make the hunters and even their dogs more alert." (Schultes,
Hofmann, and Rätsch 1998, 118)

Another similar snuff compound is *Cebil*, sometimes called *Villca*,
which is *Anadenanthera colubrina*, also containing various DMT-like compounds including bufotenine. It can be snuffed or smoked. It is made
from the seeds of a tree found in northwest Argentina. It influenced the
Tiahuanaco culture, considered the mother of Andean civilization; the shamans of the Wichi (Mataco Indians) of this region still use it today. Many
of these Indians have converted to Christianity in recent years, yet they
continue to see the *Cebil* as a holy tree, used by shamans for healing.
The psychoactive effects last about thirty minutes and begin with a feeling of heaviness, followed by hallucinations, featuring worm and snakelike
images, often entwined and coming out of the head of an oracle god.
(Schultes, Hofmann, and Rätsch 1998, 122)

These plants are included for discussion due to their long history of usage by the indigenous tribes in South America, the West Indies, and the Incas of Central Chile, for shamanic healing ceremonies and envisioning. How the ancients discovered these plants is a fascinating question. I presume it was through trial and error, over centuries, while searching for food. There were occasional visionary surprises and enjoyable intoxications. This relates to the concept of the existence of an innate human need to alter consciousness, open the veil of daily reality, and to experience the realm of the spirits and gods. I am unaware of these snuff compounds in common usage among present-day psychedelic journeyers, other than toad medicine or synthetic DMT, as previously described.

Chapter 25

Khat (Catha edulis): The Sacred Plant of Ancient Egypt

Khat or *Qat* (*Catha edulis*) is a flowering plant native to Ethiopia. It contains the alkaloid cathinone, which is a stimulant that causes euphoria, excitement, and loss of appetite. It has been used as a social custom for thousands of years, analogous to the usage of coca leaves in South America and betel nut in Asia.

As with any amphetamine-like drug, khat has abuse potential that can cause addiction and dependence. However, it remains legal in traditional cultures in Africa and the Mid-East, especially around the Red Sea region. In Yemen, it is so popular that approximately forty percent of the water supply goes toward its irrigation in this drought-stricken region. Also, it provides considerable income to the farmers that grow it. Khat addiction is not considered a serious problem in these cultures by the World Health Organization (WHO). It is estimated that five to ten million people use it daily worldwide. It is traditionally chewed by the user but also has been brewed as a tea. In Yemen, its use is so popular, it is estimated that ninety percent of the population use it, including men, women and children as young as twelve.

The Yemeni military used khat to fight with their enemy, the Houthis, a Shia movement. On a daily basis, the Yemenis will buy some from the enemy, stop battle from noon to 4 p.m. to do the khat chewing ritual, then resume fighting again. This Houthis insurgency started in 2004 and has since escalated into a full-scale civil war.

The military liken it to strong coffee or tea, which at first is stimulating, then inducing a languid, mellow, and ruminative mood conducive to deeper conversation. Its supporters do not believe it is addictive, but

225

believe it actually improves productivity by keeping the user awake and focused, much like methylphenidate (Ritalin) or amphetamines (Adderall) in our culture. Stimulants in the chemical of class phenethylamines, including cocaine, methamphetamine, and dextroamphetamine, all used in modern Western cultures, have become recreational drugs with severe abuse issues. This plant's inclusion in this discussion is to honor its sacred usage in Egypt and the region.

The most ancient use of a plant medicine to alter consciousness in recorded history within a sophisticated culture, was in Egypt. It antedated the civilizations of Sumer and ancient China, when the shamans were beginning to scratch the I-Ching oracles on burnt bones. Later, in the Gilgamesh myth of ancient Sumer, the hero sought and found a sacred plant to help in his heroic quest, as Sumerian-Babylonian cuneiform tablets tell us. (Musès 1989, 144)

In Ancient Egyptian ethnobotany, the ingestion of sacred plants was designed to impel a theurgic transmutation to enhance a spiritual experience, and not simply to get high. From accounts it is difficult to know whether an authentic visionary experience occurs with khat, like what is experienced with other entheogenic plants. Khat's euphoric effect may have been a key to the user's meditations on spirit. In psychiatry, it is known that during the hyper-stimulated state in bipolar mania, the individual often has spiritual identifications and hyper-religiosity. The khat-induced state perhaps temporarily mimics mania.

The pharmacopeia of Ancient Egypt described *Three Paths* for plant usage. The hippopotamus path were medicines for bodily therapies at the molecular body level. The second was called the divine cow path, with medicines that could lead the body into therapeutic visionary states, the in-between realm of bodily life and death (the world of Duat or Bardo), likened to *Dante's Purgatorio*. The third path was called the lion's path, beyond the body. These special elixirs were to accelerate a process beyond the molecular body level to a level of dawning, a happier and more lasting sphere, Paradiso. (Musès 1989, 155-156)

In ancient Arabic and hieroglyphic texts (dated 311 B.C.E.), khat is mentioned as "the divine shrubs to prompt the speech of star gods" and to create ". . . a spell to protect against evil beings' attacks." As a sacred plant of ancient Egypt, it was regarded as a food for the gods. (Musès 1989,

149-150) The tradition of khat was passed from the Ancient Egyptians into the Islamic pharmacopeia of Arabia by the 13th century and was used to combat depressed states.

It is an interesting aside that the Baroness Tania von Blixen (aka: Isak Dinesen), who wrote the book *Out of Africa*, on which the movie is based, used khat regularly to attain the creative states in which she wrote many of her stories. (Musès 1989, 158)

Its chemistry was identified in 1930, by O. Wolfes, as a constituent of the alkaloid cathinone, d-norisoephedrine. It is a sympathomimetic stimulant similar to ephedrine and pseudoephedrine, and also related to mescaline. It works primarily on the brain by enhancing the norepinephrine and dopamine circuits. As mentioned, cocaine and other stimulants work similarly.

These compounds in lower dosages are used medically to treat the inattentional type of attention deficit/hyperactivity disorder (ADHD) and as an occasional augmentation strategy for treatment-resistant depression, especially when there are vegetative symptoms. As a class of compounds, stimulants enhance alertness, focus, social confidence, verbosity, creativity, and euphoria, all reasons why they are commonly abused. Adverse effects may include increased blood pressure and heart rate, strokes, insomnia, increased motor activity, agitation, appetite suppression (it is frequently abused as a diet drug), constipation, and impotence (despite increased sexual arousal). At its worst, it can lead to psychosis, mania, and frequently severe paranoia, as in the paranoid speed freak.

According to the eminent psychopharmacological researcher, Stephen Stahl, M.D., the mechanism of action of the stimulant class causes an activation of the neural circuitry by enhancing the neurotransmitters norepinephrine and dopamine in the brain regions of the pre-frontal cortex and hypothalamus. This action improves attention, concentration, executive functioning, and wakefulness. Dopamine also may improve hyperactivity in patients with ADHD, by its action on the basal ganglia in the brain. (Stahl 2006, 29) The reward circuits governed primarily by dopamine may account for its euphoriant and addictive potential. Stimulants are still frequently used by combat pilots on long missions to maintain alertness and focus. Possibly, they were used in the past to enhance warriors in their prolonged and brutal battles.

My personal use of stimulants, other than caffeine, was mostly for all-nighters in college to cram for final exams. I learned a hard lesson that my perceived enhanced learning was state-dependent, and as the drug wore off by morning, I was unable to remember what I integrated for the test. But I certainly do remember the euphoria I felt watching the sunrise.

As a psychiatrist, I know stimulants are highly addictive and challenging to treat. Repeated relapses are common, and long-term remission is difficult, even with the best of treatment. Khat and coca use seem rarely to lead to such dire consequences when used in their cultural context.

Chapter 26
Coca: Stimulants

It is not within the scope of this book to provide details of stimulant usage in either ancient or modern cultures, but there are some interesting facts to be gleaned about these plants. Another honorable mention stimulant widely used is the coca plant, *Erythroxylum coca*, with its four varieties. The psychoactive alkaloid cocaine is extracted from the leaf of the coca plant. The cocaine content in the leaf is very low, between 0.25 and 0.77 percent, so the native use of chewing or brewing coca (*maté de coca*) as a stimulant does not lead to the dangers that the high potency of pure cocaine has on the brain. Coca-Cola actually used the leaf extraction in their drinks from 1885 to 1903.

The plant is mostly cultivated on the eastern slopes of the Andes and in the Amazonian jungles of Columbia, Peru, and Bolivia. It is believed its use is of great age. An origin myth "tell[s] that the first settlers arrived in a dugout canoe dragged by an anaconda and bearing a man, a woman and three plants – manioc, yajé (ayahuasca), and coca." (Schultes 1992, 98) The healthiest and hardest working Indians of the Colombian Amazon chewed enormous amounts without problems while raising crops, hunting, and fishing for their food supply. By contrast, the Indians of the Andean highland, who endured poverty and were indentured to overlords, used it as a food substitute to assuage hunger, not having time to locate or raise food. (Schultes 1992, 99) The leaves were often lightly toasted, pulverized, and mixed with an alkaline ash. During the preparation of the coca powder, tales were often recited about the origin of their race. (Schultes 1992, 106)

Its traditional medical use was primarily to overcome fatigue, hunger, and thirst. It was also effective against altitude sickness, and as an anesthetic and analgesic, for headaches, rheumatism, wounds, and sores. Its high calcium content is why it was frequently used to treat bone fractures. Coca is rich in nutrients such as calcium, potassium, phosphorus, protein, fiber, and vitamins B1, B2, C, and E. Its vasoconstrictive effects were used to reduce postpartum bleeding and nosebleeds.

Coca was also regularly used by the Inca culture in their religious rituals and within their military while fighting off the Spanish conquest. The Spaniards noticed that the Incas could not complete their work without coca. Pre-Incan cultures used coca as part of the religious cosmology of the Andean people. Offerings of it were made to the mountains (apus), the sun (inti), and the Earth (Pachamama). The reading of its leaves was also used for divination. It is unfortunate that the negative effects outweigh the positives of this plant, which is still considered sacred by the indigenous natives, causing them no long-lasting harm.

My personal forays into cocaine abuse occurred when I was younger. During the 1970s and 80s, one could not go to a party without it being offered. Despite its illegality, it was de rigueur to partake among us young professionals. My experience was a transient physical energizing feeling with euphoria. It wore off within the hour, requiring boosters of further nasal insufflation to prolong the effect, but never equaling the initial high. Although enjoyable, my heart would race, and my hands would shake with tremors.

There were never any visual experiences or visionary teachings from it for me or anyone else I knew. It was purely sensory. It was often combined with alcohol to tamp down the nervousness or with marijuana to enhance the sensory experience.

Cocaine is highly abusable, expensive, and addictive. Its pharmacological effects are similar to methamphetamine. Avoid it completely.

Chapter 27

Cannabis:
The Nectar of Delight

"Tradition in India maintains that the gods sent man the Hemp plant so that he might attain delight, courage, and have heightened sexual desires. When nectar, or 'Amrita' dropped down from heaven, Cannabis sprouted from it. Another story tells how, when the gods, helped by demons, churned the milk ocean to obtain Amrita, one of the resulting nectars was Cannabis. It was consecrated to Shiva and was Indra's favorite drink . . . Ever since, this plant of the gods has been held in India to bestow supernatural powers on its users." The Indian Vedas sang of cannabis as one of the divine nectars. (Schultes, Hofmann, and Rätsch 1998, 92-94)

Much has already been written about this ubiquitous plant, so I will provide only a summary of its remarkable historical relationship with humanity. In 1936, the classic movie *Reefer Madness* falsely described marijuana to the public as a dangerous drug, frightening people, and perhaps being one of the main reasons leading to its ban. In the late 1960s, the film reemerged and grew very popular; many of us saw this movie stoned and could only laugh. The *Reefer Madness* theory of marijuana creating widespread social problems never manifested. It was a government-based propaganda lie. At present, it is estimated that 2.7 to 4.9 percent of the population between the ages of 15 and 65 use cannabis worldwide.

Some of the many names that the cannabis plant is known by include marijuana (sometimes spelled marihuana), pot, weed, hemp, wacky tobaccy, kief, bhang (less potent leaves and seeds), and ganja (the potent flowering tops). Skunk is another name for particularly powerful weed with a pungent smell. Hashish is the concentrated resin cake form of cannabis, sometimes called charas. Cannabis can be smoked, vaped, extracted into an oil or tincture for infusion, or processed for oral consumption (edibles) in cookies, brownies, candies, food, and pills.

The most potent part of the plant is prepared from the pistillate flowering tops of the female plants. *Sinsemilla* is a term used for the potent tops before they go to seed. Since what is desired is the potent THC, located in the female plant's flowers, the male plants are usually discarded before they fertilize the flower to prevent the females from going to seed. Once seeds form, the potency of the plant rapidly diminishes.

The psychoactive ingredient is THC, or tetrahydrocannabinol, is one of 483 known compounds in this plant. There are also at least 65 other non-psychoactive cannabinoids, including CBD, or cannabidiol, which is being studied and used for pain control, sleep problems, and anxiety. There are three main plants in the family *Cannabaceae*; they are *Cannabis sativa, Cannabis indica*, and *Cannabis ruderalis.* Today, most strains combine the properties of the first two species, each with varying percentages of hybridization that have distinct psychoactive differences. Some strains are more activating (generally *sativa)*, and some more potent and sedating (*indica*), although researchers question this simple classification. *C. ruderalis* does not appear to have much psychoactivity. The addendum at the end of this chapter provides a list of the compounds found in cannabis.

The effects of cannabis vary from person to person. Users over time, by trial and error and with differences in set and setting, find the potency and qualities they prefer for getting high that resonate with their mind and body. Various strains have different potencies, with resin contents of THC from 15-25 percent. Those most informed about the properties of the numerous strains are the cultivars themselves and the employees at legal dispensaries, not actually doctors. The plant has low toxicity and is without fatal overdoses, unless combined with other dangerous drugs. However, in some branches of native shamanism, marijuana is sometimes combined with tobacco, *Datura, Brugmansia, Amanita,* or *Salvia divinorum* to augment its psychoactive effects, and these combinations may produce toxic reactions.

Marijuana's THC mechanism acts upon the cannabinoid receptors CB1 and CB2, found in the brain and peripheral nervous system. The cognitive effects occur primarily through the CB1 receptor which stimulates the release of the neurotransmitter dopamine, which may account for the pleasurable, euphoric effect. From an evolutionary perspective, it is interesting that these cannabinoid receptors existed in the brain before human usage, and therefore, may confer a survival advantage to humans and primates. This also implies that the brain synthesizes its own endogenous cannabinoid for some type of brain function or regulation. CBD works as an agonist of the 5HT-1A brain receptor, which may account for its anti-anxiety and pain-relieving effects. Cannabis is lipid-soluble and accumulates in the body's fatty tissues; the tissues slowly release THC back into the bloodstream; thus it can be detected in urine testing for many weeks.

Besides the pleasurable effects, some partakers may experience adverse effects, most commonly anxiety, paranoia, social withdrawal, decreased concentration, carbohydrate and fatty food cravings, and short-term memory issues. Also, reaction time and motor function are slowed, affecting driving skills and working with machinery. Rarely, it can trigger a psychotic response in individuals who already have this underlying predisposition. However, there is no clear evidence that it causes psychosis in the general, healthy population. Unlike alcohol, it is rare for a user to experience violent ideation or behavior. The U.S. Federal government classifies it as illegal, yet alcohol, having much greater destructive potential has been legal, before and since the brief period of Prohibition. Regarding marijuana's positive and negative effects, it is said, "It's not so much about the plant, but about the people that use it."

Marijuana does contain known carcinogens in its combustion product and its tar deposits, more so than cigarettes, perhaps because it is inhaled more deeply and for longer durations than tobacco. The question of whether or not marijuana smoking increases the risk of lung cancer remains an open question. To date, well-designed population studies have failed to find an increased risk. However, since all smoke is a lung irritant, chronic users can develop coughs and bronchitis. Animal studies have suggested that THC and CBD may have anti-tumor properties, which may account for the lack of lung cancers. Presently, there is no supporting evidence that smoking marijuana contributes to COPD or emphysema. Short-term use is associated with bronchodilation, which is useful in treating asthmatics. One other health concern is that for the first hour after smoking cannabis, heart rate and blood pressure elevate, increasing the risk of heart attacks and stroke. More research is needed about these health effects.

In addition to the euphoric high that is created, significant research and the experience of many users have brought to light the medicinal properties of the cannabis plant. As a medicine (known as medical marijuana), it can be an alternative for some people to improve anxiety, mood, sleep, pain syndromes (especially due to the CBD component), emotional trauma, glaucoma, migraines, and as an anti-nausea drug in chemotherapy. Often, it has fewer adverse effects than the benzodiazepines, antidepressants, opiates, and sleep medications that are commonly used. Despite some of the adverse effects of marijuana, it is important to remember that most medicines used in traditional medical practice also have side effects or toxic potential. This is true as well of medicinal herbs and other natural products sold without prescriptions.

Over the last few years, many states have decriminalized marijuana, either making it legal or downgrading arrests to misdemeanor charges. There are now numerous cultivars throughout the country, both large-scale and small growing operations. A current irony is that many people are still in prison, unfortunately including a disproportionate number of minorities, serving long sentences for the possession, sale, and growing of cannabis. However, many people of privilege remain free to participate in the new wave of legal marijuana proliferation and make a great deal of money.

The main pleasurable effect of marijuana is enhancement of the senses. Sounds intensify, and, accompanying this is an augmentation and appreciation of musical nuances. Appetite is activated with cravings for carbs (contributing to weight gain for chronic users). Food tastes better, smells intensify, and the sense of touch is enhanced. Many individuals experience an aphrodisiac effect with enhanced libido and erotic pleasure. Everything appears more colorful and animated. With eyes closed or in a darkened environment, beautiful visual displays can occur much as with psychedelics, but generally less intense.

Often an appreciation of the environment is enhanced, leading to an increased connection with nature, plants, and animals. For some, it helps improve pain symptoms and mood, decreases nausea, and provides an overall improved sense of well-being. Anxiety relief and stress reduction often occur. An enhancement of spiritual feelings frequently accompanies the high; this is one reason that it is used as an augmenting agent in shamanic practices. One common response to marijuana is an enhanced sense of humor, with uncontrolled giggles as a side effect. This may be one of its unheralded health benefits.

Unfortunately, the above effects do not occur for some individuals, and therefore this plant spirit is not for them. It is common for some users, after their high wears off, to feel a mental dulling, energy loss, heaviness, and sleepiness. While stoned, most people find it more difficult to concentrate, to read, or to complete focused or sequential tasks; short-term memory is diminished as well. Time feels like it slows down. The pleasurable effects occur at the expense of mental sharpness, not good for students trying to study or those in the workplace. For a person who work on an assembly line, coffee breaks with caffeine as a stimulant help them keep their focus on routine, repetitive tasks. But, if someone took a "pot" break, they would probably sit around and discuss whatever comes to mind, spacing out, not completing necessary tasks.

It would seem likely that a drug that enhances pleasure, reduces stress, pain, and boredom would be a perfect candidate for causing addiction. In reality, studies and experience indicate that marijuana is much less addictive than alcohol, cigarettes, narcotics, cocaine, or methamphetamines, especially regarding physiological dependence. However, chronic use can be psychologically addicting, for example, by allowing a person to avoid conflictual situations. It can impede developmental maturation for a young person trying to master life's demands, which require learning conflict resolution skills. Chronic users start avoiding the struggles inherent in living. It can impede the development of authentic social relationships. These are the main reasons why cannabis is not recommended for young people with developing brains. In addition, poor school performance has been associated with marijuana use among teens.

Regarding addiction, there can be withdrawal effects for chronic users who abruptly stop, but they are not as severe as the abstinence symptoms seen with alcohol, opiates, cigarettes, benzodiazepines, and amphetamines. Irritability, sleep disruption, cravings, depression, and lassitude are common complaints with abrupt stoppage of regular marijuana use.

As a psychiatrist, I have witnessed both sides of the coin. On the negative side, cannabis can cause amotivational syndromes in many chronic users. I have seen people presenting with complaints of adverse reactions, dependency on the drug, and a lack of manifesting progress in their life. By the time these patients appeared in my office, there were typically many other concurrent psychological issues. Admittedly, as a doctor, my sample was already skewed toward pathology. I have witnessed many relationships that became dysfunctional as a result of the social distancing effects of cannabis abuse. There are 12-step marijuana programs available for support, but they are rare. Complete abstinence is the only solution. Most patients with occasional use were not adversely affected. If one wants to have recreational highs, then from a doctor's perspective, marijuana is less toxic and preferable to alcohol and other drugs.

One controversy that remains is whether cannabis is a "gateway drug" to other, harder drugs such as narcotics, cocaine, or methamphetamines. There is no definitive proof of this hypothesis, but it must be acknowledged as a possibility in high-risk groups or among poly-drug users. It is more likely that other social factors are the gateway to any type of drug abuse.

Although cannabis can launch a person to other realms of consciousness, it is not in the same category as the other psychedelic drugs previously described. Navigating in daily reality is less problematic than on the more powerful hallucinogens. It can enhance creative thinking and expression for a few hours, but eventually, one becomes more somnolent and soporific, creativity becomes dulled, and one can withdraw more into their shell. I read somewhere in an old book that the musician Joni Mitchell said that marijuana made her more musically creative for the first hour of the high but then dulled her creative manifestations.

Besides the marijuana plant's uses as a euphoriant and an enhancer of sensory awareness, certain strains of *Cannabis sativa* are called hemp and have multiple industrial uses. Some products include rope, clothing, textiles, shoes, paper, insulation, bioplastics, hemp concrete, and biofuel. Hemp seeds (called akenes) contain important nutrients as a foodstuff. It is a common component of bird seed mixes. The akenes are a complete protein, high in unsaturated fatty acids, loaded with vitamins and minerals, and are a great source of iron. It can also be eaten as a leafy vegetable or made into hemp milk and juice. The fast-growing hemp plant was first spun into useable fiber fifty thousand years ago. It is completely legal, and often, its products are sold in health food stores. Hemp usually has low concentrations of THC and a higher CBD ratio; it is not considered psychoactive, although hemp is an equivalent term to marijuana in older writings.

A Fascinating History:
The Big Bhang! Historical Anecdotes

The fascinating pedigree of the cannabis plant since ancient times, in all cultures and historical periods, speaks to its power and longevity among humans. Following is a summary of anecdotes and history about this very old and beneficial plant.

Cannabis originated in central Asia, where cultivation of it may have occurred for over ten thousand years, since Neolithic times. A ubiquitous plant, it has been used as a medicine in India, China, the Middle East, Southeast Asia, South Africa, and South America. The long list of ailments for which it was used for treatment includes malaria, constipation, analgesia, dysentery, rheumatic pain, dysmenorrhea, fever reduction, inducing sleep, epilepsy, stimulating appetite, relieving headaches, and improving digestion. It was also purported to be used to treat snake bites, venereal disease, and aid in childbirth. Although this list is dated, as stated earlier, cannabis is increasingly used to alleviate a number of discomforts today. Cannabis did not come to use in the modern West as a medicine until the mid-1800s, as will be discussed later. (Grinspoon and Bakalar 1993, 3-4) "The earliest reference to the mind-altering effects from cannabis appears in the Atharva-Veda of the second millennium. B.C., when it was already regarded as one of the five sacred plants of India." (Stafford 1992, 157)

"The Tibetans considered *Cannabis* sacred. A Mahayana Buddhist tradition maintains that during the six steps of asceticism leading to enlightenment, Buddha lived on one Hemp seed a day . . . In Tantric Buddhism of the Himalayas of Tibet, *Cannabis* plays a very significant role in the meditative ritual to facilitate deep meditation and heightened awareness. . . One preparation [in India], Bhang, was so sacred that it was thought to deter evil, bring luck, and cleanse man of sin." (Schultes, Hofmann, and Rätsch 1998, 97-98)

The use of hemp was thought to have been introduced in Persia by an Indian pilgrim (A.D. 531-579), but it is known that the Assyrians used hemp incense as far back as the first millennium B.C. From Islamic influences, it eventually spread to Africa, where it is known as Kif or Dagga. It entered into the archaic native cultures in its religious, medicinal, and social contexts among the Hottentots, Bushmen, and Kaffirs, where its

237

vapors were inhaled. It was also used in the Congo by the Kasai tribes. (Schultes, Hofmann, and Rätsch 1998, 98-99)

In addition the warrior-barbarian cults, especially the Scythians, spread the use of this plant, eventually to the Greeks and Romans of classical times. The Scythians were a nomadic tribe that roamed the Russian steppes from Turkistan in the east to the Altai mountains of Siberia. They introduced hemp into northern Europe as well. Around 500 B.C., the Greek writer Herodotus described the Scythians making a steam bath with smoldering hemp seeds thrown on hot stones that "gives out such a vapor as no Grecian vapor bath can exceed; the Scyths, delighted, shout for joy." (Schultes, Hofmann, and Rätsch 1998, 94; Stafford 1992, 159) Apparently, the records state that it was probably the *Cannabis ruderalis* strain which was used by the Scythians.

Some scholars believe that cannabis cultivation may have originated in China in Neolithic times rather than in central Asia. Its psychoactive properties were known at least by 2000 B.C.E. during the reign of the legendary emperor Shen-Nung. In these early periods, there is some evidence that it was used by Chinese shamans as a hallucinogen until the demise of this practice when European contact was made. (Schultes, Hofmann, and Rätsch 1998, 94)

"Democritus [460–370 B.C.] wrote that it was occasionally drunk with wine and myrrh to produce visionary states; Dioscorides [40 – 90 A.D. and the Roman physician] Galen [129 – 200 A.D.] indicated that it was valued for its medicinal and therapeutic uses. Galen also recorded that this herb was often passed around at banquets to promote hilarity and joy." (Stafford 1992, 160) Marco Polo wrote about hemp being used for food; he described the secret order of Hashishins consuming it, explaining they used it to explore the rewards in store for them in the afterlife. In later European history, the famous Swiss physician, philosopher, and theologian, Paracelsus (1493-1541), the father of alchemy, also became aware of cannabis products and their use.

Charles Baudelaire, the 19th century French poet, believed that the creative ability could be greatly enhanced by cannabis. He wrote in *Les Paradis Artificiels*: "This marvelous experience often occurs as if it were the effect of a superior and invisible power acting on the person from without . . . This delightful and singular state . . . gives no advance warning. It is as unexpected as a ghost, an intermittent haunting from which we must draw, if we are wise, the certainty of a better existence. This acuteness of thought, this enthusiasm of the senses and the spirit must have appeared to man through the ages as the first blessing." (Schultes, 1998, 101) The French illustrator and engraver, Gustave Doré (1823-1883), also used cannabis to inspire his art.

Hemp cultivation began in the British colonies, first in Canada in 1606, then Virginia in 1611. The pilgrims brought it to New England in 1632, where its fibers were used for work clothes in pre-revolutionary times. It was also used for shamanic purposes in the sacred ceremonies of the Cuna Indians of Panama and the Cora Indians of the Sierra Madre region in Mexico. It was introduced into these cultures by early Europeans.

Modern History

The first Western physician to study cannabis was Sir W.B. O'Shaughnessy, M.D., a young professor of Medicine at the University of Calcutta. He first experimented with it on animals; once he realized it was safe, he started treating patients suffering from rabies, rheumatism, epilepsy, and tetanus (presumably by reducing muscle spasms). He returned to England in 1842 and provided the drug to pharmacists. It then began to be prescribed by doctors in England and the United States for a variety of conditions. (Grinspoon and Bakalar 1993, 4) Reports of its benefits were reported by Dr. R.R. M'Meens to the Ohio State Medical society in 1860. He compared its hypnotic efficacy to opium. In 1887, H.F. Hare recommended cannabis to reduce anxiety and to distract a patient's mind from a terminal illness and other painful conditions.

Its uses for these conditions began to decline by 1890 after the use of hypodermic syringes for injecting opiates became common and allowed for faster pain relief. Various cannabis preparations had different potencies, and therefore its effects were more erratic. Synthetic drugs for fever control (aspirin) and sleep (chloral hydrate, barbiturates) also hastened the end of cannabis as a medicine. These synthetics were more stable compounds than cannabis, but as we now know they have their own dangers. (Grinspoon and Bakalar 1993, 7-8)

The end for cannabis came when the Marihuana Tax Act was enacted in 1937 and undermined further experimentation and research. This led the Federal Bureau of Narcotics, led by Harry Anslinger, to consider the drug an addictive narcotic, and thus a cause of social problems in society. As mentioned before, the movie, *Reefer Madness* was part of Anslinger's campaign to demonize marijuana and further its illegal status. (Grinspoon and Bakalar 1993, 8)

With increasingly widespread recreational use of marijuana in the 1960s, Congress passed the Controlled Substances Act in 1970, which placed cannabis as a Schedule I drug, its most restrictive category. It meant that the drug has no medical use, a high potential for abuse, and cannot be safely used even under supervision by a doctor. (Grinspoon and Bakalar 1993, 13) This category is the same as drugs like heroin, cocaine, and methamphetamine. Efforts to downgrade cannabis to the lower Schedule II, where it could be used under medical supervision, continued to be rejected by the DEA, even though numerous states have decriminalized its usage. As we understand today, it can be prescribed by specific, certified M.D.s for various medical conditions that are not improved by standard medications.

In December 2012, Washington, closely followed by Colorado, became the first states to legalize the use and sale of recreational cannabis, and in 2013, Uruguay became the first country to legalize it. Canada made recreational consumption legal on October 17, 2018. As of this writing, these two countries are the only ones to legalize it thus far. Despite it now being decriminalized in many states, the U.S. government still considers its use illegal and can continue to prosecute people at will.

With its usage dating to the Neolithic era, it is clear cannabis is ingrained in human history as a medicine, food source, fabric, and a mind-altering drug to enhance pleasure and spiritual communion. For those interested, much more information is available from a wide variety of sources on its use, properties, and research in our present time.

Addendum: Various Chemical Compounds Found in Cannabis

THC: (*delta-9-tetra hydrocannabinol*) – Chief psychoactive component found in marijuana. Legal is some states but remains illegal federally.

CBD: (*cannabidiol*) – First isolated in 1940, this is the second-most famous chemical in marijuana. Remains legal under federal law. Used for health purposes such as anxiety, insomnia, inflammation, pain, and some types of seizures.

CBN: (*cannabinol*) – Barely noticeable in fresh cannabis, but its presence increases over time since it is a byproduct of THC oxidation. So, leave an open bag of your stash at home. Touted as a sleep aid, possible potent antibacterial, appetite stimulant, and may be helpful in delaying onset of ALS symptoms. Can be found in Kikoko's Tranquili-Tea, and other edibles.

CBC: (*cannabichromene*) – A lesser-known cannabinoid that shares the therapeutic properties of CBD and THC, but without the psychoactive impact of the latter. Being studied as a possible cancer fighter and acne inhibitor. Studied as possibly having therapeutic value as a pain blocker, anti-inflammatory, and migraine inhibitor.

Delta-8-THC: (*delta-8-tetrahydrocannabinol*) – Psychoactive like THC, although not as intense, and can be extracted from hemp, which makes it federally legal. It's now trendy and offered in gummies and vape pens.

THCa: (*tetrahydrocannabinolic acid*) – Non-psychoactive but is being studied as an anti-inflammatory, an antiemetic, and a neuroprotectant to help battle Parkinson's, as well as a cancer fighter.

THCv: (*tetrahydrocannabivarin*) – Energetic, uplifting high with reputation as sports car weed. Battles anxiety, epilepsy, Parkinson's, and is an appetite suppressant.

CBG: (*cannabigerol*) – Converts to THC and CBD as the cannabis matures. Touted for CBD effects for symptoms of inflammatory bowel disease, slows growth of colorectal cancer cells, and battles glioblastoma.

(For more information, see Tschorn 2021.)

Chapter 28
Tobacco (*Nicotiana*)

Tobacco has been used historically and in shamanic practices is considered sacred, and for this reason I have included it for discussion in this chapter. Tobacco is a sacred plant for many Native American tribes and for some South American Indian people. It is sometimes called a "treacherous and beloved poison" and is the most common addictive substance for human beings. It is "the most toxic plant regularly used by humans. . . the model of ambiguity: healer and killer, ally and seducer." (Pendell 1995, 31) Tobacco is found to be more habit-forming and harder to quit than opium, heroin, cocaine, amphetamines, benzodiazepines, and other sedatives. Yet, it is legal throughout the world largely due to its economic advantages.

Tobacco is the common name for the genus Nicotiana and is in the family of Solanaceae. As discussed previously, other plants within this family include tomatoes, potatoes, chili peppers, deadly nightshade, henbane, *Datura*, and hemlock. There are five dozen wild species of tobacco, but the main cultivated forms are *Nicotiana tabacum*, and *Nicotiana rusticum*. These have the highest content of nicotine, especially the rusticum variety. However, in cigarettes, the tabacum species is the most widely used preparation.

Nicotine is a highly addictive stimulant, harmala-based alkaloid. Pharmacologically, it is structurally similar to the neurotransmitter acetylcholine (ACh). It has a stimulating, arousing effect that can enhance learning and performance of simple tasks. It is active in both the sympathetic and parasympathetic nervous system and at the neuromuscular junction. The dried and cured leaves are consumed in cigarettes, cigars, and pipes. Also, it can be chewed, snuffed, and occasionally used as an enema. If taken as a drink or tincture, it can be extremely toxic and deadly. That is why it is often chewed and absorbed through the mucous membranes.

The World Health Organization (WHO) claims that tobacco usage is the world's single most preventable cause of death. According to the website cancer.gov, about 7,000 different chemicals are found in tobacco smoke and more than seventy are linked to cancer. Also, chemicals are found naturally in the tobacco plant itself and some are absorbed from the soil, air, and from fertilizers. Manufacturers of cigarettes use additives to enhance flavor, reduce harshness, and promote smoother burning. Ammonia substances are added to change how the nicotine can be more easily absorbed into the body.

Added sugars, when burned, become carcinogens. During the curing process, carcinogens called TSNAs (tobacco-specific nitrosamines) form within the tobacco leaves and can cause lung and esophageal cancer. The main compounds are ammonia ($NH3$), acetaldehyde ($C2H4O$), and TSNAs. Other chemicals include arsenic, benzene, and the toxic metals: beryllium, cadmium, and chromium. (If people read about all these adulterants, it is a wonder how anyone would choose to smoke.)

Additionally, hazardous gases, 1,3-butadiene, hydrogen cyanide, and carbon monoxide are formed. In addition to the nicotine, these chemicals are also deposited as tar in the lungs and promote cancer. Other than cancers, as we all know, smoking causes heart disease, strokes, COPD, including emphysema and chronic bronchitis, and peripheral vascular disease of the lower extremities, which can lead to amputation. It also increases the risk of tuberculosis, certain eye diseases, and problems of the immune system, including rheumatoid arthritis.

The bottom line: there is no such thing as safe tobacco. (See fda.gov/tobacco-products) The least harmful cigarette is Natural American Spirit products, which are certified organic, additive-free, and natural. An October 2019 study from Columbia University examining 25,000 people reports that smoking five or fewer cigarettes a day can cause almost as much lung damage as smoking two packs a day. Low tar cigarettes are no better since users usually inhale the smoke more deeply and smoke more of these cigarettes.

History

Before becoming known and consumed in Europe, tobacco had long been used in Mesoamerica and South America prior to 1492. It was more widely cultivated in the New World than maize and spread to the Old

World more quickly than any plant in history, presumably because of the nicotine's powerful addictive effects. The English settlers learned its use from the Powhatan and Opechancanough Indians in Jamestown. It soon became a successful cash crop and a favorite among sailors and mariners, who exported it to the Europeans. The early sailors told of its aphrodisiac qualities, causing women to be more passionate and active after smoking it, in contrast to its more common association as a post-coital custom. There were many reactions against the tobacco plant when it conquered Europe. In the seventeenth century, possession of tobacco became a capital offense in Russia and Germany. (Pendell 1995, 36-38)

Tobacco's religious use is still common among some northeastern Native American tribes, including the Cree and Ojibwe, where it is offered to the Creator in the sweat lodge and pipe ceremonies. Other Native Americans continue to use tobacco in various ceremonies for purification, blessing, and as a gesture of unity by passing the peace pipe to each other. They believed the smoke itself would rise to the spirit world and would serve as a conduit of communication. "The Indians say that this smoke is very wholesome for clearing and consuming superfluous humors of the brain. Moreover, if taken in this manner, it satisfies hunger and thirst for some time." (Pendell 1995, 33 – in Thevet, 1558)

The following is an excerpt from a Crow and Hidatsa Indian story, as relayed in a promotional piece from the Santa Fe Natural Tobacco Company, which makes American Spirit cigarettes. The piece is titled "The Legendary Origin of Tobacco", it speaks to the plant's mythic sources:

> *One day Starboy's wanderings brought him to the foot of the highest mountain. No one had climbed it before, but Starboy started the slow climb upward without hesitating. Somewhere near the sky, Starboy fainted. A shining silver man appeared to him. The man was a star. He told Starboy that he was his father but he spent his life traveling far beyond the earth, and he said he would not pass near the mountain again in his son's lifetime. 'And so to show my love and concern for you, my son, I will give you the gift of strength and colors of the sunset. Keep this plant with you wherever you wander, and in springtime plant it everywhere you go. Tend the scarred beds, and harvest them when they are tall.'*

With these words, the star plunged his hands into his own silver chest. When he pulled them out again, they were full of tobacco. He told Starboy that tobacco would make everyone in their family strong and free. To share the tobacco and its power, the people must be adopted into Starboy's family. Starboy listened carefully, but was too overwhelmed to speak. He nodded his head gratefully, and his father burst away from him, back to the sky."

Another vignette relayed by Santa Fe Natural Tobacco originates with the Keresan Pueblo Indians, in which Turkey Buzzard offers tobacco to the people. This occurred after a Pueblo young girl insulted the Hummingbird, bringing the tribe misfortune. Finally, the girl goes out on a quest to make amends, where she encounters the friendly Turkey Buzzard:

The girl climbed down from the cliffs and began her long, slow return, while Turkey Buzzard circled high above her. When the people from the Pueblo first saw Turkey Buzzard circling, they thought the girl was dead, but as they watched, he circled closer and closer, and they became hopeful. Finally, Turkey Buzzard arrived in the Pueblo and went straight into the kiva to talk to the People. He asked them about their offerings and prayers, which had been many and beautiful. Soon he realized they had forgotten to offer Tobacco. 'Bring sacred Tobacco, and let's make new offerings,' said Turkey Buzzard. 'When the smoke drifts up into the Sky World, the Spirits will see and remember the beauty of the rain clouds, and they will be inspired to fill the sky with them.' The People and Turkey Buzzard took Tobacco in cornhusks and walked to each corner of the village, offering Tobacco smoke to the East, South, the West, and North, and then to the center. As they did this, the fragrant and purifying smoke filled the entire village and drifted upward to the Rain Spirits...When the Spirits smelled the delicious, rising smoke, and saw its beautiful swirls drifting toward them, they softened and forgave the People.

The more potent *Nicotiana rustica* variety of tobacco may possess hallucinogenic properties and is used for shamanic practices involving the stages of shamanic initiation: sickness, death, and rebirth. In shamanism, tobacco has to do with transferring and attuning energy. An anonymous tobacco shaman states that "Tobacco is the muscle. Maybe mushrooms or the little leaves of the Shepherdess [*Salvia divinorum*] will give you seeing, but you need tobacco for the muscle, to clean the sickness out." (Pendell 1995, 39)

The term *Picietl* was the Aztec term for the inebriating magical plant thought to be *Nicotiana rustica* (or perhaps the species *glauca*). The Aztec diviners used it as they did with other psychedelic plants, including peyote (contains mescaline) and *ololiuqui* (*Turbina corymbosa*) which contains lysergic acid alkaloids. Today, Indian healers use Turkish tobacco (pisiete), which is the rustica species, for magical purposes. (Rätsch 1992, 144)

The Aztecs have been able to find the pathway to the Spirit World by offering songs when smoking tobacco. One Aztec story also relayed by Santa Fe Natural Tobacco reflects this:

> *One man was sent in search of the other Gods. He walked until he reached the western sea. Then he sat down at the edge of the World and cried out to the Gods. Tezcatilopoca, the Jaguar, heard him and took pity. Tezcatilopoca whispered to the man that he should smoke fragrant tobacco and sing the most beautiful songs he could. The man did this with all the reverence he could gather. As the delicious fragrance of the tobacco mingled with the sweetness of songs and drifted upward into the Spirit World — the Gods witnessed this and felt appreciated. These offerings tempted the Gods to follow the smoke back down to the Earthquake World, and they carried their beautiful musical instruments and played them to accompany the man.*

Nicotiana tabacum is a very important plant utilized in South American shamanism and is native to the Andes. The *payés* (shamans) use tobacco to blow smoke over a sick patient along with appropriate incantations as a curing practice or prelude for further treatments. (Schultes and Raffauf

1992, 87) Tobacco was essential training for young payés in virtually every tribe in the Colombian Amazon. Among the Yukuna tribe, a student payé would snuff tobacco in large amounts for some years to master shamanic knowledge and to prove proficiency as a healer. Among the Tukano tribes, tobacco was used by the payés to increase their knowledge and understanding of the benevolent and malevolent spiritual forces required for communication during healing seances. It was thought of as food for the spirits and that it opened the mind to understanding the wisdom of this realm. (Schultes and Raffauf 1992, 90-92)

Tobacco is a fascinating plant in the shamanic pharmacopeia. Its history reflects its ambivalence in its addictive, toxic, spiritual, and healing potentials.

Chapter 29

The LSD Story: Lucy in the Sky with Diamonds

During the Summer of Love in 1967, the album *Sgt. Pepper's Lonely Hearts Club Band* was released. I was hitchhiking through Europe that summer and when I returned to start medical school at UC San Francisco, my girlfriend introduced me to the song "Lucy in the Sky with Diamonds," an obvious reference to LSD. That summer, LSD use was in full swing throughout the world, largely due to Timothy Leary, recognized as the primary influence opening up awareness in the collective populace to psychedelic consciousness. LSD had already been in use for some time before then, but my first experience took place in 1967, while I was traveling through Istanbul. I was given a dose by someone I met at the infamous Pudding Shop, where I imbibed it late in the evening. This pudding shop was a known meeting place in old Istanbul where drugs were exchanged. (The chocolate pudding was also good.)

My experience was not a guided journey, but one filled with visions and an awe-inspiring adventure as I traipsed around old Istanbul after midnight, oblivious to any dangers. At one point I was being chased by robbers through the streets, but being young and strong, I was able to outrun and escape them. I was never the same after that LSD trip; as I started my medical training, I realized I was the only student I encountered there who had had such an experience. It was formative and opened up the "doors of perception."

LSD, d-lysergic acid diethylamide tartrate, was discovered by Albert Hofmann, a chemist who worked for Sandoz Pharmaceuticals in Basel, Switzerland. In his laboratory, he synthesized a series of ergot analogues containing lysergic acid as possible medicines, especially for use in obstetrics, geriatrics, and for migraine headaches. The twenty-fifth chemical

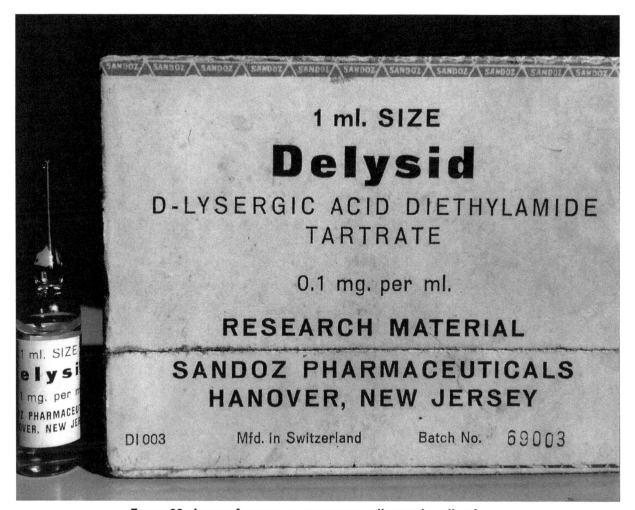

FIGURE 68. Image from an anonymous colleague's collection.

Hofmann synthesized was called LSD-25, which was being evaluated as a respiratory stimulant in experimental animals in 1938. It displayed strong uterine contractions, but the results were insufficient to continue research and Sandoz ceased testing it. LSD was marketed by Sandoz by the name Delysid (see Figure 68).

Later, in 1943, Hofmann reexamined this compound for possible other uses, and as part of the lore around this drug, accidentally spilled a drop on his finger, which apparently was absorbed into his bloodstream. Interesting things began happening, which he describes as follows:

> I suddenly became strangely inebriated. The external world became changed as in a dream. Objects appeared to gain in relief; they assumed unusual dimensions; and

colors became more glowing. Even self-perception and the sense of time were changed. When the eyes were closed, there surged upon me an uninterrupted stream of fantastic images of extraordinary plasticity and vividness and accompanied by an intense, kaleidoscopic-like play of colors. After about two hours, the not unpleasant inebriation, which had been experienced whilst I was fully conscious, disappeared. (Stafford 1992, 37)

Prior to this experience, mescaline from peyote had been the most powerful known hallucinogenic agent. LSD is about four thousand times as potent. Hofmann may have spilled about 20-50 mcg (micrograms) on to his skin. Three days later, he decided to try 250 mcg, and his experience was even more powerful, starting as he bicycled home from his laboratory. This experience lasted longer with more intense imagery, some of which was grotesque, with mind-body distortions, synesthesia, and ego loss. Later he experienced a renewed sense of life flowing through him as well as extraordinary pleasure when he walked into his garden as the sun shone through the spring rain. There was no apparent hangover effect. (Stafford 1992, 38)

By the 1950s, LSD was being actively researched as a possible psychotherapeutic agent. It was also being tested by the CIA, Army, Air Force, and Navy as an agent for intelligence and interrogation, which led to controversy. However, in 1966, curbs were placed on further research due to its widespread abuse by the general population.

In 1954, a batch of the Sandoz drug was studied in Prague, Czechoslovakia, where a medical student, Stanislav Grof, became intrigued with its effects as a possible model to study psychosis. Eventually this led to Grof's ground-breaking book, *Realms of the Human Unconscious: Observations from LSD Research*, published in 1975. Once LSD became outlawed, Grof developed a non-drug method to achieve altered states of consciousness, known as *Holotropic Breath Therapy*.

Neurochemically, LSD works on both the serotonin and the dopamine systems. It works primarily on the serotonergic 5-HT 1A and various 5-HT 2 receptor subtypes, as well as being an agonist for the dopaminergic D 2 receptors. Actually how this activation opens up the channels for consciousness expansion and spiritual experiences is unknown. The effects normally last from six to twelve hours depending on dosage, set and setting, age, and weight, but the non-peak aftereffects can last longer. There is no evidence for tolerance or addiction to this drug, but repeated frequent usage sometimes leads to behavioral dysfunction and difficulty dealing with daily reality needs and the clarity of a focused mind needed for employment and relationships.

LSD-25 is a synthesized drug and is considered to be the archetypal mind-expanding agent of the present time. As noted previously, the term psychedelic means mind-manifesting. However, there are plant-based chemicals that have been used indigenously that contain derivatives of lysergic acid. The Zapotec Indians of Oaxaca, Mexico, and the Aztecs called this medicine *ololiuqui*, derived from the morning glory plant (*Turbina corymbosa*), sometimes identified as *coaxihuitl*, or snake plant. The seeds contain the hallucinogenic compound. The morning glory seeds, along with the psilocybin mushrooms, were considered sacred by these cultures, dating back to at least 500 C.E. *Ololiuqui* in the Nahuatl (Aztec) language means round thing, which refers to the seeds of the morning glory. Notably, in our society, people who unwittingly try morning glory seeds as a substitute for LSD usually wind up feeling sick, much like solanaceous (*Datura*) intoxication.

Another morning glory variety is known as *Ipomoea violacea*, which also contains seeds containing lysergic acid, and is six times more potent than the seeds of *Turbina corymbosa*. The *Ipomoea* flowers were sometimes named heavenly blue, pearly gates, wedding bells, summer skies, and blue star. These psychoactive seeds are used primarily by the Mazatec and Chinantec Indians shamans in the Oaxaca region of Mexico.

The seeds are usually ground and placed in a gourd with water. The solid particles are strained out and the infusion is then drunk. The patient is placed in a secluded and quiet place at night, and then the shaman performs a diagnosis and divination about recovery from an illness. The usage of these medicines is considered to be "gifts from the gods." It is believed that the plant spirits will also give information about lost objects. Modern Indians have incorporated Christian elements with the pagan, not unlike the modern mixture of spiritual beliefs as used in some ayahuasca ceremonies of the Santo Daime religion in South America. (Schultes and Hoffman 1998, 170-175)

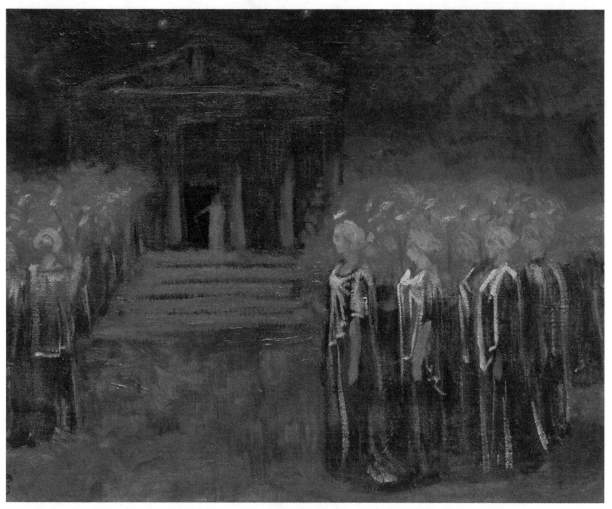

FIGURE **69.** *The Eleusinian Mysteries* **by Paul Serusier. (1888). Vision of Persephone in spring emerging from the Temple of Eleusis to the followers of the Eleusinian Mystery.**

Lysergic acid amides (ergot derivatives) have also been found in numerous other species of plants, most notably in the Hawaiian Woodrose (*Argyreia nervosa*). This is a woody climbing vine with silver foliage and violet flowers, 100-150 times more potent than morning glory seeds. It has been used as an inebriant by poorer Hawaiians and can produce a full-blown hallucinogenic experience, although more tranquil than LSD. Hangovers involving nausea, constipation, vertigo, blurred vision, and inertia have been reported. Some users feel invigorated, as though they have been on a vacation. (Stafford 1992, 98-99)

The synthetic lysergic acid diethylamide differs from the lysergic acid found in ololiuqui only by the replacement of two ethyl groups (LSD) for two hydrogen atoms. Interestingly LSD-25 is about 100 times more potent than the hallucinogenic dose of ololiuqui. The molecule of these ergot alkaloids has a tryptamine ring structure that is also found in psilocybin and the neurotransmitter serotonin. (Stafford 1992, 98-99)

Ergot (from French, meaning rooster's spur) is the name for a fungal growth, the sclerotium of a mushroom known as *Claviceps purpurea*. It is a parasite that grows on rye, barley, wheat, and some grasses. In modern medicine, ergot derivatives (non-hallucinogenic, e.g. Pitocin) are used to cause uterine contraction to enhance a stalled labor and to decrease post-partum hemorrhage after delivery. Cafergot and Bellergal are ergots used to treat migraine headaches. Hydergine is sometimes used as a treatment for geriatric cognitive enhancement.

In ancient Greece, the ergot fungus that infected the rye plant was called the sacred *kykeon* drink, presumably used in the yearly ritual of the Eleusinian Mysteries to welcome back Persephone from the underworld in Spring. This apparently caused a collective visionary state in the followers, who experienced a vision of her return (see illustration). This ergot usage during the Mysteries is a theory. (Wasson, Hofmann, and Ruck 1998, 35-37)

During the Middle Ages, the ergot parasite affecting rye caused epidemics of ergotism in people who ate bread made with infected rye. Thousands of people died. Ergotism is characterized by convulsive seizures and gangrene of the extremities. Frequently the bodily extremities would turn black and fall off. It was called St. Anthony's fire, for the patron saint founded to care for victims of ergotism, and at times known as St. Vitus dance. (Stafford 1992, 90) From the above, we can conclude that for humans, the ergot and morning glory derivatives have both poisonous as well as visionary potential.

My personal experience with LSD has been similar to that which I have had with psilocybin mushrooms. Its effects last longer and seem more electrical in quality, less organic or smooth than those of the mushroom. The visions and insights are similar, bringing both psychological and spiritual teachings. In my shamanic experiences as related earlier, it was often used in low doses as an adjunctive booster with San Pedro cactus and iboga. A negative experience (bad trip) can be quickly turned around by a change in setting, music, and a calm, experienced guide or presence.

LSD is included in the description of visionary medicines because of its rich correspondences to numerous botanicals containing similar chemistry. One can only wonder what the evolutionary function of such plant chemicals represents for the development of brain neurotransmitters and links to spiritual transcendence.

Interview with Albert Hofmann

During my time of shamanic exploration, I had the good fortune to cross paths with a psychiatric colleague, Charles Grob, M.D., with whom I shared many good conversations. He went on to become a prominent expert doing legal research into the potential psychiatric and medical uses of various psychedelic medicines, including ayahuasca, psilocybin, and MDMA. He is currently a professor of psychiatry at Harbor-UCLA in the division of Child Psychiatry. (see foreword by Dr. Grob)

Grob edited a classic book in 2002, *Hallucinogens*, which included writings from numerous prominent authors on the subject. One of the chapters recounts a conversation he had in November 1996 with Albert Hofmann, the discoverer of LSD. Hofmannn was 90 years old at the time, still in robust health. (He lived to be 102 years old, passing away in April 2008.) A discussion of the past, present, and future issues surrounding psychedelics took place; I believe it is worthwhile to include some excerpts below due to the significant insights Hofmann had about the long history of these agents. I liberally quote the interview that Dr. Grob had with Albert Hofmann. He not only describes the pros and cons of hallucinogen usage, but he provides insights into how they may enhance nature consciousness and the relationship between the material and spiritual world: (see Grob, 2002, 15-22)

"I believe that shortly after LSD was discovered, it was recognized as being of great value to psychoanalysis and psychiatry . . . and for fifteen years it could be used legally in psychiatric treatment . . . until it became part of the drug scene in the 1960s [primarily fueled by Timothy Leary]." (16)

"LSD became a drug of the street and inevitably it was made illegal . . . It is my hope that finally the prohibition is coming to an end, and the medical field can return to the explorations which were forced to stop thirty years ago." (17)

In recommending Delysid (LSD) when it was legal: "As an aid to psychoanalysis and psychotherapy . . . It was specifically stated on the package insert that the psychiatrist . . . should first test it on himself." (17)

"But as long as people fail to truly understand psychedelics and continue to use them as pleasure drugs and fail to appreciate the very deep, deep, psychic experiences they may induce, then their medical use will be held back." (18)

"And people need a deep spiritual foundation for their lives. In older times it was religion, with their dogmas, which people believed in, but today those dogmas no longer work." (18)

"This material world, made by humans, is a dead world, and will disappear and die. I would tell the young people to go out into the countryside, go to the meadow, go to the garden, go to the woods. This is a world of nature to which we belong, absolutely . . . Open your eyes, and see the browns and green of the earth, and the light which is the essence of nature . . . and realize that it is possible to experience the beauty and deep meaning which is at the core of our relation to nature." (19)

"When I was a young boy . . . I had profound and visionary encounters with nature . . . my first experiences with LSD were very reminiscent of these early mystical encounters I had had as a child in nature . . . But many people are blocked, without an inborn faculty to realize beauty, and it is these people who may need a psychedelic in order to have a visionary experience of nature." (19)

"It is important to have the experience directly. Aldous Huxley taught us not to simply believe the words, but to have the experience ourselves." (19)

"[W]e have accumulated an enormous amount of knowledge through scientific research in the material world . . . What science has brought to life is true . . . But this is only one part, one side of our existence, that of the material world . . . and matter gets older and changes, so therefore as far as our having a body, we must die. But the spiritual world, of course, is eternal, but only insofar as it exists in the moment." (19-20)

"But we must also accept that the material world is only the manifestation of the spiritual world . . . I believe that what is occurring in the material world is a reflection of the spiritual state of mankind." (20)

"If we were to read about spiritual things, it is only words. We must have the experience directly . . . Not words, not beliefs, but experience." (20)

"The pathway for this is through psychiatry . . . not the limited scope of modern biological psychiatry . . . it will occur through the new field of transpersonal psychiatry . . . These psychiatrists must become the Shamans of our times . . . But remember, the more powerful the instrument, the more the chance of damage occurring if it is not used properly . . . there were unfortunately many occasions where psychedelics were not treated with proper respect, and used the wrong way, and consequently caused injury . . . It was a great loss for medicine and psychiatry, and for mankind." (21)

"Hopefully, it is not too late to learn from these mistakes, and to demonstrate the proper and respectful way psychedelics should be used." (22)

Chapter 30

The Story of Ecstasy: MDMA, Adam and Eve

The inclusion of a synthetic drug in this overall discussion about shamanism is due to the reality that MDMA has become both widely used as a recreational drug and as a new treatment for PTSD in psychiatry. It is also utilized in healing circles to develop a sense of inner peace and conflict resolution among small groups or with couples. MDMA is known by several names, commonly Ecstasy, XTC, Molly, and Adam.

According to Ralph Metzner, the term Adam was given to MDMA by a group of West coast therapists who used this drug in underground psychotherapy. Adam is not meant to represent a man, but instead Adam and Eve as an androgynous ancestor. Adam is a highly significant symbolic figure in Gnostic and Hermetic writings. According to C.G. Jung, Adam represents the primordial and original being, the unity of life, and primal innocence in the Biblical account of the Garden of Eden. The themes are variations of returning home, finding one's original nature, celebrating one's ancestors, and feelings of connectedness with fellow human beings, animals, plants, and all the forms and energies of the natural world. It is these latter qualities that connect MDMA to the concept of Adam/Eve. (See Adamson 1985, 4-5. Note that Sophia Adamson was a pseudonym of Ralph Metzner.)

MDMA stands for the chemical 3,4 methylenedioxymethamphetamine. Its chemical structure is also related to the mescaline molecule, and its actions appear to be a hybrid, in between a pure amphetamine and a hallucinogen. However, it is not classified as a hallucinogen for it does not impart the transpersonal visionary experience typical of LSD and the other plant entheogens previously described. Instead, it is called an *empathogen*, or empathy-enhancer. It creates a sense of openness, compassion, peace, acceptance, forgiveness, healing, rebirth, emotional bonding, caring, heightened awareness, and celebration. (Adamson 1985, 1)

The experience of MDMA is overwhelmingly a positive one for most partakers, and thus it has developed a large following among party-goers and ravers. It is sometimes called the "love drug" due to its capacity to enhance a positive emotionality and closeness with others, as well as an enhanced perception of sensuality. It facilitates communication and a euphoric sense of empathy and well-being. It has been used as an adjunct in New Age spiritual practices to enhance prayer, introspection, and meditation. Although it can dissolve boundaries of hostile and traumatic feelings in users, it does not cause the ego-dissolution typical of other hallucinogens.

These properties explain why MDMA, and its similar predecessors, MDA and MMDA, have been used by various psychotherapists since the 1970s and why it is of interest in the current treatment of PTSD patients. In addition to use at parties and in psychotherapeutic settings, it is often used in casual, smaller, intimate circles for introspection, conversation, relaxation, and music appreciation, creating a loving and connected feeling tone among the participants. It promotes sensuality and pleasure, but, like all amphetamines, it may inhibit sexual performance. It may create personal and spiritual feelings, but it is definitely an empathogen and not a "cosmic experience of the godhead."

Is this drug too good to be true? Unfortunately, there can be adverse side effects from its usage; after all, it is amphetamine-based. It can produce dehydration and hyperthermia, which has caused death among rave users and at parties. It often causes bruxism (teeth grinding), jaw clenching, insomnia, elevated blood pressure and heart rate, diarrhea, anxiety, and irritability, typical of amphetamines. Frequent use can lead to addiction, dependence, tolerance, and/or withdrawal symptoms, although less than cocaine or methamphetamine. Rebound fatigue, impulsivity, anxiety, and depression are not uncommon among users. There is controversy about whether or not even moderate use may cause neurotoxicity. Impairments in cognition, learning, memory, and attention have been found in regular MDMA users. It is moderately teratogenic, known as causing neuro- and cardiotoxic effects on the fetus during pregnancy. It may also cause some damage to the serotonergic axon terminals in heavy users, but probably not casual users.

Pharmacologically, MDMA acts pre-synaptically through the release

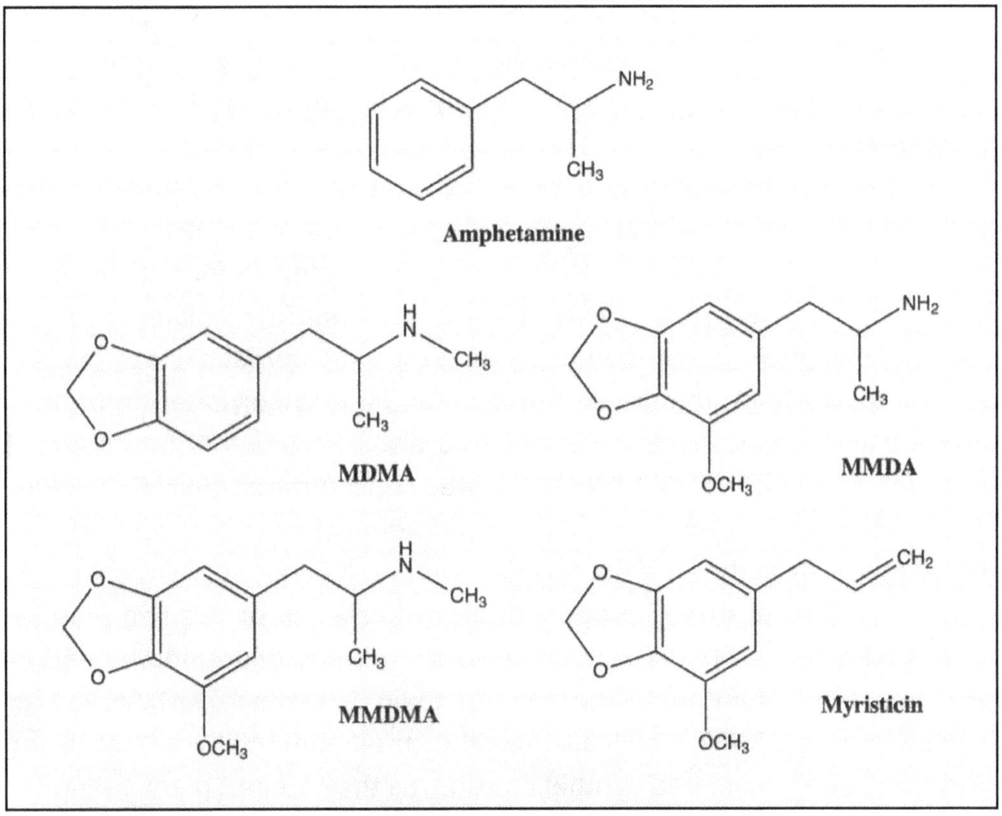

FIGURE 70. Chemical structure of MDMA and similar molecules.

of the neurotransmitters serotonin, norepinephrine, and dopamine, and to some degree, operates at the post-synaptic 5HT1 and 5HT2 serotonin receptor site. As a reminder, dopamine is a neurotransmitter connected with reward behavior and euphoria. Because of these dangers and widespread ungoverned use, the DEA banned this compound in 1985, and the FDA designated it as a Schedule I controlled substance, the most restricted category.

In 2017, the FDA began allowing research into MDMA-assisted psychotherapy, especially for the treatment of PTSD, where it shows promise. Rachel Yehuda, Ph.D. of Mount Sinai's Traumatic Stress Studies Division, has done important research in this area. The well-being it produces creates optimal conditions for processing traumatic and challenging material. In the therapeutic setting, the usual dose starts at 125 mg, followed by a booster of 62.5 mg after two hours if desired, with supervision by two clinicians. The effects can last up to eight hours. The patients usually receive two or three sessions over twelve weeks. Special training is required for clinicians who do MDMA-assisted therapy. It is found that the results can be long-term.

The history of MDMA is noteworthy as it was first synthesized and patented by the German pharmaceutical company Merck in 1912. The company was trying to develop a substance that would stop abnormal bleeding, as well as conducting research into stimulants. It was first isolated from the chemical myristicin found in nutmeg oil. When the myristicin was metabolized into MMDMA, the psychotropic potential was purported to be less potent than MDMA. Elemicin and safrole are other contributing components found in nutmeg but are at a lower concentration than myristicin. These drugs can be synthesized by the amination of myristicin and safrole, but by themselves they are not found in nature. It is not economically feasible to synthesize these compounds from sassafras or nutmeg. People have tried to mimic the effects of these stimulant compounds by eating large quantities of nutmeg, which can be toxic. In essence, MDMA and its precursor analog MDA, which also has the street name Sally, sassafras, or sassy, must be considered synthetic drugs, as they are not plant-based.

Although MDMA is an older drug, its widespread usage began in the 1980s. Its earlier sibling congener, MDA (3,4-methylenedioxyamphetamine), was more available and could usually be found through local underground dealers since the 1960s. The psychotropic effects are quite similar in that it was called the "hug-drug," and sometimes called the "Mellow Drug of America." MDA has a checkered history dating to WWII. It was studied by military and intelligence groups attempting to develop drugs to be used as truth serums or incapacitating agents for interrogation. In 1953, the army was involved in experimenting with MDA with a psychiatric patient at the New York State Psychiatric Institute, at an intravenous dose of 500 mg which proved fatal. (Shulgin and Shulgin 1992, 717)

MDMA and MDA are both stimulants, and like amphetamine, they are in the phenethylamine drug class. They share similar qualitative psychotropic effects and are considered empathogens. MDA is purportedly the more potent agent, supposedly gentler, and longer-lasting (6-8 hours) than MDMA (3-5 hours). The subjective experience may vary by the dose, set, and setting. The street drug versions are often adulterated. Since MDMA became popular, it seems to be the empathogen of choice presently in both therapeutic and recreational settings.

In the book, *Through the Gateway of the Heart*, edited by Sophia Adamson (aka Ralph Metzner), are detailed numerous accounts of the subjective experiences of these empathogens, should more information be desired.

Personal Experience

I first became aware of the healing potential of empathogens after reading the classic book, *The Healing Journey: New Approaches to Consciousness,* by the Chilean psychiatrist, Claudio Naranjo, published in 1973. It is an engaging primer to read if one is able to procure this book. Naranjo studied at Harvard and Berkeley and became a key figure at Esalen Institute in Big Sur, involved in their spiritual teaching programs. Naranjo was perhaps among the first to study the psychotherapeutic effects of MDA and MMDA. Additionally, he also researched the potentials of the drugs ibogaine and harmaline. He carried out these studies in Chile since they were illegal in the U.S. and was far ahead of his time in studying the peak experiences encountered with these drugs.

I first tried MDA around 1972, when it was given to me by a medical resident. It was an unhappy time in my life after my divorce, before I moved to Denver, where I met my present wife. I found that it helped me to ease the pain and to reconnect to loving feelings again. What endeared me the most was its enhancement of the quality of mellow lyrical music, rather than hard electric rock or psychedelic music. I first listened to Jackson Browne, Dan Fogelberg, newer Bob Dylan, David Bromberg, Jerry Jeff Walker, and J.J. Cale while high, and grew to love this style of now-classic Americana music. I found that everything seemed to flow in life in a connected way, and the rough edges and the negative "creepy crawlers" of my psyche eased.

After one year of training as a resident in radiology in L.A., I became disenchanted with this field so I quit and was promptly inducted into the Air Force and stationed in the Denver area. The Vietnam war had not yet ended. I served my two years as a general medical officer, starting out as a Captain, and then being promoted to Major toward the end of my tenure. The MDA experiences helped me reformulate my career path from studying radiology to reading more about Jung, symbolism, art, and various cultures, ultimately leading to my career in psychiatry.

I continued to experiment with MDA (I had never heard of MDMA at that time) multiple times, both alone and with small groups. Even though it truly can be called the love drug, once the effects wore off and some time passed, these connections felt misplaced and left me with a false sense of long-term bonding with these same people. The authenticity of the experience, although pleasant, did not last. I also felt the after-effects of fatigue, malaise, decreased concentration and focus, and negative cognition, all symptoms of low-grade depression. Perhaps, if a seasoned guide had led these sessions, a better integration may have occurred for me, but I was usually the guide for others.

Unlike the more potent mind-expanding psychedelics, in my experience the lessons of MDA were not enduring. The hallucinogens always provided new and variable teachings. After many experiences, I decided to abandon MDA as a teacher. Its abuse potential was more evident than its healing potential, at least for me. However, I need to credit MDA for changing my musical preferences. The musical journeys were always incredible and imprinted my psyche. Later in life, I tried MDMA several times when it became popular in the 1980s. My experiences were indistinguishable from those with MDA. The described aftereffects were also similar.

My conclusion is that there are "different strokes for different folks." What may work well with one individual may not resonate for another, which as described earlier is true of the various plant medicines. There are different spirits in each plant and chemical. What emerges may depend upon some unknown, innate affinity, or the mutual attraction between a particular "spirit-molecule" and an individual.

Currently, MDMA is phase III trials by the FDA with humans for the treatment of PTSD. It is showing some promising results, and it may someday become a legal pharmaceutical psychiatric agent, but whether the effects are long-lasting remains to be seen. As with psilocybin and other hallucinogens, it has the effect of breaking down rigid psychological barriers and creating a sense of unity from enmity. Reprogramming of the entrenched dysfunctional neural networks occurs, and the amygdala's fight or flight response is bypassed or ameliorated, so that the traumatic material can be processed objectively without the terrifying emotional accompaniment. Psilocybin and other hallucinogens also show promise in alleviating psychiatric illnesses, especially as microdosing is being tried by many who have failed traditional psychotherapeutic drugs. Rick Doblin, the founder of MAPS (Multidisciplinary Association for Psychedelic Studies), has been the leading crusader for MDMA's use legitimately for psychiatric treatment. Again, it is unclear if the medicine alone or the therapeutic support by psychedelically trained therapists creates the longer-term beneficial responses and integration—caveat emptor. It is crucial not to over-idealize any of these potential medicines as becoming the savior of mental illness, but at least there is more hope in the future.

Chapter 31
2C-B: Erotic Erox

The inclusion of 2C-B, a synthesized hallucinogen (2,5 – dimethoxy – 4 bromophenylethylamine hydrochloride) is, in part, due to my obsessive need for completeness and to its use as an adjunctive chemical to synergize with the mescaline effects of the San Pedro cactus (*Trichocereus pachanoi*) during some of the visionary journeys I described earlier. By itself, San Pedro is slow to take effect, if at all. But 2C-B is a full-on hallucinogen in its own right in the class of phenylethylamine stimulants. It can create ecstatic as well as fearsome imagery. Usually there are very colorful prismatic light patterns, sometimes kaleidoscopic, and erotic, likened to low doses of LSD.

The psychedelic chemist and explorer, Alexander (Sasha) Shulgin, synthesized this compound and described his subjective effects: "My body was flooded with orgasms – practically from just breathing. The lovemaking was phenomenal, passionate, ecstatic, lyric, animal, loving, tender, sublime. The music was voluptuous, almost three-dimensional. Sometimes the sound seemed distorted to me, underwater like . . . but I could choose to concentrate on the beauty of the music or the inadequacy of the sound's quality, and mostly chose to concentrate on the beauty." (Shulgin and Shulgin 1991, 503-506) The dosage here was 20 mg; at higher doses, such as 24 mg, he stated, "I am totally into my body. I am aware of every muscle and nerve in my body." (Shulgin and Shulgin 1991, 503-506) At even higher doses, there was more dissociation of mind and body, much like those described with ketamine. At 100 mg, he described facing his death as a unique experience and was surprised to return to the land of the living. (Shulgin and Shulgin 1991, 503-506)

At times, 2C-B is used at the end of an MDMA journey to help integrate mental and emotional discoveries. Some even advocate this combination for future use in psychotherapy once more research is done. (Shulgin and Shulgin 1991, 503-506)

It is manufactured by some clandestine labs under the name Erox.

Indeed, it produced erotic imagery and feelings for me. It had the effect of being somewhat reminiscent of a low-dose LSD/Ecstasy mixture. It seemed a bit too electrical and metallic for my taste, without resulting in any significant wisdom teachings, so I abandoned my experimentation with it. It may find use someday as a true aphrodisiac at low doses. With its stimulating effects, it also may present some danger for those with heart and blood pressure issues.

Chapter 32

Ketamine

Ketamine is a psychedelic, an antidepressant, an antianxiety agent, an anesthetic, and a club drug of abuse called "Special K" or "Vitamin K." I first became aware of ketamine through the work of John C. Lilly in the 1970s. I was a resident in psychiatry at UCLA and read his book *The Center of the Cyclone*, on his explorations of inner space. He developed the sensory isolation tank sometime in the 1950s, and he later had experiences of altered states in it using psychedelics, including LSD and ketamine. As a neuroscientific and psychonautical explorer, Lilly also became fascinated with the non-human intelligence of dolphins. Besides all of these contributions, I remember that he would periodically be hospitalized at the Neuropsychiatric Institute at UCLA for psychotic delusional episodes induced by high doses of ketamine while in the tank. At that time, I also became aware that it was used as an animal tranquilizer, so I dismissed this drug as not being practical or safe for humans.

However, this medicine was rediscovered in psychiatry around 2006 as being very useful in rapidly alleviating treatment-resistant depression symptoms (TRD) and relieving suicidal ideation. It is now being used as well for the treatment of post-traumatic stress disorder (PTSD), and other psychological issues. Since 2006, there have been over 2,000 scientific papers on its use in treating various psychiatric conditions. Initially, it was used intravenously in research settings with patients who were not responding to traditional antidepressants or adjunctive combined medication protocols. For decades, since the launching of the SSRI Prozac in January 1988, there had been no significant breakthroughs in antidepressant medications. Serotonin, norepinephrine, and dopamine had been the primary targeted neurotransmitter amines being researched for antidepressant action.

In contrast, ketamine is primarily involved with the glutamine neurotransmitter system in the brain. No one understands its mechanism of action fully, but apparently it is a partial antagonist of the NMDA

(N-methyl-D-aspartate) glutamate receptor, thus blocking glutaminergic function, allowing downstream synaptogenesis of new dendritic connections, as well as increasing neuroplasticity in the brain.

Glutamine is a prevalent neurotransmitter in the nervous system that is generally excitatory. Therefore, blocking its action is presumably sedating and calming. This mechanism does not explain how quickly it can work after an infusion. Also, its psychedelic properties may account for its clinical benefit. Ketamine seems to exert a neuroprotective function as well, which has led to the development of other NMDA antagonists used to treat dementias (e.g., memantine) after head trauma, strokes, brain hypoxia, and seizures. Naltrexone (Narcan), an opioid blocker used as an antidote for opioid overdoses, prevents the antidepressant effect of ketamine, so perhaps the mechanism of action may be mediated through the opiate receptor site. Memantine, another NMDA antagonist used in dementia, does not have an antidepressant effect.

Ketamine-assisted psychotherapy (KAP) is a new model for treatment for treatment resistant depression (TRD), post-traumatic stress disorder (PTSD), obsessive-compulsive disorder (OCD), addictive disorders, and anxiety states. According to the research psychiatrist Gary Bravo, M.D., the medicine may work by the above-noted chemical mechanism of action (blocking glutamate) by itself or by the combination of its psychedelic (ego-dissolving) or psycholytic (ego-loosening) aspects. Ketamine's psychoactive properties may enhance better access to unconscious processes leading to insight and self-acceptance. (Bravo 2021, 328) In clinical practice, some psychiatrists administer the medicine alone, but many combine it with KAP, often based on a cognitive-behavioral therapy (CBT) model.

Historically, ketamine was first synthesized in 1962 as an anesthetic, considered safer than others in use since it does not cause pulmonary or cardiac suppression; additionally, its dissociative properties created an indifference to pain. It was used during the Vietnam War as a battlefield anesthetic. It is still used for its anesthetic action in elective surgery or pain relief in the ER, usually as part of a cocktail that reduces the requirement for more potent opioids. It is chemically related (a class called arylcyclohexylamines) to the compound PCP (angel dust), which was first synthesized in 1926 but abandoned in the 1970s because of its dangerous psychomimetic (mimicking schizophrenia) effects. This class of compounds is not found in nature.

Ketamine developed a reputation within the psychedelic community throughout the 1980s and 1990s as a club and date-rape drug, and cases of addiction and dependence occurred. For this reason, it was classified by the DEA as a Schedule III drug in 1999, which allowed a more unrestricted path for research exploration. (All other psychedelics are in the Schedule I legally banned category, meaning there is a high abuse potential and no medical use.) Hopefully, this will change, but ketamine remains the only legal hallucinogen.

The psychedelic dose of ketamine is about six to ten times less than the dosages necessary for anesthesia. The psychoactive effects compare favorably to the other classic psychedelics, such as psilocybin or LSD. For patients, it is usually administered intravenously (IV) or intramuscularly (IM), but it was approved by the FDA in March 2019 as a nasal spray called esketamine, under the proprietary name, Spravato.

According to Gary Bravo, M.D., "Ketamine can bring people into non-ordinary states of consciousness [NOSC] that have the potential to disrupt rigid and maladaptive mental structures, reorient self-narratives, loosen defense mechanisms, and increase opportunities for personally meaningful experiences." (Bravo 2021, 331) There is some evidence to suggest that the dissociative and psychedelic effects correlate with therapeutic outcomes. He relates some first-person accounts of reported use, both with lower doses for depression and higher dose psychedelic sessions:

> "I felt like I traveled far away from my body and had a different perspective about my life and my problems . . ."
>
> "It is as if it is the space of death. If there is existence of consciousness after death of the physical body, this could be it . . ."
>
> "It was as if I completely understood the interconnectedness or oneness of all things . . . On returning to my body, there was an overwhelming sense of peace, as if I now understood the answers to the ultimate questions."

As with any medicine, there are possible side effects. Commonly, headaches, dizziness, dissociation, blurred vision, and elevated blood pressure may occur but usually resolve after the procedure. Longer-term effects, usually with repeated and higher dosing, can cause addiction in recreational users, cognitive deficits, anxiety, liver toxicity, and chronic cystitis with a dysfunctional bladder. Compulsive ketamine abuse seems linked to the dissociative state that some crave. Thankfully, recreational usage is low in the general population and may be declining.

The medical use of ketamine derivatives in the described psychopathologies is usually done by intravenous dosing of 0.5 mg/kg over a 40-minute infusion cycle. About 60-70 percent of treatment-resistant depressed (TRD) patients improve within 24 hours, but the remission tends to wear off after ten days for most. A treatment course of six intravenous sessions over three weeks is the typical protocol. Practitioners also use sub-lingual, intramuscular, and nasal spray dosing to maintain an extended remission. Some practitioners use the higher psychedelic dosing of 1.0 -1.5 mg/kg to optimize outcomes.

Evgeny Krupitsky conducted the most comprehensive research on *ketamine psychedelic psychotherapy* (KPP) in the former Soviet Union, starting in 1985 primarily for use as a treatment for alcoholism. He found that the patients who experienced a transpersonal experience had better outcomes than the controls, who had the typical aversive therapy. His patients experienced less anxiety and depression. Later, in 1999, he utilized KPP for heroin addiction. The high-dose ketamine patients experienced better results and fewer relapses than those on low-dose ketamine. Psychotherapy had an additional benefit in outcome. (Kolp 2014, 84-140)

Eli Kolp, M.D., was also trained as a psychiatrist in the USSR; he immigrated to the United States in 1981. He continued Krupitsky's work with multiple addictive disorders, including alcohol, drug, and food addictions. For political reasons, university facilities did not want to support or fund further addiction research with ketamine or other hallucinogens, so Kolp developed his treatment protocols in a private practice setting in Florida. He developed an extensive six-week preparatory procedure for his patients before ketamine administration. This included a whole food plant-based diet, meditation practice, contemplation of the Self and God, optimal hydration, detoxing from screen time, sedatives, stimulants, alcohol, sugar, and nicotine. Also, daily physical exercise was required. Only then was the ketamine administered first in low doses, then in the higher psychedelic doses.

Integration of the experience consisted of up to sixty hours of psycho-educational courses, including communication and relational-skills training, anger management, and transpersonal and existential group therapies. Also, art and music therapies and nutritional counseling were offered, all taking place in a residential treatment setting. No wonder he got such good results. It would be useful to carry out a controlled study with ketamine-only patients without therapeutic support and conditions. Kolp also used ketamine for his patients with treatment-resistant depression (TRD) and augmented it with an MAOI (monoamine oxidase inhibitor) antidepressant to maintain remission.

An article by Kolp and his colleagues describes four stages of ketamine dissociative states of nonordinary consciousness. The first is a mild dissociative state at lower doses, which generated a state of empathy (empathogenic) and mental relaxation, a pleasurable state. The ego remains preserved but detached in a positive state. The person can work with unresolved trauma. The second stage (intermediate) is characterized by an out-of-body experience (OBE), where one feels a separation from the body (non-corporeal consciousness), travels through space and time, and can have intense psychedelic visions and archetypal encounters. The third stage is a severe dissociative state where one has a near-death experience (NDE), moving through a tunnel, and reviewing one's life.

Using high doses, Kolp describes the fourth level as a profound dissociative state, which is ego-dissolving and transcendental (EDT), sometimes leading to a mystical experience and an identification with divinity. Sometimes meeting ancestors occurs in these last two stages, and there can be a profound death and rebirth experience. To an outsider, the person under the influence may appear to be in a catatonic state. (Kolp 2014, 84-140) These ketamine states are also typical of other psychedelics but without any attending anxiety if given in a safe set and setting. Whether these higher psychedelic doses are necessary for treating TRD and other psychopathologies is still under investigation.

Kolp describes the paradisical experience of one of his alcoholic patients that is reminiscent of other psychedelic medicines:

> *My mind left my body and I found myself in Heaven . . .*
> *flying high above the silver and gold clouds . . . in the company*

of thousands of angels who were there to guide and protect me. The music was exceptionally lovely and we were ascending higher and higher . . . eventually arriving into the Garden of Eden. The angels showed me the beauty of their home and then helped me to soar directly to the throne of Jesus... I felt Jesus's unconditional love and understood that all my sins were forgiven. He blessed me and I promised Him to never ever touch another drink of Vodka again. I then returned to my body . . . feeling joyful and full of bliss . . . and I knew–with all my heart–that I got reformed forever. (Kolp 2014, 106)

Another patient reported this experience:

My body became dissolved as an icicle in a hot water and my mind began steadily expanding as an inflating balloon. First, I got aware of the surrounding space around me and actually became the growing trees . . . and birds. . . and animals. . . and other people. . . in the range of 300-400 yards around me. This expansion did not stop. . . and my mind continued progressively getting larger and larger. . . until it embraced the entire Earth and I became aware that I am a part of the Great Mother Gaia. At that point my individual mind disappeared and became transformed into collective mind. The collective mind continued rapidly expanding to the entire Solar system. . . to the entire Milky Way galaxy. . . and eventually the entire Universe. The individual awareness of the Universal Mind and my personal Soul became part of the Universal Consciousness. God and I are One, and We are omniscient, omnipotent, and omnipresent. The experience seemed lasting for the eons. . . and all that time the awareness remained "everything is exactly as it should be" . . . "We are all One" . . . "everything is perfect . . ." (Kolp 2014, 112)

Ketamine practices have proliferated in psychiatry, both with and without psychotherapy. Because IV ketamine is expensive, approximately $2000 per session, many practitioners use IM injections to bring the cost down significantly to about $400. The nasal spray, esketamine, for ongoing maintenance, reduces the price even more. Cognitive-behavioral therapy (CBT) seems to augment the response, at least with TRD and OCD.

Questions remain about the best dosage requirements as well as the experience and training of the administering practitioner. The safety of prolonged repetitive usage needs further research since the positive effects of a ketamine session can be short-lived and with a high relapse rate in the patients with TRD. Another question is whether psychedelic dosing levels aid in the healing process as is the case with other traditional hallucinogens. If so, practitioners, including doctors, will need training in the process of assisting the navigation of non-ordinary altered states of consciousness (NOSC), other than just having a psychopharmacological understanding of the drug.

According to Kolp and Krupitsky, the mechanism of action of ketamine is the blockade of thalamo-cortical projections and activation of the interactions between the frontal cortex and limbic structures. The thalamus's primary function is to relay sensory and motor signals to the cerebral cortex. Ketamine blocks the transmission of incoming signals from all sensory modalities, which reinforces the interactions of the cognitive and emotional minds. Presumably, it removes a filter or veil between the conscious and the unconscious mind and disconnects the self from objective reality. This results in an awakening that resembles the altered states of ego dissolution transcendence (EDT) and near-death experiences (NDE) of death and rebirth.

This mechanism has been postulated for other psychedelic medicines, although this remains a speculative theory. (Kolp 2014, 110) Its agonistic effect on the opioid receptors in the brain may account for its analgesic, anti-anxiety, and euphoriant properties. It also seems to enhance dopaminergic activity, which may add to its pleasurable and reward effects.

As far as the shamanic usage of ketamine in healing circles, its current prevalence remains unclear. A startup company Silo Wellness, founded by Mike Arnold in Oregon, is trying to create a framework for psychedelic retreats for healing. In November 2020, the voters of that state approved Measure 109, which legalized therapeutic uses of psilocybin. They are first doing initial test runs with ketamine and later will introduce psilocybin and MDMA for severe psychological conditions that have been resistant to conventional therapies. These sessions take place in nature settings.

There is a long-term link between psychedelics and nature awareness. Albert Hofmann, the discoverer of LSD, stated that the medicine revealed to him "the magnificence of nature and of the animal and plant kingdom." Ralph Metzner, the psychologist, wrote, "Awareness may also expand outward into a greatly enhanced sense of interconnectedness with all life-forms in the great ecological web of life." (Kushner 2021)

Other scholars refer to the current human psychopathology as *nature-deficit disorder*. Psychedelics may be a tool that enhances a phenomenon known as nature-relatedness. Studies have shown that a stronger connection to nature benefits mental health and improves mood. (Kushner 2021) With nature-relatedness, a person's mind expands to notice and appreciate plants and animals, and the natural world comes more alive. At the Silo retreats, the ketamine sessions involve screened participants inside a cozy mountain lodge amidst nature which creates a safe container (set and setting). Ketamine's dissociative effects also bring on hallucinatory visions and ego-dissolution experiences.

The development of psychedelic-therapeutic centers may well be a wave of the future. Ketamine, being legal, would be the prototype medicine utilized, and protocols are being established. Even though ketamine is relatively safe, medicines like psilocybin and other psychedelics may become preferable alternatives because there is no addictive potential and they are less likely to be abused.

As related through personal communication with colleagues, there has been some psychonautical usage of ketamine used in conjunction with psilocybin, LSD, and MDMA. The reported augmentation experiences have been predictably out of this world. It causes a total dissolution of ego identity while the medicine itself works its healing magic on the individual in a very intense way, without the conscious participation of the patient, who becomes very dissociated. Ironically, legal prescription medicines may be harder to procure than illegal hallucinogens such as psilocybin, LSD, or ayahuasca. Eighty percent of street ketamine can be obtained from clandestine labs based in Mexico, as well as India, and China. The only time I personally took ketamine was recently as part of an anesthetic cocktail for back surgery. I did not experience psychedelic effects upon recovery, and I have never tried ketamine as a hallucinogen.

Ketamine looks promising in usage for various psychiatric conditions which are not improved by conventional psychotropic medicines and therapies. The question remains whether psychedelic doses are needed to treat the numerous disorders described or whether ketamine at lower doses with its NMDA antagonism is sufficient. As far as viability as a shamanic medicine for healing and visioning, much more study of ketamine will be needed. Whether it will achieve the psychedelic notoriety of psilocybin mushrooms, LSD, ayahuasca, or MDMA remains to be seen. It does have addictive and other side effects that may preclude increased popularity during the present-day psychedelic renaissance. Again, it is essential to emphasize preparation, treatment, and follow-up integration for any healing or visioning work with any psychedelic medicine.

I want to conclude with a report of a firsthand, non-patient experience using ketamine given to me by a friend. No dosage was given.

Before I take K, I find the time when I will be alone in my home at night. As I take K, I choose a single song on repeat that I know will open my heart, light some candles, and turn off the lights. As the K slowly begins to take effect, my mind calms down, and the chattering monkey mind stops. I slowly start to move and feel my heart opening up. I allow myself to feel the love I have for myself, my partner, and my family and friends. This love, a physical feeling, combines with the music and begins to move my body with a concentrated purity and visceral gratitude as strong and perfect as a diamond. The next day, I feel reset, and the feeling of connected love remains. I feel a little tired, but nothing like I feel after having a few drinks. Where alcohol depletes my soul and emotional energy, ketamine does not.

Chapter 33:
Ecozoic Era: Psychedelics and Nature-Relatedness

Man follows the way of the Earth. Earth follows the way of Heaven. Heaven follows the way of Tao. Tao follows the way of Nature. — Tao Te Ching

This book describes how psychedelic medicines and shamanic methods can bring about profound personal healing in the human psyche and create visionary experiences of the transpersonal realm. Humanity is a part of the natural world and all psychedelics enhance nature-relatedness. The transpersonal dimension of the human psyche is what Carl Jung defined as the collective unconscious, the repository of all the memories and knowledge about the evolution of planet earth and the cosmos. It also encompasses non-human entities within the psyche, including plants, fungi, and minerals. This realm of understanding is essential to developing a spiritual dimension in human consciousness. The relationship between the personal and transpersonal aspects of the psyche forms an ego-Self axis through which potential wisdom can be attained and integrated in the individual.

Through transpersonal psychology and psychedelic journey work, this introspective approach can realign one's values toward a healthier relationship to nature and stewardship of the Earth. Developing a positive relationship with the natural world using psychedelic and shamanic methods requires a proper intention as well as proper set and setting. Carrying out a vision quest or circle in a natural location promotes experiences of meeting nature entities. There is a rapid immersion into the prevailing ecosystem, and the spirits of nature emerge with wisdom to share. When psychedelic medicines are used in a clinical setting for healing psychological issues, the encounters with nature are less likely to be prominent.

One of the positive outcomes for me from all my visionary journeys was that of creating a profound awareness of my relationship with nature, including hearing clearly the cry of the environment degraded by human intervention. The Lakota medicine man, Black Elk, states it clearly, "We don't have to heal the Earth; she can heal herself. All we have to do is stop making her sick." However, humanity can participate in the healing process, and this is necessary. The question remains, is it possible for us to change the destructive trajectory that we humans have embraced, threatening the survival of our Earth? Politics, religion, education, and psychology are the primary influences of human change. It is much easier to intellectually describe the historical and mythological roots of our present destructive attitudes than to discuss possible solutions. It is less challenging to analyze our dilemma than to construct healing ideas and necessary behavioral changes. Without humans, the Earth will eventually heal itself, but what type of human interventions could possibly change the tides of destructive environmental changes that we call the climate crisis in the present era? The New Age must be the Age of Nature or the Ecozoic Era. (Swimme and Berry, 241-261)

Ecopsychology is a developing field of interest that studies the human need for the natural world as a critical aspect of the healing process, as well as the actions humanity can take to help restore the health of the Earth itself. A primary change that visionary work can bring about is that of replacing anthropocentric, exploitative, ego-centric attitudes toward nature with a non-dominating, eco-centric, biocentric approach. Sustainability, mutuality, symbiosis, reciprocity, understanding ecosystems, and adaptability are the watchwords that requires integration into the human value system.

Ralph Metzner outlines several eco-movement contributors, noted below, who have focused on the underlying human psychopathologies contributing to our attitude of domination and the resulting exploitation of nature (Metzner 1999, 82-91):

Anthropocentrism: Human Superiority Complex is a concept coined by Arne Naess, the originator of the Deep Ecology Platform in 1984. It implies that our attitude of superiority (ego-centricity) is equated with the right to dominate rather than to steward nature. There is tremendous resistance and reluctance to give up human moral authority, especially to non-human entities, and to give them equal value. No one chooses to give up hard-won rights, freedom, or independence.

Developmental Fixation, or arrested development, with the adolescent values of boisterousness, arrogance, and self-assertion leading to consumerism and militarism, was promoted by Paul Shepard. He called it ontogenetic crippling, its origin lying in a disruption of the infant-caregiver dynamic, leading to mistrust and insecurity.

Thomas Berry, the theologian/geologian, postulates that our species has an *autistic* (neurodivergent) attitude toward nature, with an inability to hear, see, or feel Mother Earth, as well as impaired reciprocal communication.

Addiction is another concept used in describing a process in which individuals are unable to stop their destructive behavior of the environment. Even though they perceive the negative consequences, they continue to repeat this behavior.

Narcissism is a personality disorder characterized by feelings of entitlement and a grandiose self-image, covering up underlying feelings of unworthiness and emptiness. In this outlook, the Earth owes us something, so the pursuit of consumption of resources, consumer goods, and status compensate for unconscious feelings of alienation and inferiority. Lack of accountability and projection of blame onto others are aspects of this psychopathology.

Another dynamic is called *Ecological Amnesia*. Here, modern human culture has forgotten the ways that our ancestors knew and practiced connection with the Earth. Shamanic understanding can reignite this lost knowledge. Some call this the *nature deficit disorder*.

Most psychotherapies have various treatments for some of these disorders, but they usually exclude the nature/human dynamic. In taking a psychological history, the therapist usually focuses on the individual, especially personal traumas and childhood relationships. The natural environment is rarely addressed in psychotherapy other than the places one chooses to live, work, and develop friendships and community, representing the individual's ecosystem. The present psychological modalities focus on individuals, couples, and families, but not the impacts of environmental changes on the psyche. The recent pandemic has contributed to an awareness of environmental incursions that has left many people feeling vulnerable and anxious with significant social isolation. Ecopsychology incorporates more all-encompassing issues, and hopefully, eco-oriented therapists can be trained to address environmental impacts on the human psyche. Values clarification is also a necessity of any therapy process.

Psychedelic-based therapies activate and enhance relationships with the natural world and can allow individuals to realign their values towards planetary awareness. Psychedelics foster neurogenesis and neuroplasticity, which open up new channels to expand consciousness and bring about the experience of transpersonal insights. These medicines can break down rigid old patterns of thought and behavior, thus creating new contexts for interactions with the natural world. The veil of daily consensus reality is lifted so that new connections can be made. The larger forces at work can be seen and incorporated. Nature can speak directly to the individual regarding the changes necessary to relate symbiotically with an ecosystem and its health. The integration phase of psychedelic therapy can occur instantly, or over a longer period of time, when a new outlook and value system can congeal. Psychedelics allow non-human guides, ancestors, and mythic figures to participate in the psychotherapy of individuals. They make us aware that these larger forces are at work beyond our limited human perceptions and understanding of nature and ourselves.

When contemplating the degradation witnessed in nature, it is essential to become more knowledgeable about a number of topics. Some of the crucial issues that require further understanding and integration for us to contribute to restoring the health of the Earth are as follows:

Human Pollution: The thorny issue of human pollution must be addressed in effecting positive changes regarding the climate crisis. It has been demonstrated worldwide that many pollutants are tied directly to people's current lifestyles, including home electricity, heating, air conditioning, and transportation. While we are all increasingly aware of the impacts of issues, such as plastic waste, due to immediate information available over social media and the internet, finding economically viable solutions is an extremely challenging endeavor. A more sustainable practice is the development of reusable versions of items such as bottles, containers, straws, with a return to sustainable paper products and stainless-steel containers.

Oceans: In addition to witnessing changes on the land and in the atmosphere, there is a growing awareness of the declining health of our oceans and waterways. Oceans comprise about 75 percent of the Earth's surface; they represent the source of about 50 percent of the planet's oxygen. They also serve as a significant source of binding, storing, and fixing excess atmospheric carbon pollution. In 2015, the Intergovernmental Panel on Climate Change published a special report on climate change's impacts on oceans and land and sea ice, painting a grim picture. Oceans have absorbed more than 90 percent of the excess heat from carbon; they have become warmer, more acidic, and more oxygen-depleted, resulting in devastating effects on marine species. The global sea level, which rose about six inches in the last century, is now rising more than twice as fast and could increase as much as 3.5 feet if greenhouse gases continue to build up in the atmosphere.

Due to humans' addiction to petroleum-based products, ocean ecosystems are being polluted by oil spills, non-recyclable plastics and other waste materials, killing off fish, marine mammals, turtles, and sea birds. Unregulated fishing practices have depleted many fisheries, including sardines and anchovies, which are prey for creatures higher up the food chain. We find it easier to identify with the effects on large species of whales, dolphins, sharks, and sea turtles rather than feeling sympathy for the plight of the small anchovy.

Scientists have warned for several decades that our oceans are warming due to planetary climate change, significantly altering ecosystems and causing die-offs and migrations of various sea creatures. Ocean protection organizations, such as Oceana, Ocean Conservancy, Wild Oceans, Surfrider, Sea Shepherd, and Greenpeace, are active in battling these illegal practices and supporting the use of newer sustainable fishing technologies.

The interdisciplinary understanding of ocean ecology and ocean economics is necessary to balance the food needs of the overpopulated world. Fish is recognized as healthy for humans, especially in Asian countries; however, it is crucial for consumers to realize the prevalence of seafood fraud, a practice whereby an inferior fish species is passed on as a more expensive and desirable product. Farmed fish, especially salmon, are often fed polluted fishmeal leading to fish lice. Also, they are adulterated by food coloring chemicals to turn them orange, then sold as healthy for consumers. Most salmon sushi and Atlantic salmon are farmed. Wild salmon from Alaska is the only healthy, sustainable salmon option but is more expensive. It is vital to know the source and practices associated with the fish we eat.

Food Waste: When discussing issues about climate change, very few people understand the role of wasted food's impact on the environment and the economy. According to a recent Op-Ed in the *L.A. Times*, this accounts for four percent of greenhouse gas emissions and two percent of the gross domestic product in the United States. We toss out nearly 125 billion meals a year while 45 million Americans struggle to eat. The homeless could be nourished by all this food we are wasting. Recently, the national non-profit ReFED identified more than forty solutions to help the U.S. reach the 2030 goal of a 50 percent reduction in food waste. Implementing these solutions, they estimate, will result in a 73 billion dollar annual economic benefit and the elimination of 75 million tons of greenhouse gases, the equivalent of removing 16 million cars off the road annually.

Investments in software to estimate the amount of each foodstuff a grocery store needs to stock would help decrease waste. Also, developing an infrastructure for composting scrap food would allow nutrients to be recycled into the soil. This would reduce dangerous methane gas release and promote healthier soils to sequester carbon and retain moisture. Besides wasted and uneaten foods in grocery stores and restaurants, it is estimated that households account for 38 percent of the food waste, higher than any other sector. An example of changing food waste behavior is that in West London, in 2013, an initiative called "Love Food, Hate Waste," which led to a 14 percent decline in waste over a six-month period.

These are just a few of the issues that require collective value changes to aid in the restoration of a healthy planet and avoid human extinction. They all influence the climatic and environmental crises that are now being observed, affecting our well-being.

The best practice is first to educate ourselves, listen to science, and understand the idea of ecosystems. Then, it is essential to spend time in nature to observe and to bathe in its radiance. Then each individual can decide the best way to become involved in some form of eco-activism. It is helpful to identify with some organization that promotes sustainability and conservation to protect vital ecosystems, be they on land, in oceans, or in the planet's atmosphere.

Charles Darwin and Alfred Russell Wallace simultaneously put forth the concept that evolution is based on natural selection, in which the most adaptable survive and thrive. The concept is that it is not always the strongest that survives, but the most adaptable species within a given ecosystem. This takes the view of a dance of cooperation and reciprocity rather than a competition of brute strength. Catastrophic events such as pandemic diseases, wars, and environmental disasters often cause quantum jumps in evolution where other forms of life replace the dominant species. An example is when dinosaurs were wiped out by a meteor sixty-five million years ago and replaced by mammals who inherited the Earth.

To further understand our connection to the natural world, look historically at how our pre-scientific ancestors managed the Earth. As described earlier, the study of shamanic practices in other cultures has now been appropriated and made relevant to modern society. Such practices continue to hold valid truths and to provide clues on deepening our relationship with nature. Psychedelic medicines with an intention to heal our split from the natural world represent powerful tools to aid in exploring solutions to all these environmental challenges confronting humanity. These mind-expanding medicines open up new neural pathways and connections, enabling the individual to view relationships in new ways. All psychedelic medicines promote interconnectedness and unity rather than disparity, especially within nature.

There are multiple ways to be involved as participants who still hold the Earth as our Great Mother, our source of life and sustenance. My own experiences have motivated me to develop an attitude of activism with many issues facing the natural world. What is essential to keep in mind is that psychedelics enhance ecological consciousness, which shifts perspectives and leads to action and change.

Chapter 34
Psychedelic Alchemy

What causes change? The seasons change, evolution is change, we grow and mature, there is birth and death. When we cook, we transform basic ingredients into new food chemistries with delectable tastes. How transformation actually occurs has been the great mystery for the human understanding of phenomena. Imagination allows us to travel to places unseen in daily reality. Modern psychotherapies evolved to help us understand human transformation in health and illness. Previously, the alchemists developed a symbolic system of the transmutation of matter from base to precious. Certain alchemists, notably Paracelsus, saw a deeper meaning in alchemy referring to the inner workings of the human psyche.

Jung rediscovered this alchemical symbolism as it applied to the process of individuation (psychological development) from undifferentiated unconsciousness to the discovery of the deeper Self and the Godhead residing within us all. Although there is no evidence that Jung knew about or used entheogenic plants, the chemistry of psychedelics opens the same channels of imagination that the alchemists experienced. (For more on Jung's work and influence, see Appendix 1.)

Alchemy, during the Middle Ages, studied the molecular transformations that occur within matter. It pre-dated the complex scientific chemistry of modern times. It attempted to refine base matter to its precious form, called the *philosopher's stone*, hoping to change lead into gold, and to change corruptible matter into an incorruptible, pure essence. It attempted to unite spirit and matter. In this process, the alchemist would observe images of these transitions in the alchemical flask called the *retort*. Alchemy is the projection of unconscious thought-processes, and as such, it is a precursor of modern psychological analytic therapy.

There were operations that the alchemists would perform: first separating the elements of a base material (*separatio*), then sublimating (*sublimatio*) and discriminating the spiritual component, then recombing

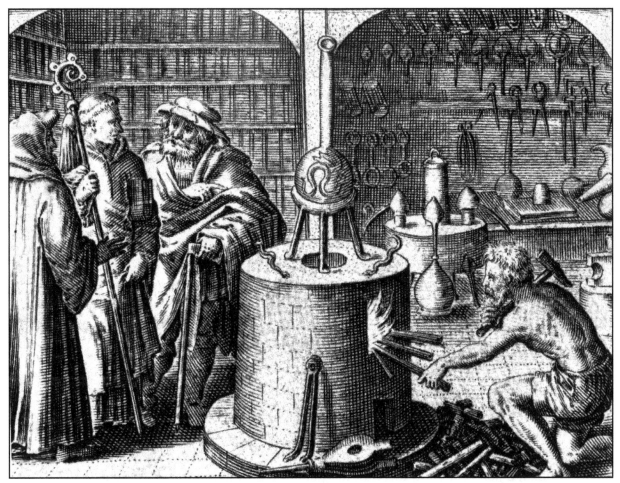

Figure 71. *Tripus Aureus*. Alchemical adept at work at the furnace and retort while the scholars contemplate philosophy. (Jaffe 1979, pg. 96)

it (*coagulatio)* into a new form uniting the spirit with matter (*coniunctio*). According to Jung, the alchemical methods corresponded to creating consciousness from an unconscious state and thus served as a roadmap for his psychoanalytical theories. Again, psychedelic medicines open awareness to the interconnectedness of previously separated, often hostile entities within the psyche; thus fostering unity, which is a type of *coniunctio*.

It is not inconceivable, but speculative, that various plant chemicals could have been used to aid visions seen within the retort by the alchemists. Various mushroom species and the ergot rye fungus, which were psychedelic, were used by shamans and others during ancient times. It also has been speculated that the famous alchemist/physician, Paracelsus (1493-1541), was well aware of cannabis and its psychoactive effects. Again, there is no definitive proof that the alchemists used hallucinogens, but the processes bear distinct similarities.

This alchemical task of taking *prima materia* (primal, undifferentiated base matter) and creating something more complex and refined is a type of evolution similar to that experienced in a psychedelic state. The prime matter of the first living molecules on earth consisted of hydrogen (H), oxygen (O), carbon (C), and nitrogen (N). With a bit of solar energy added, eventually, primordial germ cells were produced as well as the chemicals needed to make DNA, the genetic codes of all life forms.

In biology, especially embryology, it is taught that "ontogeny recapitulates phylogeny." The primordial germ cell, after inception, divides and in nine months produces a human being. During embryonic development, the fetus parallels evolution, recapitulating a worm, fishes (with gills), amphibians (which came on to land from the water), reptiles, mammals, and finally, humans. Thus, embryological development is an encapsulated form of evolution.

Every cell in the body carries DNA in the nucleus that connects these evolutionary memories as the blueprints of life. It traces back through the transformations of millions of generations. During the psychedelic experience, it is possible to recreate these stages and identify with ancestral animals. One can directly experience what it feels like to be a hungry snake, a fish breathing through its gills, or a bird flying through the sky. In the psychedelic state, the ego can become aware of the pre-life stages of molecular events within the body or with the cell. One can regress to experience atomic interactions, the subatomic state of quantum physics, and pure energy. The final transition can then lead the participant to extra-terrestrial cosmic consciousness, representing the body transmuting into light energy. Later, when the ego reconstitutes, it revisits these various states of being.

The psychedelic experience of the modern-day participant is not unlike the explorations of the ancient alchemists in delving deeper into the mysteries of life, consciousness, and self-awareness. In alchemy the emphasis is on transformation within the mineral realm, from lead to gold, but this is a perfect metaphor for finding spirit within matter.

An interesting active meditation, without psychedelic medicine, is to regress from being an adult human, back to birth, and through the various embryonic stages to the primordial germ cell, and then to the cosmic realm. The return is also important to witness—the reconstitution and incarnation of energy into matter, and the evolution of the embryo and the animal ancestors. (Fabricius 1976, 212-214) See Fig. 15.

C.G. Jung studied alchemy as an ancient form of transformational psychology, noticing that it was heavily steeped in archetypal symbolism. Jung was also a very fine artist. When one views his paintings, it can be seen that his use of vivid colors is reminiscent of present-day visionary artists; they are in themselves psychedelic in quality. This is especially true of his mandala-like paintings having a central source that emanates outwards with complex patterns. This pattern is very common in the visions people experience with sacred medicines. His paintings appear in many of his *Collected Works*, but are extensively presented in *The Red Book*, published in 2009 by Norton and Company. To my knowledge, there is no evidence or mention of Jung using any psychedelic substances. My conclusion is that Jung was a natural visionary and had expanded consciousness without any aid. His art reflects this mindset. Several examples follow.

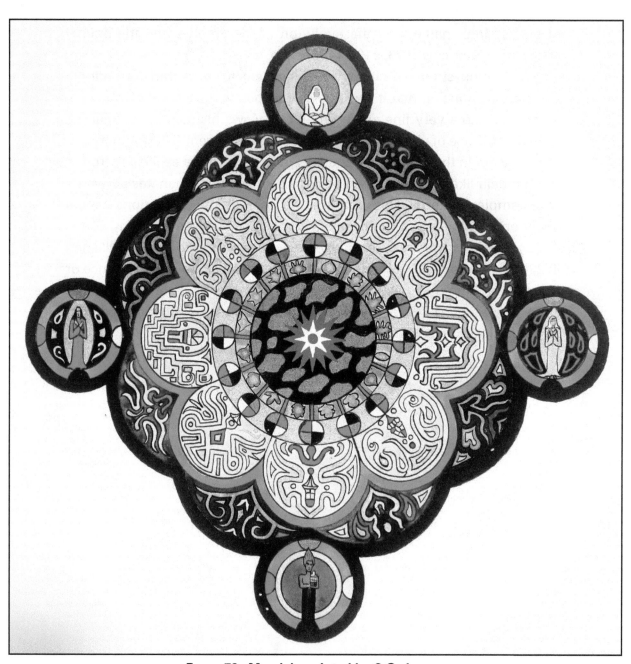

FIGURE 72. Mandala painted by C.G. Jung.
(*Red Book* 2009, 105)

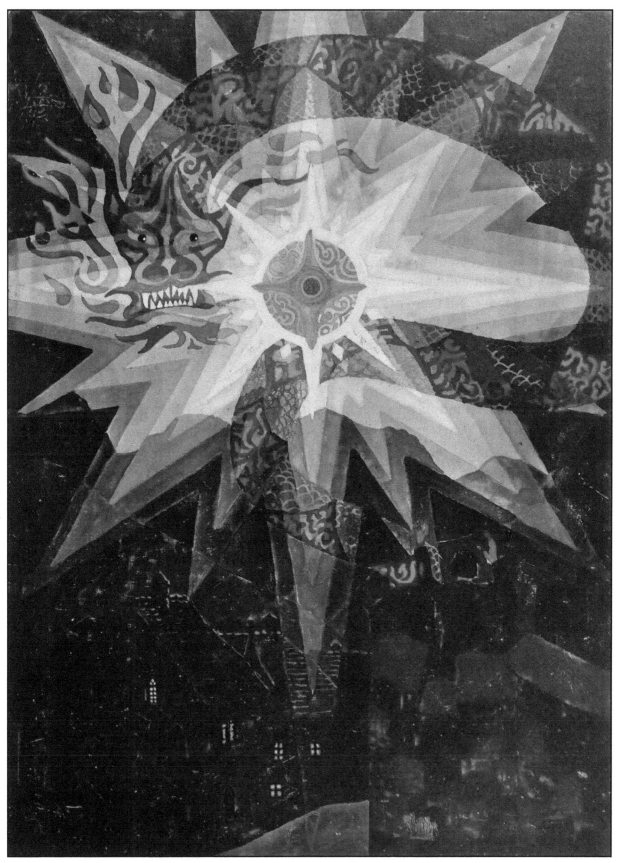

FIGURE **73. Light at the Core of Darkness** by C.G. Jung
(Red Book 2009, 129)

Conclusion

I hope this book has conveyed a first-hand account of what it is like to go through healing and visionary experiences, with the major psychedelic medicines, within carefully guided sessions. Additionally, I trust that the information about each of the entheogens has helped further your knowledge of each substance and the context in which it can be utilized. Each individual who tries a psychedelic can expect different journeys and imagery, but there are common experiences as well. One of our most shared commonalities is the interconnectedness of all life, especially in the natural world. Despite our differences in upbringing, culture, history, and degree of development, an underlying unity exists within all sentient beings at the deepest level of the psyche.

As described in these chapters, the medicines have the capacity to open expanded awareness previously hidden within the individual. They can bring about changes in underlying values as well as new behaviors of greater benefit to the person and the planet. They allow human beings to experience the divine essence of the universe as it exists in the cosmos and within Mother Earth. For some readers, the information presented may be new. For others already familiar with psychedelics, I trust that this book contains a helpful review of the literature and some fascinating stories.

Most importantly, I wish to emphasize the caution necessary in using these medicines. Knowledgeable and ethical guides are difficult to find. Each substance's purity and source are prerequisites; the proper mindset and setting are essential. I hope that the diagrams and meditations I have included help in offering examples of the structure necessary for safe, profound journey work, which is especially true if one chooses to take a medicine alone.

The knowledge of shamanic techniques is not required for taking psychedelics, but, as I have shared through my own experiences, it can serve to help orient oneself during the period of expanded consciousness, which can be daunting at times. Shamanism includes archaic techniques that have been appropriated in present times as a counterpoint to modern medical and psychological methods for understanding the psyche. Shamanism is not a religion and is not contrary to any organized religion. Without any contradiction, Christians, Jews, Muslims, Hindus, Buddhists, Pagans, and all spiritual belief systems can benefit from shamanic practices.

The essential teachings of these medicines bring about healing of personal, psychological traumas from the past and enable the development of a new vision of the future. They have the potency to break through entrenched, rigid structures in the psyche and allow for new, more functional insights to emerge, resulting in more lasting behavior change. In a word, they all help with getting "unstuck."

Personally, as I have related in these chapters, my time with psychedelic shamanic practices greatly aided the healing of my own childhood wounds, which had not been fully realized through over twenty years of psychotherapy and analysis. Significant for me is that all of these medicines enhance nature-relatedness. I learned that the natural world is erotic, not in a sexual sense, but in having a fertile, fecund, beautiful, and productive function that strives to thrive. It is not the strongest but the most adaptable species that survive. Survival is more of a dance than a competition. The most important lesson I integrated is that humans are part of nature, and as such, our survival depends on developing a symbiotic, healthy relationship with our planet.

If this book has piqued the reader's interest in trying an entheogenic medicine, please be reminded that this is an intense, heroic way of approaching expanded consciousness. A warrior's attitude is necessary to enter the psychedelic experience, during which one must confront many fears and shadow issues before transcendence can occur. It is also crucial to follow up the experience with some longer-term practice for behavioral integration. Otherwise, the lessons may be easily forgotten and lost to awareness within a short period. Developing a meditation practice, writing, artistic endeavors, and psychotherapy with a therapist knowledgeable about altered states may help integrate the necessary long-term changes that one is seeking. My intention in this book is primarily to aid in developing a working knowledge of sacred substances, not to promote their usage. I strongly recommend exploring alternatives that do not rely on these medicines, such as the vision quest model I described.

I have not included recommendations for any specific shaman, guide, teacher, or guru in this book. Part of the journey is to find one's personal guide through due diligence. It is crucial to understand that I do not know how to procure any of the described medicines and am not a source. They do remain illegal for the most part. My work with them took place many years ago within an underground movement of early dedicated explorers of consciousness. Hopefully, access will become more available as research continues to confirm the value of these sacred medicines.

Nor is this book intended as a guide to recreational usage or to the practice of micro-dosing psychedelics. Personally, I am not a proponent of such practices. If one is seeking healing for a psychological disorder, a current option is to connect with a research center using the substances within tested protocols.

I want to emphasize that despite my excursions personally into the psychedelic underground movement, I never used, discussed, promoted, or suggested using these medicines to any of my patients during my time of practicing psychiatry. I conducted my practice according to the ethical requirements of the medical and psychiatric profession and guidelines. I also never used any of the above outlined shamanic techniques with clients. I always embraced the values of integrity and ethics, whether in my practice or how I approached sacred entheogens. In my long career, I was never sued for malpractice by anyone. Yes, I was a bit of an outlaw when I left the middle of the road to dwell at the edge between the conventional wisdom and the unknown. I felt honored to be part of the new wave of psychedelic investigation to help pave the way for the eventual legal research with these medicines for healing. Whatever benefit my patients received from me was due to the integration of these psychedelic experiences combined with my knowledge of traditional psychopharmacology and other psychological/analytical training and experiences that enhanced my desire to be a healer.

Many years have passed since I participated in these psychedelic vision circles. I no longer feel any pull to repeat entheogen use. My inner development reverberated to my outer life concerns. I finally felt that I went through success's door and found security.

I hope this book has introduced the reader to the transpersonal realm of the psyche and its potential for healing personal material, as well as bringing a renewed connection with whatever you consider to be spiritual—your personal God or Nature. The interrelationships between the cosmos and the earth contain essential knowledge for humans to counteract the destruction of all life and the planet and thus participate in healing the natural world. My favorite references for further reading are the many books on the subject written by Ralph Metzner and some of the writings on or by C.G. Jung.

This book will help you structure a healing session with some orienting shamanic meditations to guide you, whether or not you utilize a psychedelic medicine. Like any form of therapy, you will have to repeat these contemplations many times to integrate a lasting behavioral change. Insights only work when you put them into behavioral action.

To end, I would like to say that psychospiritual exploration never comes to completion, but I now feel that I have come closer to the notion of "Physician, Heal Thyself." I have come to know the Universe within, experience the Divine, and become a better person. Because of this, I no longer feel the need to take more psychedelics. To paraphrase the shaman/artist Pablo Amaringo, who followed the way of plant knowledge with ayahuasca, he thought at the end of his life that he could live life more creatively and take more care of the earth. It is time now for me to pass the torch of my knowledge and wisdom to the next generation of psychonautical adventurers.

Epilogue

Wendell Berry, an environmental activist, farmer, novelist, and poet, made a telling statement to the Sierra Club in 1967, during the height of the Vietnam era. He stated that, as a member of the human race, he was "in the worst possible company: communists, fascists and totalitarians of all sorts, militarists and tyrants, exploiters, vandals, gluttons, ignoramuses, murderers." Yet he found hope through people "who through all the sad destructive centuries of our history have kept alive the vision of peace and kindness and generosity and humility and freedom."

Many years have passed since his speech, and we find ourselves again dealing with the cataclysms of war, terrorism, nuclear threat, cyber threats, pandemics, and economic and environmental destruction. Is there any hope for the future? Perhaps hope is just another word for fanciful thinking and should be associated more with the reality of activism in order for necessary change to occur. But, "hope springs eternal."

Even Jung, toward the end of his life, was uncertain about the survival of the human race after WWII and when the nuclear era began. Possessing all his inherent consciousness, Jung was not optimistic. Human beings indeed represent a paradox. On the one hand, we create beautiful art; we experience and give love. On the other hand, we destroy, dominate, and murder. We encapsulate the age-old battle of good versus evil. It seems like a race with an unknown outcome. What will prevail? Will humanity make the necessary changes fast enough to save the planet?

Another significant issue concerning consciousness remains unclear. Is there an afterlife of awareness, and is reincarnation a possibility? Many religions and spiritual belief systems promote this likelihood. My answer is that, "I don't know!" We enter the realm of beliefs, not facts. While I believe (not a fact) that there is a total ablation (annihilation) of an individual's awareness and memories at the time of death and that nothing exists once dead, I wonder: Does consciousness exist beyond the individual? My psychedelic journeys point to the strong possibility that consciousness pervades the universe independent of humanity. In this framework, human brains are like radio receivers that process this universal consciousness into human perceptions and sensations. The brain could also act as a transmitter to change the outcomes of reality.

Connected to the concept of an afterlife is reincarnation. It is a worthy hypothesis promoted by some religions. Related is the idea called karma, which represents the evolution of the psyche during a lifetime as the individual confronts necessary conflicts. In Jungian psychology, this is referred to as the individuation process. If one works through this karma, at death one achieves nirvana, and there is no need to reincarnate on earth to satisfy any further unfulfilled destiny. While there is no scientific proof that reincarnation exists, it is possible the genetic code harbors memory traces and behavioral traits of an individual and is passed down generationally. We know that DNA contains the code and memory of all life forms, from the most primitive to the most advanced.

My belief is to live this one life to the fullest and deal with whatever trials and tribulations challenge us. I try to live by the phrase of the black bluesman, Mississippi John Hurt, who states: "Don't die until you're dead." Assume this lifetime is your one chance to accomplish what you were born to do. Reincarnation, or birth, death, and rebirth, occur many times during one's lifetime as states of consciousness that can be perceived.

In case there is an afterlife and/or reincarnation exists, prepare yourself by becoming as conscious as possible when entering the beyond. Besides the difficulties that life may present, do not forget to enjoy this time on earth. As a value, developing more conscious awareness during life is essential, and psychedelics are one method that can advance this individuation process.

Biocentric theory promotes the concept that individual awareness creates material reality as we know it, in contrast to the traditional view that the physical world creates individual consciousness. Consciousness comes first. Quantum physics states that the observer can change the outcome of experiences we call reality. Psychedelic medicines, as compounds found within plants, fungi, and minerals (chemicals), are able to alter the perceptions of our radio receiver (brain) in new ways, thus permitting us to expand the frequencies received from the universal cosmic field. Therefore, these medicines actually change our observations and create a different reality beyond the consensus perceptions of most humans in their natural, non-altered state. This new reality thus gives us more choices, with the question remaining: Can this change the morality and ethics of the human being?

I believe that when properly used, psychedelic medicines attempt to communicate to us the needs of our planet, informing us about our destructive trajectory. They offer possible solutions to this dilemma. I encourage as many of us as possible to seize these insights, and change. Become your own shaman and wise elder, by any means, to participate in this transformative healing process for Mother Earth.

On a personal level, I recommend one to *slow down*, live a simple life as much as possible in the present, except to go into the past for memories and healing and into the future to get clarity of purpose and new insights. On a planetary scale, I suggest we all need to *speed up* to make the changes necessary to meet the demands of the rapid climate changes and the possible extinction of humanity.

Michael Pollan in his recent Netflix series, *How to Change Your Mind,* reiterates that with the "Psychedelic Renaissance," a container needs to exist in order to avoid the pitfalls that occurred in the 1960s with Timothy Leary's proclamations about LSD. This container needs to have wise elders at the helm, who are well-versed in the dynamics of altered states of consciousness. Whether these medicines are used individually or within a group for healing and visioning, the transcendent experience is only part of the process. Transformation or behavioral change requires an experienced psychotherapist who has also undergone the psychedelic experience and is also trained to become the healer/therapist.

Unfortunately, most traditionally trained psychotherapists are not qualified to become psychedelic guides. A new era of training and a new community of therapists hopefully will become adept in the future, and herald a new phase in mental health treatment. This is also relevant for people without mental health problems who wish to expand consciousness and have a mystical encounter.

Jung and the Transpersonal Psyche

Why include C.G. Jung in a book about psychedelics? This book reiterates the important value of experiencing the transpersonal psyche in healing and visioning, and how this can realign the human mind toward the needs of nature and preserving the Earth's health. Jung was a pioneer in describing the dynamics and experience of the transpersonal psyche, which he called the *Collective Unconscious*. It is the foundation for understanding spirituality and its application to consciousness. Jung's ideas laid the groundwork for how the transpersonal realm can heal the personal psychological issues of the individual.

My psychedelic journeys have corroborated the existence of the collective unconscious and have served to substantiate Jung's psychological theories, which include the spiritual aspects of the psyche. Prior to Jung, psychological theories emphasized the personal aspects of the unconscious as they applied to psychopathology, as described by Freud and his self-psychology-oriented followers. They considered the religious or spiritual aspect of the psyche was not relevant and that it represented wishful thinking and was neurotic. Jung incorporated this spiritual domain as being at the core of the psyche. He started with the personal psyche as a basis, and expanded the dynamics of the psyche to include the transpersonal collective unconscious. Jung "walked his talk," not only in his philosophy, but in how he lived his life, including his travels to foreign cultures.

As we all know, there is tremendous diversity in humanity with multiple cultures, languages, political persuasions, races, and religious belief systems. Jung looked to the psyche in hopes of discovering common ground beyond all these differences. The common shared experience he found is reflected in the deepest layers of psyche he called the collective unconscious. There the archetypes reside, as well as the core encounter with the godhead. There, the non-human aspects of spirit beings, plant,

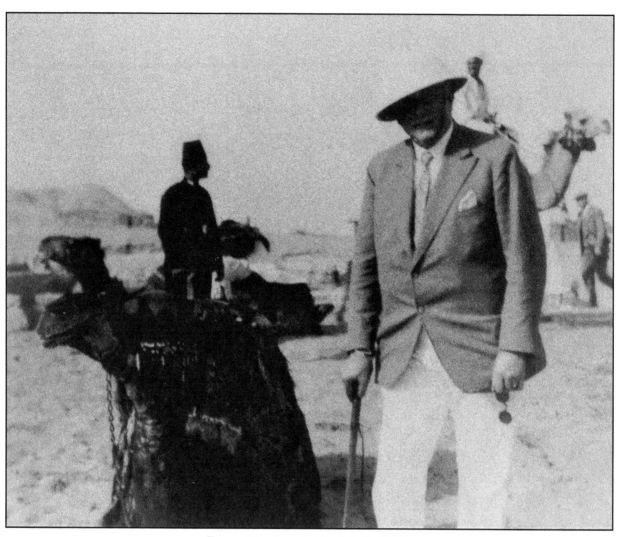

FIGURE 74. Jung in Tunisia in 1920.
(from Wehr 1989, 67)

fungal, and mineral intelligence can also be experienced. These are the realms to which I traveled through my vision quests, with and without psychedelic medicines.

Jung came to believe that his ideas were largely influenced by Western European and American thought, which was then primarily based on Caucasian, male-dominated, and scientifically evolved cultures. Modern societies were generally more removed from nature and often concentrated in cities. To corroborate his ideas about the existence of the transpersonal psyche and the archetypes, he felt the need to leave the ivory tower of intellect and European thought in order to seek an outside perspective. He decided to travel to visit civilizations that were foreign to him and less technologically evolved. These cultures dwelled closer to and were more instinctually connected with the natural world and their environments. These journeys are detailed in his autobiography, *Memories, Dreams, Reflections*; particularly in pages 238-288.

On one journey in 1920, Jung traveled to Tunisia to immerse himself in the Arab culture and stated, "my encounter with Arab culture had struck me with overwhelming force. The emotional nature of these unreflective people who are so much closer to life than we are exerts a strong suggestive influence upon those historical layers in ourselves which we have just overcome and left behind . . ." (Jung 1961, 244)

In 1924, he traveled to the Taos Pueblo in New Mexico, where he was introduced to Ochwiay Biano, known as Mountain Lake, who told him, "we are a people who live on the roof of the world; we are the sons of Father Sun, and with our religion, we daily help our father to go across the sky. We do this not only for ourselves, but for the whole world. If we were to cease practicing our religion, in ten years the sun would no longer rise. Then it would be night forever." (Jung 1961, 252) Jung also asked him why he thought whites were all mad. Mountain Lake replied, "They say that they think with their heads . . . we think here, indicating his heart." (Jung 1961, 248)

Jung called this concrete identification with the natural world the *participation mystique*, a concept first formulated by the French scholar and anthropologist Lucien Levy-Bruhl (1857-1939). This idea is explained by an unconscious identification with concrete objects or beliefs, during which reflection and logic are suspended. Unable to abstract, view reality symbolically, or use critical thinking, the individual disappears into a collective identification with a belief system as a concrete reality. It is called "magical thinking" in modern psychology.

In 1926, Jung also traveled to Mombasa on the East coast of Africa. He was introduced to the Elgonyi tribe, in the region of Mount Elgon, which worshiped the sun as god. "In the morning, when the sun comes, we go out of the huts, spit into our hands, and hold them up to the sun." This act was their true religion, all tribes worshiped *adhista*—the sun at the moment of rising. (Jung 1961, 266)

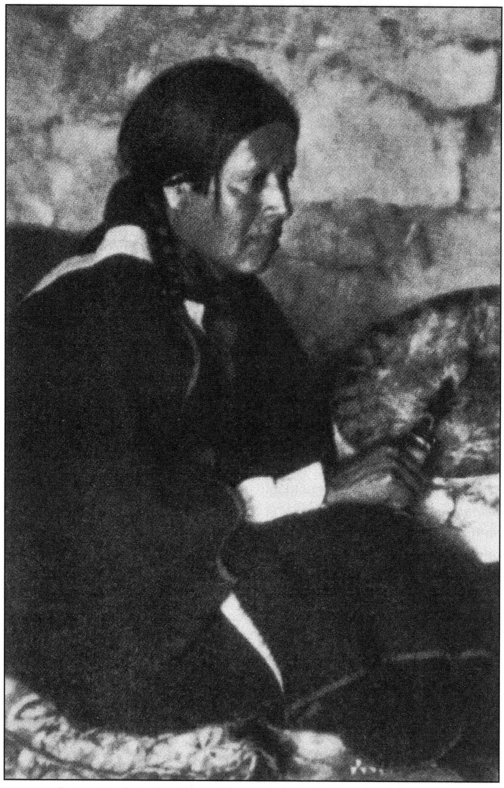

FIGURE 75. Ochwiay Biano (Mountain Lake) of Taos Pueblo, 1924.
(Wehr 1989, 63)

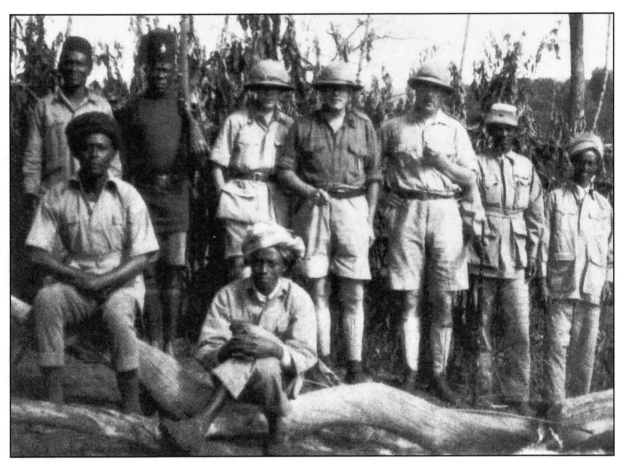

FIGURE 76. Jung in Mombasa, Africa, 1925.
(Wehr 1989, 65)

Jung embraced the direct experience of the elemental psyche which required integration, rather than relying on scholarship alone. (Direct experience rather than intellectual interpretation also occurs during the psychedelic adventure.) He found tremendous value in meeting individuals in tribes who still based their realities on myth. It was the instinct he rediscovered in the souls of humanity. These journeys had a profound effect on confirming his theories about the collective unconscious.

In addition to his travels, Jung also wanted to experience life in a more elemental, natural setting. In 1922, he bought land in Bollingen, Switzerland, on Lake Zurich. There he built the Bollingen stone tower, without any modern amenities. At Bollingen Jung could appreciate the primal, instinctive qualities that resided within himself, away from the comforts of his life and the demands of practicing analysis which meant being available to a multitude of individuals who sought after him. Thus, Jung was at his most elemental self within nature in his introspective silence. His dwelling

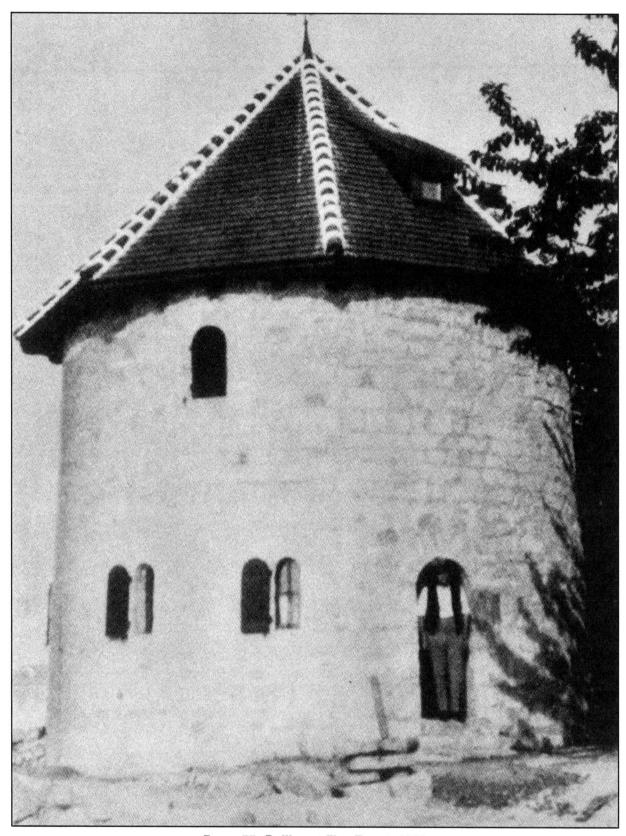

FIGURE 77. Bollingen First Tower, 1923
(from Wehr 1989, 69)

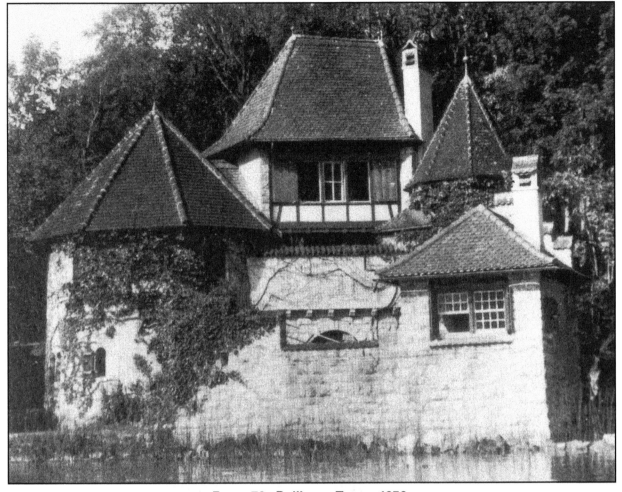

FIGURE 78. Bollingen Tower, 1956.
(from Wehr 1989, 72)

became a type of shrine to house the ancient mysteries. At Bollingen, there was no electricity, and he had to cook over a wood-fired oven. He had his own way of layering wood and kindling the fire. There he found could remain with his archaic self and the wildness within.

I encourage anyone who is interested in psychedelic journey work or immersion into the natural psyche to read some material by or about Jung. It is a basic orientation for understanding the transpersonal realms that will be experienced. It can be helpful to develop some scholarship first, as points of orientation, and then to integrate this knowledge with the experiential aspect of the vision quest model. Good primers on Jung are *Word and Image,* (Ed. Aniela Jaffe), *An Illustrated Biography of C.G. Jung*, (Gerhard Wehr), and *Man and His Symbols,* (Jung).

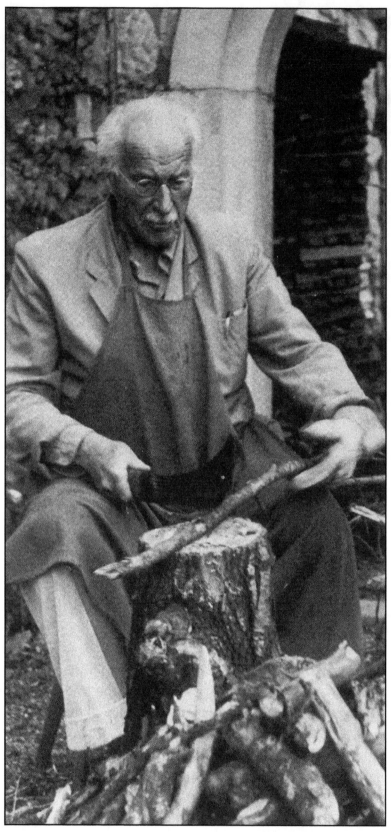

FIGURE 79. Jung chopping wood at Bollingen.
(from Wehr 1989, 71)

Nine Meditations Honoring Mutuality, Reciprocity, Interdependence, Orientation, and Balance

Consider these invocations, taught by Ralph Metzner, as useful tools for orienting oneself prior to experiencing any type of adventure into the unknown, whether or not entheogens are used. They honor the outer and inner reality of space and time, the elements, and all our relationships, invoking protection and safety on the journey. These four dimensions of space and time then enable us to experience the fifth dimension of alternate reality. These invocations can also be used during the early induction phase after taking the medicine. This is also a useful structure to contemplate during a meditation session.

(1) Four Directions and the Elements:

— We align ourselves with the powers, spirits, and allies, to help us in our lives.

— The East – The direction of the rising sun, new life, and the child.

— The South – The direction of fertility of the earth, growth, giving, and the feminine.

— The West – The direction of the setting sun, ocean, dissolving outdated structures, elder years.

— The North – The direction of the winds of change.

— The four elements of fire, water, earth, air.

(2) Spirits of Place:

— Location – habitat, name, (desert, mountains, etc.)

— Animals, plants, minerals, people – past and present who inhabit this place.

(3) Spirits of Time:

— Season, phase of the moon, time of day or night.
— Alignment of the planets and stars.

(4) Animals:

— Teach us about mobility, dynamics through movement, predator/prey, migration.
— Four-legged – mammals, live on the earth.
— Two-legged/winged – birds, live in the air, fly for perception from above.
— Swimming creatures – water, dolphins, whales, fish.
— Reptiles/amphibians – creatures that inhabit the earth and below.

(5) Plants and Fungi:

— Teach us about being fixed, growth, cultivation and regeneration.
— Provide us with food and nourishment.
— Provide us with oxygen and absorb and bind carbon (CO_2).
— Fertilize the earth through nitrogen fixing.
— Provide us with medicines and herbs for healing and pain.
— Provide us with beauty and fragrances.
— Whose flowers give us hope and inspiration.
— Provide us with visions – as teachers and expanders of consciousness.
— Communicate with other plants and animals for maintaining homeostasis.

(6) Spirits of Minerals/Stones:

— The earth we walk on, mountains.
— Stones and minerals that are needed for bones, blood, and health.
— Iron, trace metals needed for metabolic functions.
— Beauty and adornment.

(7) Ancestors:

— Physical/biological – mother/father, grandparents, children who have passed on. Focus on our reciprocity with them. Those who have gone before us want to help us with the wisdom to enable us to manifest.

- Spiritual teachers – Buddha, Jesus, Moses, Mohammed, Jung, etc.
- Gods and goddesses – mythological realm – Isis, Osiris, Shiva, Tara, Kokopelli, etc.
- Descendants – children, future beings not yet born but still in spirit world, what we want to pass on, Iroquois notion of planning for seven generations into the future

(8) Human Realm – The Circles of Relationships:

- Spouse, children, family, friends by name.
- Colleagues, other people by name.
- Collective mass of humanity, without names.

(9) Inner Orientation:

- Centering – through breath into the heart chamber, then other chakras.
- Balancing – right/left, up/down, forward/backward, six points which join at the crossroads in the heart.
- Earthing (grounding)
- Where we touch the ground with our feet and seat.
- Let the energy then come up the spinal axis through the crown and then create a sphere approximately 10-15 feet surrounding you.
- A half dome which comes back to earth in an arc.
- Opening up – of being, inner light manifesting so that an energy field of who you are surrounds you and influences other living beings that intersect with your expanded sphere.
- Ralph then reminds us that there are two forms of visions.
- Visuals come from the right brain.
- Thought forms or voice come from the left brain.
- Some individuals don't have visual imagery, which is fine.
- Also, Ralph remarks that female ancestor spirits usually enter from the left and the male ancestors enter from the right.
- Most importantly Ralph prepares us by saying:

Remember Four Things on Any Journey –

"A wise old owl once told me, when you are lost or confused on a journey, to remember…"

1) Your intention.
2) Ancestors, allies, and helpers.
3) Inner light, spirit.
4) The Earth.

In preparation for the night's journey, Ralph would share with us a short poem that came to him from the spirits about singing and chanting, which we would do during the rounds of the medicine journey:

"If you can sing the sounds that contain all the joys of your life and pains, then the song that you sing will carry away the pain until only the joy remains."

River of Time Chant:
(with drums – can be done during or at the end of the ceremony)

We come from the Sun x 4
We are born on the Earth x 4
We grow with the Plants x 4
We move like the Animals x 4
We live here as Humans x 4

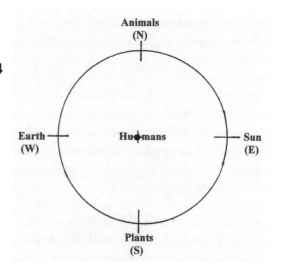

Closing Prayer – Thanking the Four Directions

We thank you Grandfather Fire for bringing us Warmth
We thank you Grandmother Ocean for bringing us Peace
We thank you Grandfather Wind for bringing us Change
We thank you Grandmother Earth for bringing us Life

Music Considerations and Inspirations

As noted throughout this book, music is essential to the journey work I have described. Ralph Metzner had a talent for choosing unique and obscure music to activate the imagination of the participants. Many shamans are also musicians who use their own vocal chanting, songs, and instruments, including the drum, rattle, flute, and guitar to drive the trance-induced imagery. All psychedelics have the capacity to create synesthesia, to change one sensory function to another in the user. Sounds can be experienced as visual images and emotional events, and can generate memories.

If you are considering a psychedelic journey, you can choose some of your favorite music to serve as a boat taking you down the stream of consciousness. I recommend choosing different musical themes for the various parts of the journey. For the induction phase, I recommend a mellow and softer meditation style of non-vocal music to help quell any initial anxiety. Once the medicine is activated and the psychedelic imagery fully emerges, music of a more rhythmic nature often enhances the experience. Later, when the imagery slows down and the teachings begin, indigenous or electronic music is often helpful. During the final phase of the session, when one begins to come down, often vocal music with emotional, devotional, or spiritual content is powerful. For the integration session, music that one can move and dance to is enjoyable.

Of course, when making a personal playlist, a process of trial and error is involved; thus, no absolute protocol exists for the sequence that best fits your nature. If you are experiencing a problematic or frightening journey, many have found that changing the music to something more meditative or soothing will dramatically alter the course of your experience. If you are uncertain about the music selections or interested in some suggestions, you will find selections I have grouped by genres. Some of these are from my private collection, and some were used by Ralph Metzner during his sessions.

Meditative:

Jonathan Goldberg – *Dolphin Dreams*
PC Davidoff – *Raku*
David Darling – *Darkwood*
Stephen Kent – *Landing (digeridoo)*
Madredeus – *O'Spirito do Paz*
Koorunba – *Walkabout*

Native American:

Carlos Nakai et al. – *Voices Across the Canyon*
Carlos Nakai, Peter Kater – *Through the Window and Walls*
Carlos Nakai, Nawang Khechog – *Winds of Devotion*
Nawang Khechog – *Karuna*
Ben Tavera King – *Visions and Encounters*
Primeaux and Mike – *Walk in Beauty*
Coyote Oldman – T*hunder Chord*

Indigenous:

Luis Panduro Vasquez – A*yahuasca Songs from the Peruvian Amazon*
Don Pedro Guerra Gonzales – S*ongs of the Plant Spirits*
Luis Eduardo Luna – *The Songs the Plants Taught Us*
Guadalupe de la Cruz Rios – *Kupuri: Huichol Songs and Music*
Inti-Illimani – *Arriesgare la Piel*
Hamza El Din – *Escalay (The Water Wheel), A Song of the Nile, Eclipse*

African:

Ladysmith Black Mambazo – *The Ultimate Collection*
Babatunde Olatunji – *Dance to the Beat of My Drum, Drums of Passion*
Seleshe Damessae – *Tesafaye: A Future Hope*
Ayub Ogada – *En Mana Kuoyo*
Geoffrey Oryema – *Exile, Beat the Border*

Electronic:

Steve Roach, Michael Stearns, Ron Sunsinger – *Kiva*
Steve Roach, Robert Rich – *Soma*
Steve Roach, Byron Metcalf – *The Serpent's Lair*

Steve Roach – *World's Edge, Magnificent Void, Dreamtime Return*
Robert Rich – *Rainforest*
Terry Oldfield – *Spirit of the Rainforest*
Michael Stearns – *Planetary Unfolding*
David Parsons – *Tibetan Plateau, Himalaya, Yatra*
Tuu – *One Thousand Years, All Our Ancestors*
Klaus Wiese – *El Hadra: Mystic Dance*

Rhythmic:

James Asher – G*lobalarium, Feet in the Soil, Tigers of the Raj*
Trance Mission – *Trance Mission, Meanwhile*
Skeleton Woman – *Flesh and Bone*
Reinhard Flatischler – *Schinore, Layers of Time*
B Tribe – *Spiritual, Spiritual*
Nomad – *Nomad*

Drumming:

David and Steve Gordon – *Sacred Spirit Drums*
Prem Das – *Journey of the Drums*
Outback – *Dance the Devil Away*
Bridgewalker Drummers – S*hamanic Journey Multiple Drumming*

Devotional:

Noirin Ni Riain and the Monks of Glenstal – *Vox de Nube*
Krishna Das – *Pilgrim Heart*
Rasa – *Devotion*
Ravi Shankar – *Concert for Peace, Chants of India, The Sounds of India*
Pandit Bhimsen Joshi – *Vocals*
Loreena McKennitt – *The Visit, The Mask and the Mirror*
Enya – *Watermark, Shepherd Moons*
Sheila Chandra – *Weaving My Ancestor's Voices, The Zen Kiss*
Djivan Gasparyan – *I Will Not Be Sad in This World*

My Recorded CDs:

Doc Bones and the Rattlesnakes; ...*Outlaws and Lovers*; ...
The Road You Choose

Personal Note:

Although the above music list is trance and indigenous-oriented, the outcome of my own musical trajectory led me to a creative state where I developed my musical skills with singing, guitar, banjo, harmonica, digeridoo, and hand drumming. The genres that I gravitated toward were Americana, folk, country-rock, bluegrass, blues, and old-time mountain music, not exactly psychedelic, but very rooted to the earth, which I call "Roots Music." I went on to make three albums in Nashville and play multiple local gigs near where I live. I didn't make it to Carnegie Hall, but I enjoyed myself and met many other musicians as friends and singing partners. Check out my music and band called "Doc Bones and the Rattlesnakes." That is where my muse led me, and I thank my psychedelic years for the inspiration to create artwork, music, and now writing. Psychedelics alone may not necessarily cause change, but they create options and choices and pressures one to express inner soul yearnings. It helped me overcome career burnout and depression by making me aware that life is about balancing meaningful work, relationships and manifesting creativity.

Microdosing Psychedelics

A recent trend (circa 2022) arousing significant interest and curiosity is the usage of small doses of psychedelics for treating depression and anxiety. Unfortunately, traditional psychiatric drugs such as antidepressants, especially SSRIs, are only effective in treating approximately 50% to 66% of patients. The rest have only partial responses or are treatment-resistant, requiring more complicated medicine regimens. Frequently, side effects preclude patients from continuing these regimens, or they complain that the drugs cause them to feel emotionally blunted. However, the majority of people taking antidepressants do not complain about feeling suppressed and are grateful for improvement in their social and work functionality, mood, stress tolerance, and anxiety levels. Benzodiazepines used for anxiety continue to be problematic, since they can be addictive and difficult to discontinue; they are prescribed much less frequently at the present time.

Since this practice became known, many people have chosen to try microdosing, if traditional treatments have been ineffective. Small doses of about one-tenth to one-twentieth of the full psychedelic doses are usually administered every other day to twice per week. Anecdotally, many people report alleviation of dysphoric symptoms and improved positive cognition and daily functionality. A major drawback of microdosing is that unfortunately, the psychedelics being used remain illegal. Presently, a number of trials are underway in research settings to determine efficacy and dosage protocols. The psychedelics being investigated for microdosing purposes are primarily psilocybin and LSD. As mentioned previously, MDMA, DMT derivatives, ketamine, and ibogaine are being studied at various dosages as treatments for various psychological disorders.

Microdosing is currently being tried extensively in various industries, especially in the Silicon Valley, for the purpose of amplifying creativity, productivity, and cognitive abilities. Whether this informal practice will prove useful and become common in the workplace is not certain; it certainly has the potential for unsupervised abuse and could result in an outcome reminiscent of the Timothy Leary era. Microdosing does not bring about the full psychedelic experiences described in this text. However, it seems to "light up" the brain to experience things differently and more positively but without the visual displays, teachings, and spiritual connections necessary for a deeper exploration of the psyche.

Although intriguing, more studies need to be undertaken to assure the safety and efficacy of microdosing. James Fadiman, Ph.D., a transpersonal psychologist and writer on the topics of psychedelics and spirituality, is a leading proponent of microdosing. He and Robert Frager created the California Institute of Transpersonal Psychology, now renamed Sofia University. Since this book does not emphasize microdosing, more detail should be sought by the experts who address this approach.

Figure Credits

Front Cover – *Peyote Vision*
Artwork by the author,
Graphic Design by Geoffrey Shester

Fig. 1 – *Young Alex* (photo – Shester collection)
Fig. 2 – *First-year medical student* (photo – Shester collection)
Fig. 3 – *Medicine Wheel* (Metzner/Shester)
Fig. 4 – *Cosmos Mandala* (Shester)
Fig. 5 – Bufo (*Incilius*) alvarius (Wikimedia commons)
Fig. 6 – *Zabka* (Michael Garfield – michaelgarfieldart.com)
Fig. 7 – *Six Directions Journey* (Metzner/Shester)
Fig. 8 – *Janus Model of Integration* (Metzner/Shester)
Fig. 9 – *Yggdrasil* (Cici Artemisia – ciciart.com)
Fig. 10 – *Cosmic tree,* as shared by Ralph Metzner
Fig. 11 – *Ten Sefiroth: Mystical Tree of God* (unknown/Shester)
Fig. 12 – *Meditacion Amazonica* – (Victor Guerra Pinedo)
Fig. 13 – *Ten Chakra System* (artist – unknown)
Fig. 14 – *Tree of Life Diagram* (Metzner/Shester)
Fig. 15 – *Well of Remembrance Meditation* (Metzner/Shester)
Fig. 16 – *Jaguar Ayahuasca* (ARUTAM Association)
Fig. 17 – *Ayahuasca Healing* (Anderson Debernardi)
Fig. 18 – *Energia Felina, 2014* (Jheff Au)
Fig. 19 – *The Face of the Lover Through All Time* (Shester)
Fig. 20 – *Lo Masculino y lo Femenino* (Victor Guerra Pinedo)
Fig. 21 – *Eros Within Nature* (Shester)
Fig. 22 – *Three Types of Sorcerers* (Pablo Amaringo)
Fig. 23 – *Purging Toxicity* (Shester)
Fig. 24 – *Instinct and Consciousness Integrating* (Shester)
Fig. 25 – *Shamanic Sacra-Mental Spaces* (Felix Pinchi Aguirre)
Fig. 26 – *Ayahuasca Admixture* (Banisteriopsis and Psychotria) – (Awkipuma– Wikimedia Commons)
Fig. 27 – *Banisteriopsis caapi Vine of the Soul* (photo – newsweek.com)
Fig. 28 – *Yana Shipiba Puma* (Jorge Ramirez)

Fig. 61 – *La Danse du Sabbat-Dore* (Émile Bayard, Public domain, via Wikimedia Commons)

Fig. 62 – *Shrunken Head – Tsantsa* (from Harner 1972, 138)

Fig. 63 – *Amanita muscaria mushroom* (photo – unknown)

Fig. 64 – *Shaman with Amanita Miter* (photo- educateinspirechange.org)

Fig. 65 – *De Sma Skovnisser* (Eska Beskow from Rätsch and Mueller-Ebeling 2003, 10)

Fig. 66 – *The Forager, 2020* (daniellecaners.com)

Fig. 67 – *Yopo being snuffed* (from Schultes 1998, 118)

Fig. 68 – *Delysid – LSD* (photo – from Shester colleague)

Fig. 69 – *The Eleusinian Mysteries* (Paul Serusier)

Fig. 70 – *Chemical Structure of MDMA*

Fig. 71 – *Tripus Aureus* (from Jaffe 1979, 96)

Fig. 72 – *Mandala painting* (from CG Jung 2009, Red Book, 105)

Fig. 73 – *Light at the Core of Darkness painting* (from CG Jung 2009, Red Book, 129)

Fig. 74 – *Jung in Tunisia 1920* (from Wehr 1989, 67)

Fig. 75 – *Ochwiay Biano (Mountain Lake) of Taos Pueblo 1924* (from Wehr 1989, 63)

Fig. 76 – *Jung in Mombasa 1925* (from Wehr 1989, 65)

Fig. 77 – *Bollingen First Tower 1923* (from Wehr 1989, 72)

Fig. 78 – *Bollingen Tower 1956* (from Wehr 1989, 72)

Fig. 79 – *Jung Chopping Wood at Bollingen* (from Wehr 1989, 71)

Fig. 80 – *The Shaman* (Roger Garner) — In memory of my wise artist friend, Roger Garner, who produced this drawing for me just before his death.

Fig. 81 – *Old Man River* (Shester)

Back Cover – *Emergence of the Anthropos*
Artwork by the author,
Graphic Design by Geoffrey Shester

Acknowledgments

Unlike a parent who raises a person and provides food, shelter, and love, a mentor's function is to be a teacher, coach, guide, and a person who fosters the soul's development. Parents are generally too subjective and emotionally involved in their roles and can hinder, rather than help, their children in realms they are not versed in, such as music, the arts, or sports. A caring mentor can be more objective and a better initiatory teacher.

During my formal education, my teachers and coaches were my mentors. After my medical and psychiatric studies, I was interested in learning about dreams, so I studied with various Jungian analysts. They included James Kirsch, the co-founder of the Jung Institute in Los Angeles, who knew and worked with Carl Jung. My other notable analysts were Jack Sanford, Robert Johnson, Jan Clanton-Collins, Katie Sanford, and Edward Edinger. Of course, C.G. Jung was my primary mentor in understanding transpersonal psychology.

I also sought mentors including Robert Bly, Michael Meade, Robert Moore, James Hillman, John Stokes, and others to learn more about men. They ran week-long workshops in wilderness settings as part of the Mythopoetic Men's movement, which emerged in the late 1980s and peaked in the 1990s.

My interest in shamanism led me to participate with a Native American (Navajo) peyote medicine man, Spirit Eagle, from Shiprock, New Mexico. I also participated in a shamanic workshop with Michael Harner. My primary mentor was Ralph Metzner for over twenty years. He had a way of integrating the traditional shamanic methods with modern psychology, making it most relevant to my practice and interests. I had several music teachers who helped me develop my guitar and banjo skills. It is fascinating that my interest in roots music is archetypal to the people's land, which attracted me to this genre.

I gratefully acknowledge the above significant influences in my life and those not noted. Most important is my family, who gave me suggestions, technical advice, editing, and design. They are my wife, Judith, and my two sons, Geoff and Blake. I am grateful to my psychiatric colleague and renowned psychedelic researcher, **Charles Grob, M.D.,** who contributed the foreword. I was so pleased to have **Regent Press** enthusiastically agree to publish this book under **Mark Weiman's** guidance. He has also published numerous works of Ralph Metzner and other distinguished authors.

I also want to thank **Cathy Coleman, Ph.D.,** who supported and encouraged me to publish this book to honor her husband, Ralph Metzner. She wrote the preface and is also is a psychedelic researcher.

I would also like to acknowledge the plants, fungi, and chemicals that have opened up the doors to a greater perception of understanding consciousness. Some of these may know more about us than we know about ourselves. Also, I thank my ancestors and spirit guides for helping me along my path of development.

I want to acknowledge and credit the Native and indigenous peoples of the world whose wisdom, visioning, and healing practices have contributed greatly to modern Western knowledge.

I am also grateful and want to thank the participating artists listed in the "figure credits," who permitted me to display their visionary artwork. Many are from the Visionary Art Center in Pucallpa, Peru. Please look them up and support their art.

I would like to specially acknowledge two close friends for their encouragement and support for this book, **Nitza** and **Drew**

Even though I created and wrote this book in its entirety, I realized that it takes a village to manifest it through publication. I had superb editors help with my rough drafts to become a finished product I can share.

Thomas Lane – principal developmental and structural editor
Judith Shester – copy editor and proofreader
Ricki Oldenkamp – copy editor, proofreader, and diagram graphics
Kristina Maria Reva – beta reader and contributing editor
Ralph Chaney – photography
Geoffrey Shester - photography and graphic design
Blake Shester – computer and technical advisor

Bibliography

Adams, Francis. *The Seven Books of Paulus Aegineta.* Translated from the Greek. 3 vols. London: Sydenham Society, 1844.

Adamson, Sophia, ed. *Through the Gateway of the Heart: Accounts of Experiences with MDMA and Other Empathogenic Substances.* San Francisco: Four Tree Publications, 1985.

Anderson, William. *Green Man: The Archetype of Our Oneness with the Earth.* London: HarperCollins, 1990.

Arrien, Angeles. *The Four-Fold Way: Walking the Paths of the Warrior, Healer, and Visionary.* San Francisco: Harper, 1993.

Berry, Thomas. *The Dream of the Earth.* San Francisco: Sierra Club Books, 1988.

Bishop, Peter. *The Greening of Psychology: The Vegetable World in Myth, Dream, and Healing.* Washington, DC: Spring Publications, 1990.

Bravo, Gary. "Ketamine." In Grob, Charles and Jim Grigsby, eds. *Handbook of Medical Hallucinogens.* New York: Guilford Press, 2021.

Bucke, Richard Maurice. *Cosmic Consciousness.* New York: Penguin, 1901.

Burdick, Alan. *Out of Eden: An Odyssey of Ecological Invasion.* New York: Farrar Straus and Giroux, 2005.

Buhner, Stephen Harrod. *Plant Intelligence and the Imaginal Realm.* Rochester, VT: Bear and Co., 2014.

Carus, Louise, ed. *The Real St. Nicholas: Tales of Generosity and Hope from Around the World.* Wheaton, IL: Quest Books, 2002.

Castaneda, Carlos. *The Teachings of Don Juan.* Berkeley: University of California Press, 1968.

Charing, Howard G., Cloudsley, Peter, and Amaringo, Pablo. *The Ayahuasca Visions of Pablo Amaringo.* Rochester, VT: Inner Visions, 2011.

Clendenen, Avis, *Experiencing Hildegard: Jungian Perspective.* Asheville, NC: Chiron Publications, 2009.

Cordy-Collins, Alana. "Chavin Art: Its Shamanic Hallucinogenic Origins" in *Pre-Columbian Art History: Selected Readings*," eds. Alana Cordy-Collins and Jean Stern. Palo Alto, CA: Peek, 1977, 353-361.

Da Silva, Arjuna. "Stalking the Spirit of Ibogaine." *Psychedelic Illuminations* 1, no. 7, 1995, 24-26.

Davis, Wade. *One River: Explorations and Discoveries in the Amazon Rain Forest.* New York: Simon and Schuster, 1996.

Diamond. Jared. *Guns, Germs, and Steel: The Fate of Human Societies.* New York: Norton and Co., 1999.

Doblin, Rick, ed. Multidisciplinary Association for Psychedelic Studies (MAPS) *Quarterly Newsletter, passim.*

Edinger, Edward F. *Ego and Archetype: Individuation and the Religious Function of the Psyche.* N.Y: G.P. Putnam and Sons for the C.G. Jung Foundation for Analytical Psychology, 1972

———. *Anatomy of the Psyche: Alchemical Symbolism in Psychotherapy.* Illinois: Open Court Publishing Co., 1985

Eisler, Riane. *The Chalice and the Blade.* New York: HarperCollins, 1987.

Eliade, Mircea. *Shamanism: Archaic Techniques of Ecstasy.* Bollingen Series LXXVI. Princeton, NJ: Princeton University Press, 1972.

Eliot, T.S., *The Complete Poems and Plays: 1909-1950.* New York: Harcourt Brace, 1971.

Fabricius, Johannes. *Alchemy: The Medieval Alchemists and Their Royal Art.* Copenhagen: Rosenkilde and Bagger, 1976.

Fadiman, James, Ph.D. *The Psychedelic Explorer's Guide: Safe, Therapeutic, and Sacred Journeys.* Rochester, VT: Park Street Press, 2011.

Gimbutas, Marija. *The World of the Goddess.* YouTube video, 1:42:44. 1990. https://www.youtube.com/watch?v=GMutw5CNiRQ.

Goldsmith, Edward. *The Way: An Ecological Worldview.* Boston: Shambala, 1993.

Gore, Al. *Earth in the Balance: Ecology and the Human Experience.* Boston: Houghton Mifflin, 1992.

Gottlieb, Adam. *Peyote and Other Psychoactive Cacti.* Berkeley, CA: Ronin Publications, 1997.

Green Earth Foundation. *Newsletters, passim.*

Grey, Alex. *Sacred Mirrors: The Visionary Art of Alex Grey.* Rochester, VT: Inner Traditions International, 1990.

Grinspoon, Lester and James B. Bakalar. *Marihuana: The Forbidden Medicine.* New Haven, CT: Yale University Press, 1993.

Grob, Charles, ed. *Hallucinogens: A Reader.* New York: Jeremy Tarcher/ Penguin, 2002.

Grob, Charles, and Grigsby, Jim (editors). *Handbook of Medical Hallucinogens.* New York: Guilford Press, 2021.

Grof, Stanislav. *Realms of the Human Unconscious: Observations from LSD Research.* New York:

Viking Press, 1975.

———. *The Adventure of Self Discovery.* Albany: State University of New York Press, 1988.

Groff, Stanislav and Christina Groff. *The Stormy Search for the Self.* Los Angeles: Jeremy Tarcher, 1990.

Halifax, Joan. *Shamanic Voices: A Survey of Visionary Narratives.* New York: E.P. Dutton, 1979.

———. *Fruitful Darkness: A Journey Through Buddhist Practice and Tribal Wisdom.* New York: Grove Press, 1993.

Hammerschlag, Carl A. *The Dancing Healers: A Doctor's Journey of Healing with Native Americans.* San Francisco: Harper, 1989.

Handwerk, Brian. "From St. Nicholas to Santa Claus." *National Geographic*, December 25, 2018.

Harari, Yuval Noah. *Sapiens: A Brief History of Humankind.* London: Vintage, 2011.

Harner, Michael. *The Jivaro: People of the Sacred Waterfalls.* New York: Doubleday Natural History, 1972.

———. *Hallucinogens and Shamanism.* London: Oxford University Press, 1973.

———. *The Way of the Shaman.* New York: Harper and Row, 1980.

Hellinger, Bert. *On Life and Other Paradoxes.* Translated by Ralph Metzner. Phoenix, AZ: Zeig, Tucker, and Thiesen, 2002.

Hesse, Erich. *Narcotic and Drug Addiction.* N.Y.: Philosophical Library, 1946.

Hesse, Hermann. *Siddhartha.* N.Y.: New Directions, 1957.

Hillman, James and Michael Ventura. *We've Had a Hundred Years of Psychotherapy and the World's Getting Worse.* San Francisco: Harper San Francisco, 1992.

Huxley, Aldous. *The Human Situation.* New York: Harper and Row, 1977.

———. *The Doors of Perception* and *Heaven and Hell.* New York: Harper and Row, 1990.

Jaffe, Aniela, ed. *C.G. Jung: Word and Image.* Bollingen Series XCVII. New Jersey: Princeton University Press, 1979.

———. ed. *Memories, Dreams, Reflections.* New York: Pantheon Books, 1961.

James, William. *The Varieties of Religious Experience.* New York: Signet, 1958.

Johnson, Will. *Yoga of the Mahamudra: The Mystical Way of Balance.*

Rochester, VT: Inner Traditions, 2005.

Jung, C.G. *C.G Jung Speaking: Interviews and Encounters.* Edited by William

McGuire and R.F.C. Hull, Bollingen Series XCVII, Princeton University

Press, 1987.

———. *Collected Works 8: The Structure and Dynamics of the Psyche.* Bollingen Series XX.

Princeton, NJ: Princeton University Press, 1960

———. *Collected Works 10: Civilization in Transition.* Bollingen Series XX. Princeton, NJ: 1964.

———. *Collected Works 11: Psychology and Religion.* Bollingen Series XX. Princeton, NJ: Princeton University Press, 1958.

———. *Collected Works 12: Psychology and Alchemy.* Bollingen Series XX. Princeton, NJ: Princeton University Press, 1968.

———. *Collected Works 13: Alchemical Studies*. Bollingen Series XX. Princeton, NJ: Princeton University Press, 1968.

———. *Collected Works 14: Mysterium Coniunctionis*. Bollingen Series XX. Princeton, NJ: Princeton University Press, 1970.

———. *C.G. Jung Letters, Vol.1*. Edited by Gerhard Adler and Aniela Jaffé. Bollingen Series XCV: 1, Princeton University Press, 1973.

———. "Psyche and Nature, Book 1 and 2: Journal of Archetype and Culture." *Spring* 75 and 76 (Fall 2006).

———. *The Psychology of Kundalini Yoga: Notes of the Seminar Given in 1932 by C.G Jung.* (Sonu Shamdasani, Ed.), Bollingen Series XCIX. Princeton, NJ: Princeton Univ. Press, 1996.

———. *The Red Book.* Edited by Sonu Shamdasani. New York: Norton and Co., 2009.

———. *The Vision Seminars: Book I and II.* Washington, DC: Spring Publications, 1976.

Kharitidi, Olga. *Entering the Circle: Ancient Secrets of Siberian Wisdom Discovered by a Russian Psychiatrist.* San Francisco: Harper, 1996.

Kimmerer, Robin Wall. *Braiding Sweetgrass: Indigenous Wisdom, Scientific Knowledge, and the Teachings of Plants.* Minneapolis MN: Milkweed Editions, 2013.

Kolp, Eli et al. "Ketamine Psychedelic Psychotherapy." *International Journal of Transpersonal Studies*, 33(2), 2014: 84-140.

Krieg, Margaret. B. *Green Medicine: the Search for Plants That Heal.* New York: Bantam, 1966.

Kushner, David. "Inside a Psychedelic Health Retreat." *Outside Magazine*, Sept./Oct. 2021. https://www.outsideonline.com/health/wellness/psychedelic-nature-therapy-ketamine-anxiety-depression/.

Lamb, F. Bruce. *Wizard of the Upper Amazon.* Boston: Houghton Mifflin, 1974.

Lanza, Robert. *Biocentrism: How Life and Consciousness are the Keys to Understanding the True Nature of the Universe.* Dallas, TX: Benbella Books, 2009.

Lauck, Joanne Elizabeth. *The Voice of the Infinite in the Small: Revisioning the Insect – Human Connection.* NY: Swan-Raven and Co., 1998.

Lawlor, Robert. *Voices of the First Day: Awakening in Aboriginal Dreamtime.* Rochester, VT: Inner Traditions, 1991.

Lawlor, Sean. *5-MeO-DMT: Light and Shadow in the Psychedelic Toad. Psychedelic* Times(article): November 20, 2019.

Luna, Luis Eduardo and White, Steven F., eds. *Ayahuasca Reader: Encounters with the Amazon's Sacred Vine.* Santa Fe, NM: Synergetic Press, 2016.

Luna, Luis Eduardo, and Amaringo, Pablo. *Ayahuasca Visions: The Religious Iconography of a Peruvian Shaman.* Berkeley, CA: North Atlantic Books, 1991

Matthews, John. *The Celtic Shaman: A Handbook.* Rockport, MA: Element Books, 1991.

McGaa, Ed [Eagle Man]. *Mother Earth Spirituality: Native American Paths to Healing Ourselves and Our World.* San Francisco: Harper, 1989.

McKenna, Dennis. "Of Apes and Men," in *Fantastic Fungi,* ed. Paul Stamets. San Rafael, CA: Earth Aware, 2019), 152-154.

McKenna, Terence. *Food of the Gods: The Search for the Original Tree of Knowledge.* New York: Bantam, 1992.

———. *True Hallucinations.* San Francisco: Harper, 1993.

Metzner, Ralph. *The Well of Remembrance: Rediscovering the Earth Wisdom Myths of Northern Europe.* Cambridge MA: Shambala, 1994.

———. *The Unfolding Self: Varieties of Transformative Experience.* San Rafael, CA: Origin Press, 1998.

———. *Ayahuasca: Hallucinogens, Consciousness, and the Spirit of Nature (Editor).* New York: Thunder's Mouth Press, 1999.

———. *Green Psychology: Transforming Our Relationship to the Earth.*

Rochester, VT: Park Street Press, 1999.

——— . *Teonanacatl: Sacred Mushroom Visions* (Ed.). El Verano, CA: Four Trees Press, 2004.

——— . *Alchemical Divination: Accessing Your Spiritual Intelligence for Healing and Guidance.* El Verano, CA: Green Earth and Regent Press, 2009.

———. *Worlds Within and Worlds Beyond.* El Verano, CA: Green Earth and Regent Press, 2013.

———. *Allies for Awakening: Guidelines for Productive and Safe Experiences with Entheogens.* Berkeley: Regent Press, 2015.

———. *Ecology of Consciousness: The Alchemy of Personal, Collective, and Planetary Transformation.* Oakland, CA: New Harbinger Publications, 2017.

Moore, Robert, and Douglas Gillette. *The Magician Within: Accessing the Shaman in the Male Psyche.* New York: Morrow, 1993.

Musès, Charles. "The Sacred Plant of Ancient Egypt" in Christian Rätsch, ed. *Gateway to Inner Space: Sacred Plants, Mysticism, and Psychotherapy.* Dorset, UK: Prism/Unity Press, 1989, 143-59.

Myerhoff, Barbara G. *Peyote Hunt: The Sacred Journey of the Huichol Indians.* Ithaca, NY: Cornell University Press, 1974.

Naranjo, Claudio. *The Healing Journey: New Approaches to Consciousness.* New York: Ballantine, 1973.

Narby, Jeremy. *The Cosmic Serpent: DNA and the Origins of Knowledge.* New York: Tarcher/Putnam, 1999.

Nicholson, Shirley ed. *Shamanism.* Wheaton, IL: Theosophical Publishing House, 1987.

Noble, Vicki. *Shakti Woman: Feelin Our Fire, Healing Our World – The New Female Shamanism.* San Francisco: Harper, 1991.

Oaklander, Mandy. "Inside Ibogaine, One of the Most Promising and Perilous Psychedelics for Addiction." *Time,* April 5, 2021. https://time.com/5951772/ibogaine-drug-treatment-addiction/.

Ott, Jonathan. *Pharmacotheon: Entheogenic Drugs, Their Plant Sources and History.* Ridgefield, WA: Natural Products Co., 1993.

———. *Ayahuasca Analogues: Pangaen Entheogens.* Ridgefield, WA: Jonathan Ott Books, 1994.

Patnaik, Naveen. *The Garden of Life: An Introduction to the Healing Plants of India.* New York: Doubleday, 1993.

Pendell, Dale. *Pharmacopoeia: Plant Powers, Poisons, and Herbcraft.* Berkeley: North Atlantic Books, 1995.

Plotkin, Mark J. *Tales of a Shaman's Apprentice: An Ethnobotanist Searches for New Medicines in the Amazon Rainforest.* New York: Viking, 1993.

Pollan, Michael. *How to Change Your Mind: What the New Science of Psychedelics Teaches Us About Consciousness, Dying, Addiction, Depression, and Transcendence.* New York: Penguin Press, 2018.

———. *This Is Your Mind on Plants.* New York: Penguin Books, 2021.

Ponting, Clive. *A Green History of the World: The Environment and the Collapse of Great Civilizations.* New York: Penguin Books, 1991.

Powers, Richard. *The Overstory.* New York: Norton, 2018.

Psychedelics Revisited. ReVision: The Journal of Consciousness and Change, Vol. 10, No. 4, Spring, 1988.

Rätsch, Christian, ed. *Gateway to Inner Space: Sacred Plants, Mysticism, and Psychotherapy.* Dorset, UK: Prism/Unity Press, 1989.

———. *The Dictionary of Sacred and Magical Plants.* Dorset, UK: Prism/Unity Press, 1992.

Rätsch, Christian and Claudia Mueller-Ebeling. *Shamanism and Tantra in the Himalayas.* Rochester, VT: Inner Traditions, 2000.

———. *Pagan Christmas: Plants, Spirits, and Rituals at the Origin of Yuletide.* Rochester VT: Inner Traditions, 2003.

Reichel-Dolmatoff, Gerardo. *Amazonian Cosmos: The Sexual and Religious Symbolism of the Tukano Indians.* Chicago Ill. University of Chicago Press, 1971.

Renterghem, Tony van. *When Santa Was a Shaman: The Ancient Origins of Santa Claus and the Christmas Tree.* St. Paul, MN: Llewellyn Publications, 1995.

Robinson, Kim Stanley. *The Ministry of the Future.* New York, NY: Orbit, 2020.

Roszak, Theodore. *The Voice of the Earth: An Exploration of Ecopsychology.* New York: Touchstone, 1993.

Sandner, Donald. *Navajo Symbols of Healing.* New York: Harcourt Brace Jovanovich, 1979.

Schenk, Gustav. *The Book of Poisons.* Translated from the German by Michael Bullock. New York: Reinhart, 1955.

Schultes, Richard Evans. *Hallucinogenic Plants: A Golden Guide.* New York: Golden Press, 1976.

Schultes, Richard Evans and Richard F. Raffauf. *Vine of the Soul: Medicine Men, Their Plants and Rituals in the Colombian Amazon.* Santa Fe, NM: Synergetic Press, 1992.

Schultes, Richard Evans, Hofmann, Albert. *Plants of the Gods: Their Sacred Healing and Hallucinogenic Powers.* Rochester VT: Healing Arts Press, 1992.

Schultes, Richard Evans, Hofmann, Albert, Rätsch, Christian. *Plants of the Gods: Their Sacred Healing and Hallucinogenic Powers,* revised edition. Rochester VT: Healing Arts Press, 1998.

Seed, John et al. *Thinking Like a Mountain: Toward a Council of All Beings.* Philadelphia, PA: New Society Publications, 1988.

Serrano, Miguel. *C.G. Jung and Hermann Hesse: A Record of Two Friendships.* New York: Schocken Books, 1966.

Shamanism: The Transpersonal Dimension. ReVision: The Journal of Consciousness and Change. Vol. 13, No. 2, Fall, 1990.

Sharon, Douglas C. and Christopher B. Donnan. "The Magic Cactus: Ethnoarchaeological Continuity in Peru," *Archaeology* 30 no. 6 (1977), 374-381.

Sheldrake, Merlin. *Entangled Life: How Fungi Make Our Worlds, Change Our Minds, and Shape Our Futures.* New York: Random House, 2020.

Sheldrake, Rupert. *The Rebirth of Nature: The Greening Science of God.* Rochester, VT: Park Street Press, 1991.

Shulgin, Alexander and Ann Shulgin. *PIHKAL: A Chemical Love Story.* Berkeley, CA: Transform Press, 1991.

———. *Tihkal: The Continuation.* Berkeley, CA: Transform Press, 1997.

Sierra: The Magazine of the Sierra Club, passim.

Smith, Huston. *Cleansing the Doors of Perception: The Religious Significance of Entheogenic Plants and Chemicals.* New York: Jeremy Tarcher/Putnam, 2000.

Snyder, Gary. *The Practice of the Wild.* New York: North Point Press, 1990.

Sociedad para la Preservation de los Plantas del Misterio. *The Salvia Divinorum Grower's Guide.* N.p.: Spectral Mindustries, 1998.

Somé, Malidoma. *Ritual Power: Healing and Community.* N.p.: Swan/ Raven and Co., 1993.

Stafford, Peter. *Psychedelics Encyclopedia,* 3rd edition. Berkeley, CA: Ronin, 1992.

Stahl, Stephen. *Essential Psychopharmacology: The Prescriber's Guide.*

New York: Cambridge University Press, 2006.

Stamets, Paul, *Psilocybin Mushrooms of the World: An Identification Guide.* Berkeley, CA: Ten Speed Press, 1996.

———. ed. *Fantastic Fungi: How Mushrooms Can Heal, Shift Consciousness, and Save the Planet.* San Rafael, CA: Earth Aware, 2019.

Stevens, Jay. *Storming Heaven: LSD and the American Dream.* New York: Perennial Library, 1988.

Strassman, Rick, M.D. *DMT The Spirit Molecule: A Doctor's Revolutionary Research into the Biology of Near-Death and Mystical Experiences.* Rochester, Vermont: Park Street Press, 2001.

Swimme, Brian, and Berry, Thomas. *The Universe Story.* San Francisco: Harper Collins, 1994.

Tart, Charles, ed. *Altered States of Consciousness.* New York: Anchor Books, 1972.

Thevet, Andre. *Les Singularitez de la France Antarctique....* 1558.

Tschorn, Adam. "Deep Into the Weed," *Los Angeles Times,* April 17, 2021.

Tucker, Mary Evelyn, and John Grim. *The Worldviews and Ecology.* London: Bucknell Press, 1993

Underhill, Evelyn. *Mysticism.* New York: E.P. Dutton, 1961.

Valadez, Mariano and Susana Valdez. *Huichol Indian Sacred Rituals.* Oakland, CA: Dharma Enterprises, 1992.

Villoldo, Alberto and Stanley Krippner. *Healing States: A Journey into the World of Spiritual Healing and Shamanism.* New York: Fireside, 1986.

Villoldo, Alberto. *The Four Winds: A Shaman's Odyssey into the Amazon.* San Francisco: Harper, 1991.

Walsh, Roger and Frances Vaughn, eds. *Beyond Ego: Transpersonal Dimensions in Psychology.* Los Angeles: Jeremy Tarcher, 1980.

Wasson, R. Gordon. *Soma: Divine Mushroom of Immortality.* New York: Harcourt Brace Jovanovich, 1972.

Wasson, R. Gordon, Albert Hoffman, and Carl Ruck. *Road to Eleusis: Unveiling the Secret of the Mysteries.* Los Angeles: Hermes, 1998.

Wehr, Gerhard. *An Illustrated Biography of C.G. Jung.* Cambridge, MA: Shambala, 1989.

Weil, Andrew. *The Natural Mind: A New Way of Looking at Drugs and Higher Consciousness.* Boston: Houghton Mifflin, 1973.

———. "The Stoned Ape Theory," in *Fantastic Fungi,* ed. Paul Stamets (San Rafael, CA: Earth Aware, 2019), 155.

Wier, Jean. *Histoires, Disputes et Discovrs. Vol. II.* Paris: Bureau du Progres Medical. Originally published 1660.

Wilhelm, Richard. *The Secret of the Golden Flower: A Chinese Book of Life.* Foreword by C.G. Jung. New York: Harcourt, Brace and World, 1962.

Woodroffe, Sir John. *The Serpent Power.* Madras, India: Ganesh and Co.,1973.

Wulf, Andrea. *The Invention of Nature: Alexander von Humboldt's New World.* New York: Vintage Books, 2016.

Zimmer, Heinrich "Sir Gawain and the Green Knight" in *The King and the Corpse,* Bollingen Series XI. Edited by Joseph Campbell. Princeton, NJ: Princeton University Press. 1973, 67- 95.

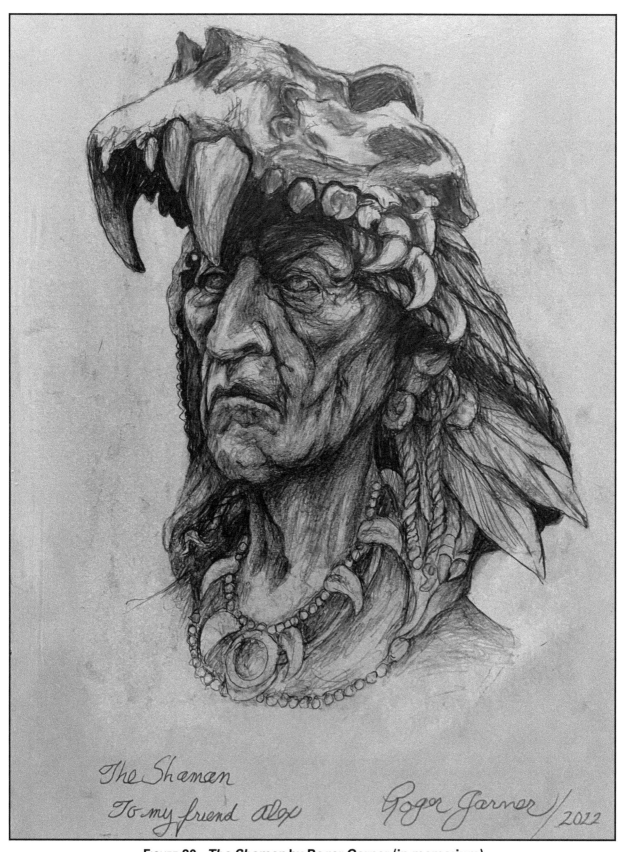

The Shaman

To my friend Alex

Roger Garner / 2022

FIGURE 80. *The Shaman* by Roger Garner (in memorium)

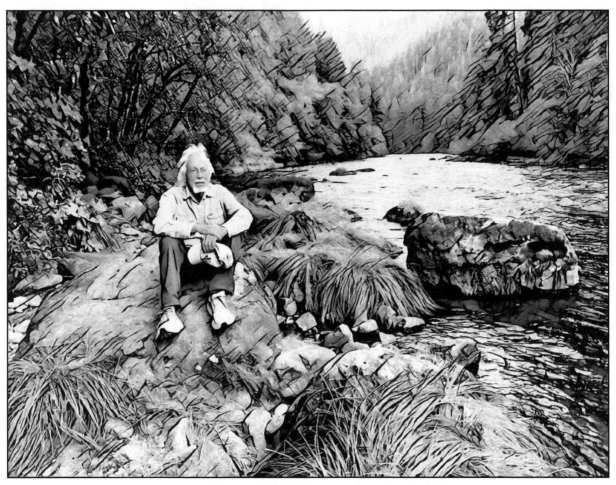

FIGURE 81. *Old Man River* (Shester)

Thank you for reading my book.
I hope you enjoyed it and found it worthwhile.
Best to you all,
— Doc

9 781587 906343